MW01670587

Epidemics and Pandemics

Epidemics and Pandemics

From Ancient Plagues to Modern-Day Threats

VOLUME 2

Joseph P. Byrne and Jo N. Hays

GREENWOOD™

An Imprint of ABC-CLIO, LLC

Santa Barbara, California • Denver, Colorado

Copyright © 2021 by ABC-CLIO, LLC

All rights reserved. No part of this publication may be reproduced, stored in a retrieval system, or transmitted, in any form or by any means, electronic, mechanical, photocopying, recording, or otherwise, except for the inclusion of brief quotations in a review, without prior permission in writing from the publisher.

Library of Congress Cataloging-in-Publication Data

Names: Byrne, Joseph P., author. | Hays, J. N., 1938- author.
Title: Epidemics and pandemics : from ancient plagues to modern-day threats / Joseph P. Byrne and Jo N. Hays.
Description: Santa Barbara : ABC-CLIO, LLC, [2021] | Includes bibliographical references and index. | Contents: v. 1. — v. 2. — Set.
Identifiers: LCCN 2020026560 (print) | LCCN 2020026561 (ebook) | ISBN 9781440863806 (v. 1 ; hardcover) | ISBN 9781440863813 (v. 2 ; hardcover) | ISBN 9781440863783 (hardcover) | ISBN 9781440863790 (ebook)
Subjects: LCSH: Epidemics—History. | Communicable diseases—History. | Diseases and history.
Classification: LCC RA649 .B97 2021 (print) | LCC RA649 (ebook) | DDC 614.4/9—dc23
LC record available at https://lccn.loc.gov/2020026560
LC ebook record available at https://lccn.loc.gov/2020026561

ISBN: 978-1-4408-6378-3 (set)
978-1-4408-6380-6 (vol. 1)
978-1-4408-6381-3 (vol. 2)
978-1-4408-6379-0 (ebook)

25 24 23 22 21 1 2 3 4 5

This book is also available as an eBook.

Greenwood
An Imprint of ABC-CLIO, LLC

ABC-CLIO, LLC
147 Castilian Drive
Santa Barbara, California 93117
www.abc-clio.com

This book is printed on acid-free paper ∞

Manufactured in the United States of America

To those across the globe who are working so hard, and often at great risk, to make daily life during the COVID-19 pandemic tolerable and perhaps even possible.

—Joseph P. Byrne

To Drs. Michelle Carlon, Daniel Torres, and Donald Nash, who contributed perhaps more than they realized to my completion of a work about epidemiology, and to Roz, with thanks and love.

—Jo N. Hays

Contents

VOLUME 2

1

Malaria in Ancient Rome

WHEN AND WHERE

Malaria was a frequent malady in the ancient Roman world. In many ways, it was more an endemic disease than an epidemic one, but its certain significance for Roman society, its dramatically seasonal character, and the wide geographical variations in its incidence, all suggest epidemic may be appropriate. Many points about its history in the ancient Mediterranean, however, remain controversial or uncertain, and so this discussion concludes with a number of unresolved issues. A strong case can be made that malaria affected the demography of the Roman world, perhaps stunting economic productivity, contributing to agricultural change, depopulating some regions and changing the social system of others, and occasionally diverting the course of political and military history.

Malaria in at least some forms was apparently found across the Mediterranean area from an early period of ancient Roman history, certainly by the fifth century BCE. Its outbreaks were highly seasonal, beginning in July, with the number of cases peaking in September; subsequent deaths rose through the fall months, before subsiding by December.

Its incidence varied widely from one region to another. In general, malaria concentrated in low-lying areas, below about 500 meters above sea level. In Italy some regions were thought by the Romans to be especially dangerous, and probably were. Such regions included much of southern Italy, the island of Sardinia, the Pontine Marshes to the south of Rome, and the low-lying regions of coastal Etruria to the northwest. In the city of Rome itself, the low valleys that lay between the hills, and the lands along the river Tiber, were fever-ridden.

SIGNIFICANCE

A modern historian has put the case for the importance of malaria in the ancient Roman world thus:

> Malaria enormously increased mortality levels, sharply reduced life expectancy at all ages, and significantly altered the age-structures of human populations in Europe

> in the past, wherever it became endemic. However, occurrences of malaria tended to be highly localized. . . . Consequently malaria generated enormous regional variations in demographic patterns in early modern Europe. In view of the compelling evidence from ancient sources for the endemicity [of malaria] in large areas of central and southern Italy . . . the comparative evidence from early modern Europe suggests that such major regional variations in demographic patterns should have occurred in Roman Italy. There is no doubt whatsoever that that is exactly what happened. (Sallares 2002, 269)

If Sallares is correct, malaria played a major role in the depopulations of important regions during the long period of Roman rule. The populations of southern and coastal Etruscan lands fell off after about 300 BCE; by the first century CE, the population of the once-fertile Pontine Marshes had collapsed. Malaria also contributed to elevated death rates in indirect ways; it interacted with both gastrointestinal troubles (such as dysentery) and respiratory ones (such as tuberculosis). Pregnant women were particularly vulnerable to it, as were their babies, many of whom suffered from low birth weight. The city of Rome itself was especially malarial, for reasons discussed in the "Background" section.

The ravages of malaria altered the way some Italian lands were used. In some cases, lands became so malarial that laborers could not be employed on them in summer; as a result, they were given over to pasture of animals. In other places, the farming population fled as environmental conditions made their lands more disease-ridden; if those lands stayed in cultivation, they may have been worked by slave labor instead, the slaves having less choice in the matter.

The Roman historian Tacitus suggests some ways in which malaria might have interfered with military affairs. The soldiers of Vitellius (one of four emperors in the chaotic year 69 CE) were thus weakened as they occupied Rome:

> Amidst the allurements of the city and all shameful excesses, they wasted their strength in idleness and their energies in riot. At last, reckless even of health, a large portion of them quartered themselves in the notoriously pestilential neighborhood of the Vatican; hence ensued a great mortality in the ranks. The Tiber was close at hand, and their extreme eagerness for the water and their impatience of the heat weakened the constitutions of the Germans and Gauls, always liable to disease. (Tacitus 1942, 532)

Speculations have been made about larger political consequences of malaria. To choose one example: Did its presence discourage the complete conquest of Italy by Attila, the king of the Huns, in the fifth century? As the historian Kyle Harper puts it, "the heartland of empire was a gauntlet of germs" (Harper 2017, 196).

Malaria was undoubtedly a presence in Roman life and death, and its overall significance no longer remains in doubt. (See "Unresolved Historical Issues" section.)

BACKGROUND

Some understanding of the modern beliefs about malaria will clarify both the role the disease played in ancient Rome and the relevance of the environmental background that characterized ancient Rome. Malaria is caused by one of several related parasitic microorganisms. In ancient Rome three of these were apparently present, those now called *Plasmodium falciparum*, *Plasmodium vivax*, and *Plasmodium malariae*. All cause intense fevers that strike periodically with debilitating effects on the body. The fevers from the first two microorganisms are called *tertian* fevers (meaning they appear every third day, counting inclusively; if fever day one is a Monday, fever will reappear on day three, Wednesday), while *Plasmodium malariae* leads to a *quartan* fever pattern (every fourth day). Of these three versions of malaria, that from *Plasmodium falciparum*, sometimes called malignant tertian fever, is the most serious; infection with it may last upward of a year and is often fatal. Malaria from *Plasmodium vivax* (benign tertian) is less serious but can persist for several years. Quartan fever may become utterly chronic, lasting one's whole life. Multiple infections by more than one type are possible; it is also possible that a previous *Plasmodium malariae* infection may lessen the effects of *Plasmodium falciparum*.

These microorganisms are found in mosquitoes that belong to the large genus called *Anopheles*, which includes hundreds of species, only some of which carry the parasites. Those different species may inhabit different environments, and that fact contributes to the wide regional variations in malaria incidence. But most often *Anopheles* mosquitoes are found around bodies of stagnant fresh water: pools, fish ponds, puddles, drainage ditches, and swamps. In Italy the mosquitoes generally are not (and presumably were not) found higher than about 500 meters above sea level.

The ancient city of Rome offered a number of such environments. The banks of the Tiber frequently flooded; much of the city lay in valleys between its famous seven hills, and mosquitoes favored those low lands; while the densely settled city's population favored irrigated gardens. And Rome adjoined other areas of Italy that had an ancient reputation as feverish, the lands of Latium and Etruria with many low-lying and swampy grounds.

The Romans undertook active projects in the landscape that contributed to creating malarial environments. Their intensive development of croplands in Etruria and Latium involved widespread deforestation. That in turn diminished the absorption of rainwater by foliage, which meant higher underground water tables and greater likelihood of flooded lowlands and marshes. The Romans were especially famous for their road building, and many of those projects disrupted drainage patterns and created new wetlands.

And the expansion of the great city of Rome represented further opportunities for both mosquitoes and *Plasmodium* parasites. Ancient Rome's population was perhaps one million, and its people lived in very crowded conditions, great numbers of them in the valleys between hills; mosquitoes had many (and easy) choices of people to infect. Rome was furthermore a huge magnet for in-migration, and people perhaps native to regions where malaria was not endemic flocked into the city where it certainly was. And people left Rome as well, perhaps carrying malaria infections with them to other places. Sallares refers to the city as a "population sink" in which malaria collected and from which it might drain elsewhere (Sallares 2002, 277); Harper claims that "the Roman Empire was an unintended experiment in mosquito breeding" (Harper 2017, 87).

HOW IT WAS UNDERSTOOD AT THE TIME

The Romans—and the Greeks from whom they adopted many of their beliefs about disease—were familiar with fevers, which had been clinically described (with some precision) both by the authors of the Hippocratic Corpus (fifth century BCE) and by later writers. Some of those fevers are clearly tertian and quartan malaria. About the causes of those fevers less agreement existed. Some followed the Hippocratic writings and blamed an imbalance of the body's humours:

> Continued fever is produced by large quantities of the most concentrated bile. . . . Quotidian fever is caused by a large quantity of bile, but less than that which causes continued fever. . . . Tertian fever lasts longer than quotidian fever and is caused by less bile. . . . Quartans behave similarly to the tertians but last longer, as they arise from still less of the heat-producing bile and because they give the body longer respites in which to cool down. (*Hippocratic Writings* 1978, 270–271)

The Roman understanding of fevers also might include a conviction that such ailments had divine (or perhaps demonic) origin. Roman (and Greek) thought about diseases included both natural explanations (such as the humoral theory quoted earlier) and supernatural ones; no clear distinction was made between the two modes, and they often flowed seamlessly together in medical explanations.

Some Romans believed that a quartan fever in the late summer or autumn was a good omen for future health. And since (according to modern beliefs) a *Plasmodium malariae* infection may protect against later *Plasmodium falciparum*, such Roman thinking may have been wise.

On an indirect level, the Romans understood that some environments were unhealthy and urged that they be avoided if possible. Such thinking went back at least to the fifth century BCE. Hippocratic text *Airs, Waters and Places*, which associated diseases with environments. Following its counsel, such later authors as the Roman engineer Vitruvius (of the first century BCE) and the slightly later Greco-Roman geographer Strabo feared swamps and marshes as feverish territory.

RESPONSES

Direct medical or therapeutic responses to malarial fever were few and generally limited to bed rest. The possibly divine origin of fevers led to people wearing amulets that might ward off an attack.

The environmental beliefs of the Romans led to a number of indirect responses to malaria that actually had some effect. Roman homeowners were urged to avoid swampy lands and river banks and to place homes on higher ground where winds might blow. In some cases, such advice was rooted in aesthetics more than in fear for health; marshes might contain unpleasant smells. For much the same reason, Romans regarded mosquitoes as pests and used fumigants and skin repellants against them. But no evidence exists that the Romans associated mosquitoes with disease transmission.

UNRESOLVED HISTORICAL ISSUES

Little doubt now exists about the significance of malaria in ancient Rome, but many questions remain about its complex relation to the eventual catastrophic collapse of Roman society in the sixth and seventh centuries CE. By the second century CE, the Roman Empire had erected a seemingly successful and prosperous Mediterranean world, highly urbanized and interconnected by roads, shipping lanes, and harbors, and that had reached out to its African and Asian neighbors. What role did malaria play in its dissolution?

Answering that question will involve more precise estimates of population, mortality, and causes of death in different times and places. In the past, studies of the importance of malaria in ancient Rome relied heavily on the documented effects of the disease in later periods of history, especially of Italy itself. More recent research has been able to analyze bones and teeth to learn about nutrition, diet, and growth at different periods and ages, and hence about possible causes of death. The rapidly developing science of recombinant sequencing of past DNA samples of both humans and microbes has made possible increasingly precise identifications of diseases. Recent and ongoing scholarship may therefore answer with greater precision such questions. (See also volume 2, chapter 2.)

REFERENCES

Harper, Kyle. *The Fate of Rome: Climate, Disease, and the End of an Empire.* Princeton, NJ: Princeton University Press, 2017.

Hippocratic Writings. Edited by G. E. R. Lloyd. Translated by J. Chadwick et al. London: Penguin, 1978.

Sallares, Robert. *Malaria and Rome: A History of Malaria in Ancient Italy.* Oxford: Oxford University Press, 2002.

Tacitus. *The Complete Works of Tacitus.* Translated by Alfred J. Church and William J. Brodribb. New York: Modern Library, 1942.

SUGGESTED ADDITIONAL READING

Jackson, Ralph. *Doctors and Diseases in the Roman Empire.* Norman: University of Oklahoma Press, 1988.

Shaw, Brent D. "Seasons of Death: Aspects of Mortality in Imperial Rome." *Journal of Roman Studies* 86 (1996): 100–138.

2

First Plague Pandemic, 541–747

WHEN AND WHERE

In 541 a devastating epidemic began spreading through the Mediterranean lands and adjoining western Asia. It first appeared at Pelusium, at the eastern edge of the Nile delta of Egypt. From there, it reportedly moved both west to Alexandria and east to Palestine and from there into Syria and Asia Minor; from Alexandria, it quickly reached Constantinople by sea. By 544 it had spread as far west as Italy and Tunisia. Thus began a period of about 200 years when epidemics repeatedly moved through an area bounded by England and Ireland to the north, the Iberian Peninsula to the west, the Sahara to the south, and Persia to the east; some of the episodes may have involved the civilizations of south and east Asia as well. Historians have documented a number of subsequent epidemic episodes in that period.

The first of these epidemics (541–544) has been called the Plague of Justinian, since it occurred in the reign of the (eastern) Roman emperor Justinian (527–565); the name has sometimes been extended to the entire 200-year period of the recurring epidemics as well. Modern authorities (Biraben and LeGoff 1975; Stathakopoulos 2004; Harper 2017) have identified differing numbers (between 15 and 20) of recurring waves of the pandemic between 541 and 747.

Any notion of the mortality involved in these epidemics remains largely speculative. Witnesses, notably the contemporary authors Procopius and John of Ephesus, claimed that in the 541–544 epidemic 5,000, and at times 10,000, people died daily in Justinian's capital city, Constantinople; John of Ephesus said that the total death toll in the city may have been 300,000. But any figures at all should be regarded skeptically. It is more certain that the death toll was simply very high; in the Second Plague Pandemic, especially its initial Black Death in 1346–1352, perhaps as many as 50% of populations in affected areas died, and similar mortality may have characterized the Plague of Justinian as well.

SIGNIFICANCE

This series of epidemics may properly be called a pandemic, for it affected a very wide area of the world in a repeated series of attacks. As such it was one of the great epidemic disasters of history, the first of the three pandemics of the disease bubonic plague. Of the three plague pandemics, it is the least known, and many of its effects on the societies of its time are only now being considered by historians. The social, economic, cultural, and political impact of its disruption may have contributed to the transitions between the ancient and medieval periods of Western history. The period between about 540 and about 750 saw the failure of the final attempt to maintain a unified Roman control of the Mediterranean; the dramatic rise of Islam in west Asia, northern Africa, and parts of Europe; the acceleration of the divergences between eastern (Greek) and western (Latin) Christianity; and the progressive localization of the economies, political systems, and societies of western (Latin) Europe. All those sweeping changes occurred against the backdrop of persistent epidemic disasters.

BACKGROUND

Plague is now regarded as a specific disease, the product of a microorganism called *Yersinia pestis*. It is enzootic, or habitually present, in communities of wild rodents. Its path to humans is now thought to be an indirect one that begins when its wild rodent hosts suffer epizootic, or "epidemic," levels of mortality; that drives their attendant fleas to seek new hosts, which they may find in "commensal" rodents such as rats that accompany human communities. The microorganism most frequently reaches a human when carried by a flea from its now-commensal rodent host. Once loose in the human bloodstream as a result of the flea bite, the microorganism causes a high fever and the characteristic swelling of lymph glands (in the groin, armpit, neck, or behind the ear) called *buboes*; if untreated with antibiotics this bubonic form of plague may be fatal in perhaps 60% of its cases. The lethal microorganism may also be conveyed directly to the lungs by droplets in the air, and that infection of the lungs leads to the form of plague called *pneumonic*, which can spread from one person to another via the respiratory system. In past plague epidemics, the pneumonic form has almost always been very rapidly fatal.

This understanding of plague, and its relation to rodents and fleas, developed in the period after 1890. It lays out certain preconditions for a plague epidemic. Humans must be in contact with an infected population of rodents and must be living in places where fleas can flourish. Since most rodents don't move very far or very fast in their lifetimes, the spread of an epidemic from one place to another depends on human traffic moving rodents (and fleas), perhaps by sea or perhaps in caravans and other means of overland trade.

Historians have come to understand that the period of the Plague of Justinian was one of very active and extensive commerce, especially by sea. Contemporary witnesses of this plague pandemic spoke of its movement from seaports inland.

HOW IT WAS UNDERSTOOD AT THE TIME

To the people of the sixth, seventh, and eighth centuries, only the act of an angry God could explain the colossal disaster of the plague. Procopius, the Greek historian who was a contemporary of Justinian and of the first pandemic, dismissed attempts to find natural explanations as inadequate for such a universal calamity. Other and later commentators agreed. John of Ephesus, a sixth-century Monophysite Syrian, lamented "over those of many cities which God's wrath turned into, as it were, a wine-press and pitilessly trampled and squeezed all their inhabitants within them like fine grapes" (*Chronicle* 1996, 74). Reports of supernatural apparitions preceded the disease; victims saw visions in dreams before they fell ill; "many people saw bronze boats and figures sitting in them resembling people with their heads cut off" (*Chronicle* 1996, 77). In 589 the visitation of plague in the city of Rome was heralded by a flood, accompanied by serpents and a dragon that swept through the city.

The contemporary descriptions of the disease's symptoms support the notion that the affliction was bubonic plague. The disease struck suddenly with a high fever; the buboes, or swellings, appeared in the groin, the armpits, behind the ears, or in the thigh; black spots might appear in the skin, especially the palm; the victims slipped into a coma or became delirious; death frequently followed within a few days. Epidemics in individual cities were reported as lasting about four months, three of them a period of particularly intense mortality and morbidity.

The epidemic also seemed to bear moral lessons. Was it God's penalty for human sins? When survivors tried to profit from the possessions of the deceased, it was reported that they were inevitably stricken with the plague themselves. But what especially survives in the contemporary accounts is a sense of horror. John of Ephesus repeatedly used the wine-press image:

> Noble and chaste women, dignified with honour, who sat in bedchambers, now with their mouths swollen, wide open and gaping, who were piled up in horrible heaps, all ages lying prostrate, all statures bowed down and overthrown, all ranks pressed on upon another, in a single wine-press of God's wrath, like beasts, not like human beings. (*Chronicle* 1996, 90)

In later outbreaks of the pandemic, in the seventh and especially the eighth centuries, consciousness grew of the disease as a more discrete entity, apart from a general God-sent pestilence. Syriac and Arabic sources began using separate terms for the disease responsible for the epidemics, and descriptions became more identifiably those of bubonic plague.

RESPONSES

The speed and severity of the plague epidemics left contemporaries helpless. The remedies of the Hippocratic and Galenic traditions of the ancient Greco-Roman world called for attention to diet, rest, and bathing, and watchful waiting by the physician, but cases of plague would be resolved (often fatally) before any such remedies could take effect. Some physicians lanced buboes when they appeared, with uncertain results. Although Procopius found no evidence that the disease was contagious, he also noted that caregivers suffered from the hardships their labors entailed. Generally, the prognoses of physicians were not reliable; Procopius reminded his readers that the disease proceeded from "no cause which came within the province of human reasoning" (Procopius 1914, 463).

In the first plague epidemic, of the 540s, the government of the Roman Empire (by then long established at Byzantium, or Constantinople) found its main task to be the disposal of corpses. The government allotted public money for digging mass graves and generously paid those hired to dig them. Boats were filled with the dead whose remains were dumped overboard at sea. The boats would then return for another grim load. People took to wearing name tags on their arms when they left their homes so that they might be identified if they were stricken.

In the sixth, seventh, and eighth centuries, religious responses overlapped with medical and political ones, but they did not seem to work either. Exorcisms failed, although belief in demons as causal agents persisted. One group of people feared as demons were those monks and other clerics with shorn tonsures; according to John of Ephesus, some people took fright at their approach and avoided them. In Constantinople, rumors led many to hurl pitchers out of their windows, believing that such action would chase the disease away; John of Ephesus argued that such rumors were themselves the work of demons.

Above all, the First Plague Pandemic seemed to have left people stunned: as if drunk, "stupefied and confused," said John of Ephesus (*Chronicle* 1996, 97). Flight, if it were at all possible, was a common reaction.

EFFECTS

Witnesses agreed that the immediate effect of these plague visitations was catastrophic. Social confusion and economic paralysis resulted. All work ceased. Shops closed for lack of workers and customers. Fields were abandoned, crops remained unharvested, fruits fell rotten to the ground, and flocks and herds wandered untended in fields and pastures. Elite members of society remained unburied when their servants predeceased them. Since those who appropriated the property of the dead seemed especially vulnerable, legitimate heirs refused their inheritances, fearing the consequences of apparent greed. At least for a time, many survivors vowed to amend their ways and return to a pious life; but when the disease passed, they reverted to their old habits.

Over the roughly 200-year period of the pandemic some attitudes toward it changed. In the Islamic world (the eastern and southern Mediterranean became Muslim in the seventh and eighth centuries), a new religious interpretation of the epidemic gained hold by the mid-eighth century, one that saw plague as a mercy and a martyrdom sent by Allah, not a punishment. Earlier Muslims had regarded plague as a product of Allah's anger and they had fled (as Christians had done); the new interpretation urged resignation in the face of God's will. There may have been some evolution of Christian responses as well. In Frankish Gaul, the Virgin Mary received increased veneration, perhaps from those who sought maternal succor from epidemic ravages.

Much evidence exists for the serious demographic impact of the pandemic, although certainly no population figures of any sort can be trusted. Contemporaries spoke of deserted villages in the wake of plague visitations. More recent archaeology has uncovered dense burial sites. Also interesting, although indirect as evidence, is the relative scarcity of new buildings, especially public ones, in the period after about 540. Rural construction, and the creation of new settlements, also seemed to have stopped or slowed after that date. The Syrian city of Antioch, devastated by an earthquake, was rebuilt, but on a smaller scale than it had occupied earlier; it evidently was built for a smaller population. In the Visigothic Spanish kingdom, another piece of evidence suggests a demographic crisis: attacks on the Jews by the Christian rulers stopped, perhaps because all the survivors were needed regardless of their "heresy." Some evidence also exists for attempts to force laborers to remain on specific pieces of land. In times of labor shortages, workers might be tempted to move away in search of better conditions or pay, and the massive depopulation caused by an epidemic would have created labor shortages on a grand scale. Rural depopulation had another important effect, this one political: plague epidemics coincided with periods of crisis in the finances of the Byzantine Empire. Did those crises stem from a loss in the taxable base of the society? Were there fewer peasants, lowered levels of production, and less tax revenue? Still another political effect may have been military; Justinian's epic wars against enemies both to the west and the east had to be carried on with reduced forces. But perhaps his Persian and Germanic foes faced the same demographic crisis.

UNRESOLVED HISTORICAL ISSUES

Many aspects of the first great plague pandemic remain unsettled and may never be known. For a start, its geographical origins are still in dispute. Contemporary opinion believed it first appeared in Egypt, and that opinion has been used to connect its origins with Africa. Some features of what is known about the evolution of the causative microorganism, *Yersinia pestis*, may also argue for its African ancestry. But the balance of evidence from paleomicrobiology now favors an Asian origin, and the existence of the sea trade routes from Asia through the Red Sea makes an Asian (or Indian) origin even more likely. Historians have especially focused on the great city of Constantinople, with its huge demand for exotic goods brought from all over the known world, as an important point of diffusion for an epidemic. Alexandria, the seaport from which much of the grain consumed by Mediterranean communities was distributed, played a similar role.

Trade was clearly an important factor in the plague's spread. These epidemics seemed to have reached new places by sea and then diffused inland from the seaports. But other loci of transmission existed at times; for example, when the pandemic belatedly reached England (in the seventh century) monasteries apparently played the role of "seaport" as centers of plague diffusion. Factors in addition to trade could put people (and their accompanying rodents and insects) in motion. Harper (2017) has recently drawn a picture of a sixth-century Mediterranean world under siege from a multiplicity of natural forces: earthquakes, the onset of a "little ice age" triggered by volcanic eruptions in southeast Asia in 536, and the relentless force of epidemics, some of long-standing pressure (malaria, tuberculosis, diarrhea, and dysentery), now joined in 541 by the overwhelming bubonic plague. All that could—and did—result in nomadic movements of peoples, some fleeing plague, some searching for new sources of food when their crops were destroyed. Did those movements help trigger the first epidemic in 541? Warfare might also have forced population movement in the sixth, seventh, and eighth centuries, the last two of which were marked by the dramatic expansion of Islam as Muslim conquerors spread outward from the Arabian Peninsula.

Some questions may remain about another previously unsettled point: the identification of the actual disease. Contemporary descriptions of it clearly suggest bubonic plague. Several arguments that have been raised against that diagnosis have largely been settled. Bubonic plague is primarily a disease of rodents, which affects humans only when they accidentally encounter rodent fleas. Rodents move slowly and never very far, but we easily account for a disease's rapid movement from city to city when we remember that humans could carry rats (and their fleas) very far in their ships, caravans, and especially their grain stocks. The patchy spread of the disease within a particular town or village accords well with a transmission from rodent to human by way of an insect. If a disease was spread through the air (as smallpox and tuberculosis are) its effects should be much more generally felt, while all plague epidemics seem to erratically affect people in some homes or workplaces, and not others. Careful archaeology has now uncovered evidence of the presence of black rats (*Rattis rattis*) in sixth-century Mediterranean lands. And finally, the evidence from paleomicrobiology has established a positive identification of *Yersinia pestis* in the tissues of bodies from the sixth, seventh, or eighth centuries and hence the diagnosis of bubonic plague as the cause of the Plague of Justinian.

Other unresolved questions remain about the pandemic's precise chronology. The first great wave of 541–544 remains the best documented. Modern authors (see the "When and Where" section) basically agree on 10 other episodes: 557–561, 570–574, 588–592, 597–601, 618–619, 626–628, 639–640, 683–687, 694–700, and 743–747. (These dates contribute to the belief that the intervals between epidemic surges in plague pandemics lengthen over time.) The scarcity of written evidence (at least relative to later periods of history) has made identification of specific times and places of the pandemic difficult. In fact, the apparent frequency of plague in Constantinople, Antioch, and Rome, for example, may reflect the relatively rich documentation of such places. As has been true of many epidemics, likely high mortalities in rural settlements have gone unrecorded.

Finally, the true long-term effects of this pandemic remain a matter of speculation. Some (e.g., Russell 1968) believe that it marked the end of the world of antiquity and the beginning of medieval times. Without the epidemic of 541–544, Russell argued, Justinian would have been able to reconstruct the broken Roman Empire. The recent work of Harper (2017) about the role of climate change casts doubt on such arguments, and historians continue to see pieces of apparently contradictory evidence. Did new churches constructed in the sixth century speak for a still-vibrant economy? Or did their appearance illustrate a change in values, as survivors became more pious? Not all cities dramatically contracted after 541. Did their relatively continued strength illustrate general vitality or the patchy nature of the pandemic? Did the pandemic represent a major discontinuity for the lands it affected or were its effects only short term for societies that quickly regained their routines? And some lands affected by the pandemic, especially some in the East, recovered more quickly than others. (See also volume 2, chapter 5, "The Black Death Begins the Second Plague Pandemic, 1346–1352.")

REFERENCES

Biraben, J.-N., and Jacques LeGoff. "The Plague in the Early Middle Ages." In *Biology of Man in History*, edited by Robert Forster and Orest Ranum, 44–80. Baltimore, MD: Johns Hopkins University Press, 1975.

Harper, Kyle. *The Fate of Rome: Climate, Disease, and the End of an Empire.* Princeton, NJ: Princeton University Press, 2017.

John of Ephesus. *Chronicle, Part III* (Preserved in Pseudo-Dionysius of Tel-Mahre). Translated and edited by Witold Witakowski. Liverpool: Liverpool University Press, 1996.

Procopius. *Works*, vol. I, *History of the Wars*, books I and II. Translated by H. W. Dewing. Cambridge, MA: Harvard University Press, 1914.

Russell, J. C. "That Earlier Plague." *Demography* 5 (1968): 174–184.

Stathakopoulos, Dionysios. "The Justinianic Plague Revisited." *Byzantine and Modern Greek Studies* 24 (2004): 256–276.

SUGGESTED ADDITIONAL READING

Another Source Account

Paul the Deacon. *History of the Langobards.* Translated by William D. Foulke. Philadelphia: Department of History, University of Pennsylvania, 1907.

Modern Works

Little, Lester K., ed. *Plague and the End of Antiquity: The Pandemic of 541–750.* New York: Cambridge University Press, 2007.

McCormick, Michael. *Origins of the European Economy: Communications and Commerce, A.D. 300–900.* Cambridge: Cambridge University Press, 2001.

Raoult, Didier, and Michel Drancourt, eds. *Paleomicrobiology: Past Human Infections.* Berlin: Springer-Verlag, 2008.

3

Smallpox Epidemic in Japan, 735–737

WHEN AND WHERE

In 735 CE a serious epidemic, almost certainly smallpox, began in the seaport region of Dazaihu on the north coast of the Japanese island of Kyushu. Its severity was quickly recognized by the Japanese government. Perhaps by the end of 735, and certainly by 736, the epidemic had spread to the main island of Honshu. It may have been carried from Kyushu to Honshu by the returning party of an emissary who had planned to negotiate better relations with Korean states. When he died en route, his party returned to Honshu, spreading smallpox through the Inland Sea area as they went. The entire island of Honshu was affected by 737, especially the western and southern provinces.

Contemporary clinical descriptions support the belief that smallpox was responsible for this epidemic. So too does the use of contemporary Japanese (and Chinese) terms for the ailment, terms that specifically differentiate smallpox from measles, which (on the basis of the clinical descriptions) might be another possibility.

Total mortality in the epidemic may have been as high as one-third of the population of Japan, with some areas experiencing a staggering mortality of 60%. Unusually good public records (censuses, tax records, land records) make such estimates possible for modern scholars; most epidemics from such an early period have not left such a clear record.

SIGNIFICANCE

The great smallpox epidemic of 735–737 was the most severe in a series of epidemics that (in the view of the historian W. W. Farris) plunged Japan into a prolonged cycle of underpopulation and lagging economic growth, a cycle that persisted until the thirteenth century. More immediately, it may have played a role in the new emphasis placed on Buddhism by the emperor who ruled Japan at the time, Shōmu.

BACKGROUND

Smallpox, an acute viral infection, had been a frequent companion of humans since the earliest civilizations. While certain identification of individual epidemics is difficult, it was, for example, the likely cause of the so-called Plague of Thucydides that struck Athens in 430–427 BCE, named for the Greek historian who recorded it. While Japan had suffered earlier epidemics, including likely smallpox visitations, its island location shielded it from constant disease pressure from its neighbors and a generation or two might separate one epidemic from the next. Each new epidemic therefore attacked a population that mostly lacked immunity from any previous exposure, so its mortality might be unusually high. Two further circumstances contributed to the severity of the epidemic of 735–737. Japan's population had apparently grown rapidly earlier in the eighth century; as the density of rural settlement increased, so too did the opportunities for the spread of an airborne disease such as smallpox. And the years immediately preceding the epidemic had been ones of widespread harvest failure; the Japanese population may have been poorly nourished in 735.

The Japanese political situation in the early eighth century helps explain the relative wealth of information we have about this epidemic. In response to the advance of the Chinese T'ang Empire and the victory of anti-Japanese forces in Korean states, the Japanese government attempted to strengthen its central control of the country. That involved adopting government practices used by the Chinese, including the careful collection of population, tax, and land-holding records. The results were unusually (for the time) complete sets of demographic data.

HOW IT WAS UNDERSTOOD AT THE TIME

The epidemic was generally understood as punishment sent by gods, either the traditional Shinto gods angered by the spread of Buddhist beliefs and images or Buddhist gods reacting to Shinto-inspired attacks on such images.

An order by the government's Council of State in 737 thoroughly describes the appearance and course of the disease. In doing so, it is very much in the tradition of contemporary Chinese medical systems and beliefs. Sufferers of the epidemic displayed red swellings and blotches on the skin, fever, thirst, and diarrhea with black or bloody stools.

RESPONSES

The Japanese government reacted to the epidemic on three levels. First, it attempted to provide care for the sick by sending medicines (probably herbal remedies based on Chinese beliefs) to communities stricken by the disease. Second, it offered assistance to entire communities by allowing exemptions from some forms of taxation and eventually ordering a grain dole sent to afflicted provinces. (The grain dole was an especially serious step, one taken only in grave emergencies.) At the end of 735, the government also extended a general amnesty to the entire population, a traditional Confucian response to trouble. Third, the state addressed the underlying religious causes of the epidemic. Prayers were ordered, provincial governors were commanded to perform propitiatory rites, Buddhist monks read sacred texts, and the ruler, Shōmu, showed signs of greater Buddhist devotion. By 748 a colossal statue of the Buddha had been erected in the capital, Nara.

More immediate medical responses to the sickness included wrapping patients in hemp or silk, keeping them warm, restraining their movements, and compelling them to eat.

UNRESOLVED HISTORICAL ISSUES

This epidemic is unusually well documented, so that most of the unresolved issues concern its role in larger trends in Japanese history. W. W. Farris, a careful modern student of the epidemic, used it to support an interpretation of the growth (or lack thereof) of the medieval Japanese economy (Farris 1985). He argued that the 735–737 catastrophe critically lowered the Japanese population and that subsequent epidemics repeatedly throttled any long-term demographic recovery. The sparse Japanese population was caught in a cycle in which abandoned land, dispersed settlements, and poor technology all meant continuing underdevelopment, which in turn discouraged population growth. According to Farris, this cycle of poverty was only broken when smallpox finally became endemic in the thirteenth century, which broke the epidemic cycle of attacks on an unexposed population. If this interpretation is correct, the smallpox epidemic of 735–737 assumes an important role in the history of medieval Japan.

REFERENCE

Farris, William Wayne. *Population, Disease, and Land in Early Japan, 645–900.* Cambridge, MA: Harvard University Press, 1985.

SUGGESTED ADDITIONAL READING

Hopkins, Donald R. *The Greatest Killer: Smallpox in History.* Chicago: University of Chicago Press, 2002. (Orig. pub. 1983 as *Princes and Peasants: Smallpox in History.*)

Jannetta, Ann Bowman. *Epidemics and Mortality in Early Modern Japan.* Princeton, NJ: Princeton University Press, 1987.

Twitchett, Denis. "Population and Pestilence in T'ang China." In *Studia Sino-Mongolica: Festschrift für Herbert Franke*, edited by Wolfgang Bauer, 35–68. Wiesbaden: Franz Steiner Verlag, 1979.

4

Leprosy in Medieval Europe

WHEN AND WHERE

The disease called *leprosy* was very widespread in medieval Europe, especially (but not only) between about 1000 and about 1350. In those years, apparently large numbers of institutions for the isolation of lepers were created, although some confusion existed between "leprosaria" and more general charities for the sick. The incidence of leprosy (as it was then understood) seemingly began to decline in the years after about 1250; by about 1350 many of the institutions devoted to it had shrunk in size or even closed. By about 1500 leprosy was unusual in Europe, except in isolated portions of Scandinavia. No reliable estimate of the number of sufferers or of mortality rates is possible, but the number of *leprosaria*, as the institutions were called, may have been in the thousands.

The victims of the disease might suffer gradually worsening lesions of the skin, sometimes leading to bone damage, deformations, and loss of extremities. The repellant appearance of those sufferers certainly contributed to the horror the disease inspired and to the social stigmatization of its victims, as well as to the contemporary (and subsequent) emphases on it.

SIGNIFICANCE

Medieval leprosy affords perhaps the Western world's clearest and most dramatic example of the relationships between disease, social stigmatization, and theological interpretations. Fear of lepers became very deeply rooted in Western society; the word "leper" ultimately acquired (in English) a more general and symbolic meaning: "a person who is shunned, especially on moral grounds," says the *New Shorter Oxford English Dictionary* (1993), which quotes the [London] *Sunday Express* by way of illustration: "There are lepers in every prison—child molesters, rapists."

BACKGROUND

Diseases called leprosy had a long and complicated history in the ancient and medieval worlds. The ancient Hebrews discussed, especially in the book of Leviticus, the presence in their midst of *tsara'ath*, a "repulsive scaly skin disease" (as translated by Hulse 1975). That condition was perhaps identical with medieval leprosy, and the Hebrews' discussion of the rituals to be performed when one was diagnosed with it entered into later Christian attitudes toward leprosy. The ancient Greeks also described similar diseases, which they called *elephantiasis* and sometimes *lepra*. Early Islamic authors described two such diseases, one probably identical with medieval leprosy, the other what is now called elephantiasis. In the early medieval West, some comments on leprosy began as early as the eighth century.

Some confusion about the term for the disease played an important role in medieval attitudes toward it. Medieval Christian scholars equated the disease known to them with the ailment subject to the ritual isolation prescribed in Leviticus, rendering (perhaps incorrectly) the Hebrew *tsara'ath* as their leprosy.

HOW IT WAS UNDERSTOOD AT THE TIME

In equating the Hebrew "repulsive scaly skin disease" with their leprosy, medieval Christian writers imposed on it the notion that the disease was divine punishment for the wrongdoing, or sins, of the sufferers. The ancient Hebrews had not emphasized wrongdoing or sin as much as a neglect of divine ordinances about cleanliness, a neglect that required rituals to appease God's anger. Priests of the community made the diagnosis of the signs of ritual uncleanness and prescribed the isolation and other rituals of atonement to be performed. Medieval Christians followed Leviticus in assigning a diagnostic role to the clergy. But for medieval Christian authorities, the issue was more mortal sin than uncleanness, and the punishment was far more permanent and less amenable to atoning by ritual. The sin most often held responsible for leprosy was lust, although gluttony was sometimes blamed.

By the thirteenth century, medieval physicians occupied a more prominent role in diagnosis, and they more often interpreted the cause of the disease within the framework of the humoral medicine derived from ancient Greek authors, especially Galen and the body of writings attributed to Hippocrates. That approach believed that diseases resulted from imbalances in the four humours (blood, phlegm, yellow bile, and black bile) that coursed through the body. Diseases that related to passion, or lust, were associated with disorders and imbalances of blood, and some symptoms of leprosy seemed to confirm that association, especially the reddish lesions of the skin and the cracked and bleeding gums. But by the fourteenth century, medical opinion began to relate the disease more with another humour, black bile, and so associated it less with lust and more with melancholia and depression. That view marked a weakening of the moral failure interpretation of the disease that had dominated earlier medieval responses.

Fears of contagion were also evidently very old, as the isolation demanded by Leviticus illustrates, and they remained an important (if inconsistent, as the next sections will suggest) aspect of the medieval understanding of the disease.

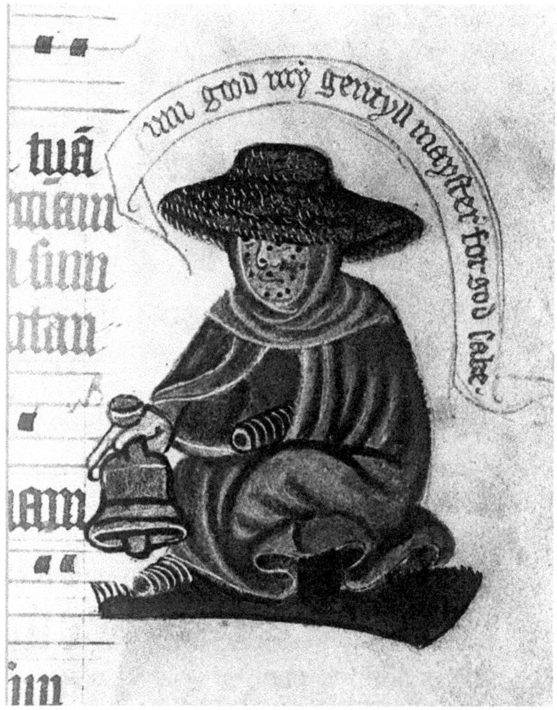

A leper with a disfigured face and amputated limbs rings a warning bell, from an English music sheet, c. 1400. By that date, the incidence of leprosy in Europe was declining. (Wellcome Library)

RESPONSES

In the centuries (between the eleventh and the fourteenth) when leprosy was at its peak, the most widespread responses to it were the leprosaria, institutions or communities for lepers on the outskirts of towns and villages. Sufferers were exiled to such communities after public accusations led to an examination (by a priest and increasingly a physician) found them to be leprous. A ritual, formalized in 1179 by the Third Lateran Council, followed that symbolically severed the victim from his or her home community, in effect pronouncing the victim dead, an impression reinforced by throwing cemetery earth on the sufferer. The ritual forbade contact with the living and prescribed a distinctive costume and a bell that would warn others of the leper's approach. It included such orders as "I command you when you are on a journey not to return an answer to anyone who questions you, till you have gone off the road to leeward, so that he may take no harm from you," and "I forbid you to touch infants or young folk, whosoever they may be, or to give to them or to others any of your possessions." The victim was then led to the leprosarium that would henceforth be home. (Translations of the terms of the 1179 ritual are reprinted in Brody 1974, 66–67; Richards 1977, 123–124.)

Leprosaria varied considerably in size, elaborateness, and even wealth. Some—probably most—were a miserable collection of a few huts; others were larger and more substantial. In some cases, the lepers were allowed to accumulate their worldly possessions in the institution. Some leprosaria demanded a fee collected by the administrators; most were heavily dependent on charity. Leprosaria were originally (and usually) under church control, but in the later centuries of the epidemic lay political authorities assumed more power over them.

Medieval authorities held out little hope of a cure, so that diagnosis of leprosy often amounted to a life sentence. A life of religious penance, parallel with the devotions of a monastic order, was urged for the lepers; confession, as one modern writer (Palmer 1982, 85–86) notes, was an important therapeutic tool in the medieval West, not just for leprosy. At times, the residents of leprosaria were the objects of fierce and deep prejudices. In the early fourteenth century, for example, King Philip V of France directed murderous local attacks on lepers. Their isolation in separate communities, and the accusatory process that brought them there, made them logical targets of blame for all sorts of imagined crimes.

UNRESOLVED HISTORICAL ISSUES

On one level—perhaps the most obvious—medieval society punished lepers for their sins, which were held to be the ultimate cause of the disease. They were isolated from the society, stigmatized, and might lose legal standing as humans; in some cases, their surviving spouses might remarry, for the ritual symbolically buried them in a cemetery.

In practice, however, medieval treatment of (and response to) lepers betrayed many uncertainties. The bans that prohibited lepers from touching things, passing people on one side of the street, handling water and food, having contact with children, and the like were often simply ignored or only enforced sporadically. Perhaps, therefore, many medieval people continued to recognize and respect their friends and former neighbors. Some evidence suggests, moreover, that medieval religious attitudes were mixed as well. Had God punished lepers for their sins or had he singled them out for special grace? Jesus had suffered. Were the lepers in some way replicating that suffering? Should they be stigmatized or venerated? Medieval writings suggest that both approaches were followed in different times and places.

The fear that leprosy was contagious led to other ambiguities. That fear was clearly very ancient, as the provisions for isolation in Leviticus illustrate. In the later medieval period, medical opinions increasingly emphasized the contagious nature of diseases, perhaps as convictions about the contagious nature of plague strengthened in the fifteenth century (see subsequent chapters on plague). If leprosy were spread by contagion, how did the moral failure argument apply? Did the disease only spread to the impure of heart? In some cases, lepers were allowed to continue to live with their uninfected spouses in the leprosaria. Were those spouses at risk, if the disease was as contagious as the rituals of separation suggested?

The identification of the leprosy of the Middle Ages remains uncertain. Modern leprosy is now usually called Hansen's disease, thought to be the product of a microorganism, *Mycobacterium leprae*, identified in 1873 by Gerhard Hansen, a Norwegian microbiologist. Hansen's disease may result in the deformations described in medieval accounts, but other diseases might account for them as well, including, for example, syphilis and yaws (whose existence in medieval Europe is at best unproven). Other skin ailments, such as psoriasis, might have been responsible for milder cases of medieval leprosy. Modern opinions about Hansen's disease hold that it is only very slowly and erratically contagious, that its symptoms may vary widely, and that those symptoms usually develop very slowly.

Some solid evidence suggests the existence of Hansen's disease in medieval Europe. Bone deformations characteristic of that disease have been found in skeletons in some Danish cemeteries known to have been set aside for lepers. The wide variety of symptoms of Hansen's disease, and the unclear pattern of contagion that it follows, both are consistent with the differing and ambiguous medieval responses to it. But clearly medieval diagnoses may have categorized a number of complaints under leprosy, especially in view of the moral connotations of that disease. People unpopular in a village community or people with a powerful enemy might have been so diagnosed.

Also unresolved is why the apparently high level of infection of leprosy in the period between about 1000 and about 1350 subsequently declined. That decline roughly coincided with the onset of the second plague pandemic, but that may have been coincidental. Perhaps the deaths of caregivers for leprosaria left their populations more vulnerable, and so more likely to die more rapidly of all causes; the subsequent depopulation would result in the closing of leprosaria, our main measure for the decline in the incidence of the disease.

A more likely cause for the decline in medieval leprosy was a corresponding rise in the infection rates of pulmonary tuberculosis. The causative microorganisms of Hansen's disease and of pulmonary tuberculosis are closely related—both give rise to mycobacterial diseases. Further, they may share important cross-immunities, in which infection by one prevents infection by the other. If pulmonary tuberculosis (a far more immediately contagious infection than Hansen's disease) became more widespread in the late Middle Ages, the waning of leprosy might be explained. Another possibility is that leprosy affected male fertility, and so those people genetically susceptible to it were bred out of the population.

Leprosy, or Hansen's disease, persisted in some parts of Europe (especially in Scandinavia) well into the nineteenth century. It was also prevalent in tropical regions, particularly those under Western imperial rule, which included Pacific Islands, among them Hawaii. Hence, tropical medicine came to study leprosy as well as such diseases as malaria and yellow fever. It continues to infect world regions where poverty is widespread or locally severe. The countries with the greatest number of new 2016 cases are now India (with two-thirds of recent infections), Brazil, and Indonesia.

REFERENCES

Brody, Saul N. *The Disease of the Soul: Leprosy in Medieval Literature.* Ithaca, NY: Cornell University Press, 1974.

Hulse, E. V. "The Nature of Biblical 'Leprosy' and the Use of Alternative Medical Terms in Modern Translations of the Bible." *Palestine Exploration Quarterly* 107 (1975): 87–105.

New Shorter Oxford English Dictionary. Oxford: Clarendon, 1993.

Palmer, Richard. 1982. "The Church, Leprosy and Plague in Medieval and Early Modern Europe." In *The Church and Healing*, edited by W. J. Sheils, 85–86. Oxford: Basil Blackwell, 1982.

Richards, Peter. *The Medieval Leper and His Northern Heirs.* Cambridge: D. S. Brewer. 1977.

SUGGESTED ADDITIONAL READING

Demaitre, Luke. *Leprosy in Premodern Medicine: A Malady of the Whole Body.* Baltimore, MD: Johns Hopkins University Press, 2007.

Demaitre, Luke. *Medieval Medicine: The Art of Healing from Head to Toe.* Santa Barbara, CA: ABC-CLIO, 2013, esp. 102–109.

Edmond, Rod. *Leprosy and Empire: A Medical and Cultural History.* Cambridge: Cambridge University Press, 2006.

5

The Black Death Begins: The Second Plague Pandemic, 1346–1352

The Black Death, and the Second Plague Pandemic that it commenced, remains the most significant and most disputed disease event in human history. As this chapter discusses, historical controversy continues about many of its main features. Since the Black Death is inextricably connected to the Second Plague Pandemic (1346–1844), this chapter will also refer to the history of that pandemic.

WHEN AND WHERE

The Black Death

The earliest clearly documented appearance of what would become the Second Plague Pandemic occurred in 1346, in the Mongol territory called the Khanate of the Golden Horde: south of the Don River, west of the Volga River, north of the Caucasus Mountains, between the Caspian and the Black Seas, in lands now in southern Russia. In 1347 the disease began to spread rapidly, following seaborne trade routes, which carried it first from the Crimean Peninsula across the Black Sea to Constantinople. From Constantinople, the epidemic also moved inland into western Asia Minor. More dramatic were its overseas jumps. From Constantinople, sea traffic in 1347 carried plague to Cyprus; Alexandria (on the coast of Egypt); Crete and southern Greece; Dubrovnik, Split, and Venice on the Adriatic; Sicily and the toe of Calabria; Sardinia and Corsica; and Pisa and Genoa in northwest Italy. Further shipping from Genoa spread the disease to Marseille (in southern France), and from there the plague reached Mallorca before the end of the year.

By 1348 the plague reached many of the most densely settled areas of both Muslim and Christian worlds. In some cases, seaports served as nodes from which the disease moved inland: along the eastern Mediterranean and up the Nile from Alexandria; into the interior of Tunisia and Algeria from Tunis; into Italy from Pisa, Genoa, and Venice; into southern France from Marseille and Narbonne.

But the plague also continued to reach across the sea, notably from Bordeaux. That port was apparently first affected overland, from the French Mediterranean lands. From Bordeaux, shipping rapidly carried plague along the Atlantic coast of Europe: to La Coruña into northwestern Iberia, to Rouen and up the Seine to Paris, to Weymouth and Bristol and hence across southern England, and to the east coast of Ireland. Yet another 1348 seaborne jump took the plague from London to Oslo.

During 1349, plague epidemics moved into Mesopotamia, Morocco, southern Iberia, the central and northern areas of France that had not been touched in 1348, northern England, the whole of Ireland, southern Germany and central Europe along the Danube, and a variety of northern German cities as well. Further sea transit occurred as well: from London to the Orkney and Shetland Islands, and to Bergen; from Oslo into the Baltic to Danzig. By 1350 virtually all of western and central Europe had been affected, for in that year the plague reached Scotland, Sweden, the Netherlands, the balance of northern Germany, and the Bohemian and Moravian lands. The final eastward overland movements of the Black Death then took place: Poland and the Baltic lands in 1351; Novgorod, Smolensk, and Kiev in 1352, and Muscovy in 1353. In that year, the epidemic apparently died out in Europe, North Africa, and western Asia.

The epidemic had therefore completed something of a clockwise loop that began in southern Russia in 1346 and reached back into central Russia seven years later.

This epidemic resulted in enormous mortality rates in the areas it infected. For many years, historians accepted a total mortality of between 30% and 40% of the population in the years between 1346 and 1353. In individual places, the epidemic usually lasted three or four months, and much of the dreadful toll occurred in that brief span. A more recent (and thorough) review of the Black Death (Benedictow 2004) argues that if anything those estimates are too low and suggests that mortality rates across Europe may have approached 60%, with some variation between different economic groups (somewhat lower for householders) and regions (somewhat lower in urban northern Italy, where a more elaborate administrative system provided some help). If Ole Benedictow is correct, perhaps 50 million Europeans (of a total population of 80 million) may have died between 1346 and 1353. Mortalities in western Asia and North Africa may have been comparable.

The experiences of individual places illustrate the sudden devastation that the epidemic brought. In the Egyptian region of Asyūt, about 6,000 individuals ordinarily paid land tax; during the Black Death that number plunged to 116. In Chambéry, France, 403 households existed in 1348; by 1349 there were only 184. In the Italian commune of San Gimignano, a population of about 11,400 in 1332 had fallen to about 4,500 in 1349. The number of wills proved in London courts increased by a factor of *fifteen* between 1348 and 1349.

Only much later (apparently in the seventeenth century) did this terrible episode come to be called the Black Death, although the Latin phrase *atra mors* that led to its use went back to classical antiquity. No clear connection exists between the phrase Black Death and any of the symptoms of the disease. In the fourteenth century, witnesses most often simply spoke of a great pestilence or a great plague.

Contemporaries left many descriptions of the disease. One of the best known was that of the Italian author Giovanni Boccaccio (1313–1375), who structured his great *Decameron* around the epidemic's events. According to Boccaccio:

> For in the early spring of the year we have mentioned, the plague began, in a terrifying and extraordinary manner, to make its disastrous effects apparent. It did not take the form it had assumed in the East, where if anyone bled from the nose it was an obvious portent of certain death. On the contrary, its earliest symptom, in men and women alike, was the appearance of certain swellings in the groin or the armpit, some of which were egg-shaped whilst others were roughly the size of the common apple. Sometimes the swellings were large, sometimes not so large, and they were referred to by the populace as *gavòccioli.* From the two areas already mentioned, this deadly *gavòcciolo* would begin to spread, and within a short time it would appear at random all over the body. Later on, the symptoms of the disease changed, and many people began to find dark blotches and bruises on their arms, thighs, and other parts of the body, sometimes large and few in number, at other times tiny and closely spaced. These, to anyone unfortunate enough to contract them, were just as infallible a sign that he would die as the *gavòcciolo* had been earlier, and indeed it still was.
>
> Against these maladies, it seemed that all the advice of physicians and all the power of medicine were profitless and unavailing. . . . At all events, few of those who caught it ever recovered, and in most cases death occurred within three days from the appearance of the symptoms we have described, some people dying more rapidly than others, the majority without any fever or other complications. (Boccaccio 1972, 50–51)

Some particular characteristics of the epidemic related to seasons, ages, and social groups affected, and its speed of movement by land, by sea, and through rural or urban areas. Generally, the spread of the disease coincided with warm weather, and cold weather slowed or stopped it. There were, however, exceptions to that. Although the disease attacked all levels and ages of the population, children and the poor suffered at least marginally higher mortality rates, partly owing to greater vulnerability to other infections because of their inadequate nutrition and the lack of social networks to care for the sick (see the "Background" section). The disease spread much more rapidly by sea than it did overland (there is a brief discussion of modern beliefs about the epidemiology of bubonic and pneumonic plague, in the "Background" section). And the disease apparently moved more rapidly, and dangerously, through rural villages than through dense cities (again, see the "Background" section).

The Later Stages of the Second Plague Pandemic

While the great Black Death epidemic receded by 1353, the disease had become established in both Europe and the Muslim world, and a long period ensued when plague was always a menace. According to one tabulation (by Biraben 1975, 1:363–449), plague was present in *some* European location every year between 1347 and 1670. Over those several centuries, plague flared in repeated epidemics, many of them serious by any reasonable standard, and dwarfed only by the Black Death. The first such epidemic occurred in the early 1360s and is sometimes called the *pestis secundus* (second plague); another spread widely through Europe in the middle 1370s. Such widespread outbreaks recurred at generally widening intervals into the seventeenth century, although plague might be found somewhere at any time. Some studies have attempted to discover a predictable rhythm in the reappearance of plague epidemics over those centuries.

This prolonged pandemic ended at different times in different places, and subsequent historical accounts have given different end dates depending on their regional or national focus. In the years after 1670, plague visited Europe only sporadically; for many historians the Second Plague Pandemic ended in 1722, the date of plague's last appearance in western Europe. But the plague persisted in eastern Europe and in Muslim lands. A serious epidemic shook Moscow in 1771; Tunisia suffered a major epidemic between 1818 and 1820, and the disease remained in Egypt until 1844.

The end of the Second Plague Pandemic, therefore, was a ragged affair and not clearly defined. The Second Plague Pandemic may more clearly be separated from the third by geography than by dates. While the Second Plague Pandemic was flickering out in western Asia in the early nineteenth century, another zone of plague infection had taken root in Yunnan, in south China, by the 1770s; from that epicenter would grow the Third Plague Pandemic, beginning in the 1860s.

The reasons for the disappearance of the Second Plague Pandemic remain controversial, and they are discussed in the "Unresolved Historical Issues" section. Specific episodes of the Second Plague Pandemic are treated in separate chapters in this volume: "Plague in Italian Cities, 1630s," "Plague in London, 1665," "Plague in Marseille, 1720–1722," and "Plague in Moscow, 1771."

SIGNIFICANCE

The Black Death epidemic was a demographic event of nearly unique significance. The sudden loss of perhaps 50–60% (or even "only" 30%) of the population of Europe, North Africa, and western Asia created dramatically different economic, social, political, and cultural situations. Apart from the actual toll of the Black Death, one important other question remains unresolved: for what period in the subsequent Second Plague Pandemic did the population of Europe (and the Near East) remain low? That is, did population levels start to rebound fairly quickly (by the 1370s, for instance), or did the repeated shocks of later plague epidemics hold those levels down until the sixteenth century? This chapter accepts the latter argument, that the persistent pressure of epidemic-related mortality maintained the significantly lower population levels of 1353 into the early sixteenth century at least. The effects of the Black Death were therefore reinforced by the continuing pandemic, making it impossible to separate the significance of the Black Death from that of the Second Plague Pandemic as a whole.

Much of that significance stems from the contrasts between the pre– and post–Black Death worlds. In the early fourteenth century, Europe was at the end of a prolonged period of population growth, one that had begun no later than the twelfth century. By the mid-thirteenth century, the continent's population had perhaps reached a limit; the available land and agricultural technology could feed no more, and they only fed those numbers with difficulty. The economic (and social) situation therefore reflected a world of labor surplus, land shortage, and food shortage—low wages, high rents, and high prices.

Apparently, the rapid population growth that created those circumstances began leveling off, or even slowly reversing, in the early fourteenth century. But the Black Death epidemic between 1347 and 1353 turned those circumstances inside out. Landlords suddenly lacked tenants or laborers for their lands; employers lacked employees; sellers of goods lacked buyers. Rents (and other conditions imposed on tenants) fell; wages rose; and prices fell. These changes did not happen neatly or immediately, both because (in the immediate wake of a three-month epidemic) production of food or other goods might fall even more sharply than demand for them and because employers and landlords could use political power to delay changes unfavorable to their position (e.g., see the "Responses" section).

The changes happened nevertheless, and clearly better economic conditions for the majority of the population resulted. Wages had risen with respect to prices. Circumstances of land tenure improved for peasants; while serfdom had been in decline in western Europe anyway, the Black Death may have ended it in many areas, as landlords were forced by the new conditions to stop demanding labor services and to free peasants from ties to their land.

The greater prosperity enjoyed by many contributed to changing consumption patterns. Before the Black Death, many people had to devote a disproportionate share of their income to basic food, especially grain. After 1353, as grain prices (and rents) fell while wages rose, greater varieties of foods (and clothing) were within reach. And producers of goods (and agricultural producers as well) responded to the situation. With labor more expensive and the prices they received for grains falling, landowners might concentrate on goods that both required less labor and for which markets now existed: for example, a landlord might convert grain fields to pasture, which both needed fewer hands and produced goods (e.g., meat or wool) that customers could now better afford.

The new supply-demand situation of labor also encouraged greater efficiency of production. The pre–Black Death economy had little incentive to save on labor costs; surplus population made labor cheap. The Black Death—and the continuing demographic pressure of the ongoing pandemic—coincided with a remarkable period of technological innovation, which likely was *not* coincidental (see the "Unresolved Historical Issues" section).

These economic and technological changes formed important links in the evolution of a new society in the late medieval and early modern centuries. The variety of consumer goods increased, as did the efficiency of their production because new technologies appeared. Distinctions between medieval and modern societies are generally artificial and exaggerated, but the Second Plague Pandemic was an important—perhaps *the* important—engine of change between the fourteenth and seventeenth centuries.

The Black Death epidemic, in particular, shifted Western attitudes toward authority on several levels. Obviously, the authority of landowners and employers declined with their economic position; lords lost their grip on serfs. And because much Western political authority rested with those who controlled land, traditional political authority suffered as well, if only because many ruling groups depended on revenues (either from production or from taxation) derived from land ownership or control. With the Second Plague Pandemic, governments sought to diversify their sources of income, just as landowners tried to diversify their crops and products.

Whether the Western church lost authority is not so clear, although many factors must have weakened it. The church lost a high proportion of its clerics to the Black Death; their evident powerlessness in the face of the epidemic, and the fact that some of them behaved ignobly, called that authority into question. The sudden death of a priest could leave a village without spiritual succor, and his rapidly ordained successor might be untrained or lack a calling. The church, too, depended heavily on income from land. But at the same time the epidemic called forth evident and deep popular piety (see the "How It Was Understood at the Time," "Responses," and "Unresolved Historical Issues" sections).

Was the social fabric torn by the Black Death? Did people give way to hysteria? Did routines break down? Did the society become obsessed by images of death? Some evidence suggests that all of those things occurred, but much countering evidence exists as well (see the "Responses" and "Unresolved Historical Issues" sections). Certainly, huge numbers of individuals (of whatever social rank) experienced colossal personal tragedies involving the sudden loss of loved ones. A cold economic analysis might suggest that many such survivors were better off than they had been before 1347. But to a person mourning a spouse and three children that must have been cold comfort indeed.

In the course of the Second Plague Pandemic, attitudes toward the disease (and by extension toward all diseases) underwent some important changes, and the experience of the epidemics certainly played a role in that evolution. Generally and gradually, thinkers placed less emphasis on the role of God and God's wrath, and more emphasis on causes that might be controlled by direct human action without God's intercession. Led by northern Italian city-states, governments began taking a more active role in resisting disease, and their public health bureaucracies, quarantines, and isolation facilities may ultimately have diverted the Second Plague Pandemic from their borders. (See the "How It Was Understood at the Time," "Responses," and "Unresolved Historical Issues" sections as well as volume 2, chapter 9.)

BACKGROUND

The preponderant historical opinion now believes that the Black Death, and the subsequent several-centuries-long pandemic, involved the disease called plague. Since the 1890s, plague has been understood as an infection by a microorganism called *Yersinia pestis.* (The microorganism was originally called *Pasteurella pestis*, and that term is found in older books on the subject.) That microorganism is ordinarily found in communities of burrowing rodents, persisting in what is called a "maintenance" phase, *enzootic* (that is, endemic) in animals that are relatively

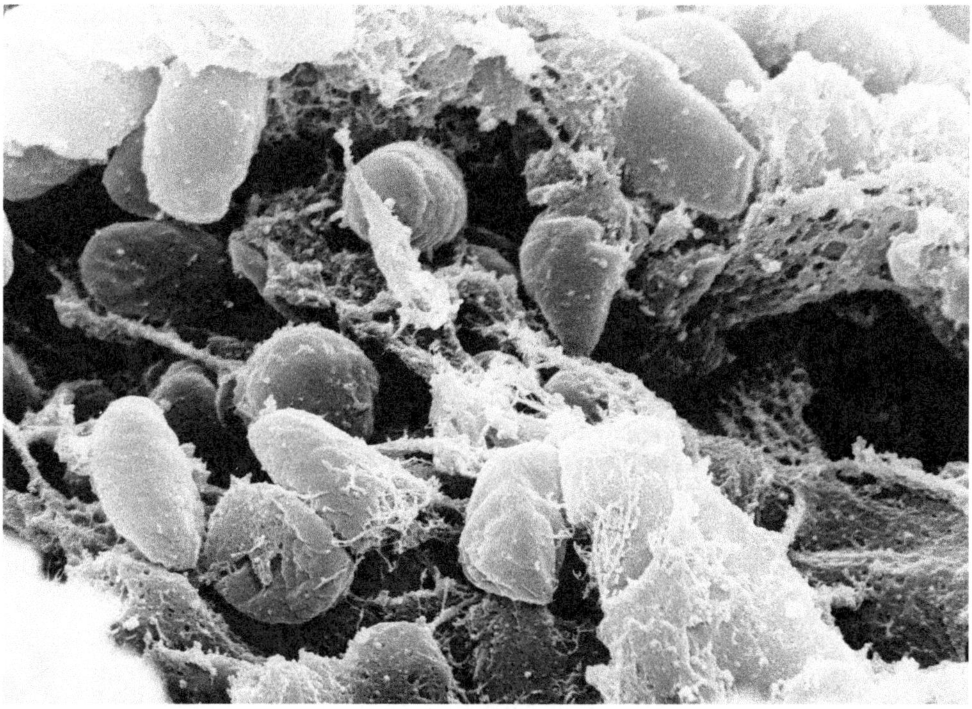

An electron micrograph shows a mass of *Yersinia pestis*, the bacteria that causes plague. Since 1994, advances in the field of paleomicrobiology have settled long-held doubts that *Yersinia pestis* is, indeed, the pathogen responsible for the plague. (Rocky Mountain Laboratories, NIAID, NIH)

resistant to it. When insects carry the organism to more susceptible, commensal, rodents (that may live closer to humans), an "amplifying" phase in which the disease becomes *epizootic* (epidemic) results in which rodents die. Most often a human case of plague results when an insect such as a flea carrying *Yersinia pestis* alights on (and bites) a person; that is most likely to occur when rodents are dying and the fleas seek new hosts.

The form of plague that then results is called bubonic plague, named for the characteristic swellings, or buboes, that form around lymph glands in the groin or armpit. Other forms of plague are pneumonic plague and septicemic plague. The first of those results from an infection of the lungs by *Yersinia pestis*, the latter from an infection of the bloodstream. Pneumonic plague may develop from a bubonic infection carried to the lungs through the bloodstream, or from the direct inhalation of droplets carrying *Yersinia pestis*, coughed up by another person already infected.

An epidemic of plague might therefore involve several different possible modes of transmission of the disease. The death of a large number of infected rodents might lead their fleas to seek new hosts and to find them in humans. Human fleas might pass the microbes from one person to another (although this possibility is controversial). And the pneumonic form of plague may be passed from person to person through the respiratory system.

If the prevailing historical view is correct, then clearly facts about rodent populations, insect populations, and their relationships to human settlements are important to the background of the Black Death and of the succeeding pandemic. The rodent long believed responsible for the pandemic in Europe and the Near East was the black rat (*Rattus rattus*), apparently present in large numbers in the medieval world. It is a commensal species, sharing food (and much else, including living quarters) with human settlements. More recent scholarship has argued that a variety of rodents have been involved, and a likewise greater variety of insects could be found in addition to the rat flea (*Xenopsylla cheopis*) and the human flea (*Pulex irritans*).

The more rodents (and insects) existed, the greater the likelihood that a plague outbreak in the rodent population might be transmitted to humans. Medieval cities, villages, and farms all provided rats with close human companionship, and as Benedictow (2004) argues, rats (and fleas) were probably more numerous, per capita, in rural surroundings than in urban ones. A greater variety of rodents also existed in such rural areas, putting them at an even greater proportional risk. So too were women because they likely spent more of their time in houses and around food, and hence, in more proximity to household rats.

Several important potential limits on the spread of the disease (as described earlier) certainly existed. Rodent colonies ordinarily do not move very far or very fast. Bubonic plague seems a disease that is transmitted to humans almost accidentally. The rapid spread of plague through a human community seems to depend on direct human-to-human transmission, and that in turn requires either the infective capacity of the human flea (a contested point) and/or a widespread pneumonic plague infection. But the pneumonic form of plague is almost uniquely fatal, both rapidly and invariably. A person infected by pneumonic plague will not live long enough to travel any distance.

How then did plague move so swiftly across Europe and the Near East in the years after 1346, and how did it achieve its staggering rates of morbidity and mortality? Different forms of human traffic played an important role, for while rats in villages may not move far or fast, ships carry them from one port to another. We have seen (in the "Where and When" section) how plague was diffused across the Mediterranean and along the Atlantic coast of Europe by sea. The density of seaborne commerce was an important aspect of late medieval economic life; the early urban areas of northern Italy in part flourished as a result of their sea connections with the civilizations to their east, while Flanders (the other prime medieval urban center) depended (to a lesser extent) on Atlantic coastal traffic.

The size of the ships' crews, especially in the Mediterranean, played an important part in the diffusion of plague, as Benedictow (2004) has emphasized. Large numbers of rowers manned Mediterranean galleys, and many of those vessels also carried military men to defend against pirates. Crews were therefore large enough to sustain a chain of plague infections through a voyage and still have enough men to bring the ship to port.

Another significant trade system was that of grain. Around granaries and mills all over Europe farmers and merchants gathered, traveling to and fro with cargoes of the prime food of rats. Rats also gathered around the granaries and mills, and while the rats might not have traveled overland with the merchants, fleas certainly did; some fleas even live off grain. The nearly universal traffic in grain, both by sea and overland, therefore was a crucial diffusing mechanism in the spread of both the Black Death and the later episodes of the Second Plague Pandemic.

Merchants were, of course, not the only significant groups of travelers in the fourteenth and later centuries. Armies frequently moved through the landscape, for war was nearly endemic. (And armies could themselves be formidable diffusers of disease.) Pilgrimages carried still other numbers of people and fleas across long distances.

By the beginning of the fourteenth century, medieval Europe's population had increased to the point where food supplies were often stretched thin, and several major periods of famine occurred, especially in the decade of the 1310s. Involved was what Bruce Campbell (2016) has called the Great Transition that occurred between the late thirteenth and late fifteenth centuries, which brought significantly colder temperatures and erratic weather fluctuations and hence serious declines of agricultural productivity. Many people therefore suffered from malnutrition at the time of the Black Death, and a weakened human frame was more likely to succumb to a plague infection. It may also be true that malnutrition played a role in other infections that occurred simultaneously with the plague outbreaks; not all the catastrophic mortality of 1346–1352 was due to plague. And if plague wiped out the adults in a family (or even simply reduced their ability to earn income), the children might suffer from subsequent neglect and malnutrition, and thus be weakened in the event of onslaught of other diseases.

HOW IT WAS UNDERSTOOD AT THE TIME

The Black Death

The great epidemic of 1347–1353 was such a vast event that (at least on some level) Christian and Muslim thinkers alike could only explain it as a product of the will of God. Why did God choose to send the pestilence? For Muslims the answer was relatively clear: the plague was a "mercy and a martyrdom" (Dols 1977, 23) for the faithful, who were urged to regard death from plague as a martyrdom on a par with death in battle. (As we will see shortly, not all Muslims agreed with this teaching.) Christian thinkers tended to regard plague as a punishment sent by God to scourge sinful humanity. Although the scale of the epidemic made it difficult to say that only some wicked individuals had been singled out, opinions ranged from a general punishment for the evils of the time, through God's particular wrath at the clergy for their failings, on to fears that a love of indecent clothing had sparked divine ire. That is, in general, Christian attitudes embodied some notion of guilt, perhaps collective, perhaps individual, as an essential explanation of the epidemic.

Fourteenth-century thinkers did not stop there, however; having decided that ultimately the plague came from God, they then asked by what means, or mechanism, did the disease reach the human body. The answers to that question linked God's supernatural powers with natural forces that human reason could understand. Most often a *miasma*, a fatal corruption of the air, was seen as the immediate cause. Perhaps, as the medical faculty of the University of Paris argued in October 1348, that miasma had its origins in astrological events: an unfortunate "configuration of the heavens" (quoted in Horrox 1994, 159) led to atmospheric corruption. Other possible sources of miasma were considered as well, including poisonous vapors from swamps, from volcanoes, from fissures in the earth caused by earthquakes, or given off by unburied corpses.

These miasmas affected the human frame because the body transformed air (and food and drink) into the humours whose balance assured health, and the "spirits" that carried those humours through the body. Corrupt air became corrupt humours and spirits. For those ideas, Christians and Muslims alike relied on earlier ancient Greek conceptions, especially the Hippocratic writings and those of Galen, both of which related disease and health to the atmosphere. Air (the element whose qualities were hotness and wetness) was intimately related to blood, one of the four humours, so that bodies especially liable to this particular corruption included those that were hot and moist already: people who exercised too much, practiced sex actively, bathed frequently, babies, and women.

Corrupted air was not the only cause considered, for the epidemic called forth a variety of other explanations of secondary causes. Supernatural beings were seen by some. In the Muslim world, *jinns* might be thought the agents of plague, and Christians too feared such witches as "la Mère Peste." For some, plague was spread not by supernatural agents but by malicious individuals who poisoned wells. (In some Christian communities, Jews were especially suspect; see the "Responses" section.)

Even as early as the Black Death, some began to believe that the great pestilence might be spread by contagion from one person to another. That thought led to the further idea that the way to escape the disease was to escape the infected, by fleeing from their presence. (Categories of cause were not always clearly maintained. A belief in miasma was for some consistent with contagion, if—for instance—the diseased created the miasma in their environment; flight might also escape a corrupt environment, but most believers in miasma thought it was universal, not local.) The idea of contagion made greater headway in the Christian world; for most Muslims, flight was an act of defiance of Allah's will, and Allah's will worked through a universal miasma, not a particular contagion. Some Muslim authorities—notably Ibn al-Khatīb—did argue for contagion, however.

The Succeeding Second Plague Pandemic

The interlocked themes of God's wrath and environmental corruption persisted in subsequent centuries, but they gradually gave way to stronger convictions about the role of contagion, and to fears of potentially infectious agents.

Starting in northern Italian city-states, governments created boards of public health in direct response to the continuing presence of plague, and those bodies took actions that illustrated the changing beliefs. Contagion was to be halted by controlling the movement of people and by isolating the sick. Infectious agents were carefully disposed of, whether they were the possessions of plague victims, the corpses of the victims, or the dogs and cats thought to be bearers of disease. In some cases, these beliefs associated plague with social disorder (or the threat of it) among the lower orders and the poor; the understanding of plague was therefore framed within social and political presuppositions (see the "Responses" section).

Galenic interpretations persisted as well, but the humoral interpretation of plague shifted its focus from blood to black bile. This had an impact on therapies offered by physicians (see the "Responses" section).

In general, the growing emphasis on contagion was part of a gradual rise of secular, as opposed to religious, explanations of the disease. The two (secular and religious) were not sharply divided in most minds, however, until at least the eighteenth century. Some examples of the tensions and ambiguities that could arise between the two may be seen in accompanying chapters about specific plague epidemics during the Second Plague Pandemic.

RESPONSES

The Black Death

Perhaps the most widespread responses in both Muslim and Christian societies were religious. Supplications, prayer services, and processions were all held. The Black Death evidently spurred popular piety in both Europe and the Near East, although (as mentioned earlier) its effects on the position of religious authorities were mixed. Generally, Muslim religious leaders met less criticism than Christian ones did. An unclear boundary separated appeals to religion and appeals to magic. Prayers were offered to saints, the Virgin Mary, or Allah; exorcisms and incantations were directed at evil spirits or *jinns.*

Another frequent response was flight, undertaken (especially) by those who could afford it. The atmospheric theory of the plague's cause led many to seek the "purer" air of mountain country. Perhaps the most famous literary account of the Black Death is Boccaccio's *Decameron*, in which a group of Florentines flee their plague-stricken city in 1348 and tell stories to divert themselves on their journey to purer air. Pope Clement VI did not exactly flee, but he isolated himself in his Avignon palace, surrounded by fires to purify the air around him. And while orthodox Muslim teaching discouraged flight (as an action undertaken to avoid Allah's will), the Mamlūk sultan fled Cairo at the height of the Black Death in 1348.

The magnitude of the epidemic left healers largely helpless. Physicians in the Galenic tradition (in both Muslim and Christian worlds) tried those remedies that their humoral understanding of the disease suggested, which especially meant bleeding (since the disease was thought, at this stage at least, to be an imbalance of blood). Some physicians (and other healers) attempted to lance the buboes that characterized the disease. Other medical advice stemmed from the idea that atmospheric corruption conveyed the disease. People were therefore urged to seek fresh air, and when (as was usually the case) that was impractical, they were to press pouches of sweet-smelling herbs over their noses and mouths. Some medical men urged attention to diet, and others (also arguing from humoral principles) cautioned against excitement for fear that would increase body heat; preferably one should adopt a quiet, moderate life.

Governments responded to the epidemic on several fronts. Some measures addressed what were seen as causes, or at least as behavior that made the epidemic worse. For example, if a love of luxury led to unhealthy immoderation, then such profligate habits should be curbed. Some cities, following that argument, passed sumptuary laws that forbade (or heavily taxed) conspicuous displays of wealth and fashion. That was one way in which God's anger might be appeased.

Governments also moved to counter the upward pressure of wages and the countering fall in prices and rents. Perhaps the best-known example of such an effort was the English Statute of Labourers of 1351, which attempted not only to freeze wages but to roll them back:

> Whereas, to curb the malice of servants who after the pestilence were idle and unwilling to serve without securing excessive wages, it was recently ordained by our lord the king . . . that such servants, both men and women should be bound to serve in return for salaries and wages that were customary in those places where they were obligated to serve during the twentieth year of the reign of our said lord the king, that is to say, five or six years earlier. (Stephenson and Marcham 1937, 225)

The twentieth year of Edward III's reign was 1346, before the Black Death and resultant rise in wages. Such moves clearly reflected the interests of the powerful and wealthy in fourteenth-century Europe. So too did efforts to restrict the movement of laborers (who hoped by moving to find a place where their skills were in even greater demand) from one place to another.

In some cases, the traditionally powerful and wealthy may also have felt challenged by groups newly enriched by the changed economic circumstances, and their fears may have been another motive behind the passage of sumptuary laws. In the Italian city-state of Siena, post–Black Death sumptuary laws were aimed at curbing the fancy-dress displays of the newly rich.

Certainly, one response to the epidemic of the Black Death was a sudden desire to enjoy whatever few short days of survival people might have. Boccaccio put the matter clearly:

> Others took the opposite view [from those who urged moderation], and maintained that an infallible way of warding off this appalling evil was to drink heavily, enjoy life to the full, go round singing and merrymaking, gratify all of one's cravings whenever the opportunity offered, and shrug the whole thing off as one enormous joke. Moreover, they practiced what they preached to the best of their ability, for they would visit one tavern after another, drinking all day and night to immoderate excess. (Boccaccio 1972, 52)

Against that hedonism were set some remarkable examples of self-denial and self-scourging. The processions of the Flagellants represented perhaps the most dramatic social response to the Black Death. Such processions occurred in Germany and the Netherlands in 1348 and 1349, as the epidemic approached. Groups of people undertook processions from town to town; when such a group reached a town, its members would assemble in a central place and ritually scourge themselves with nail-embedded thongs, while the townspeople gathered around. The Flagellants, punishing themselves, replicated Christ's sufferings and thus seemed to offer themselves as a sacrifice for the sins of all.

Great excitement, sometimes becoming mass hysteria, followed the Flagellants. Their relationships with authority, both political and clerical, were often tense. They seemed to usurp the roles of clergy, and their appearance sometimes touched off bursts of anti-clerical feeling, with attacks on churches and priests. In some cities—notably Frankfurt, Mainz, Cologne, and Brussels—the coming of the Flagellants touched off savage massacres of the local Jews, as furious and fearful Christians sought scapegoats for the plague that advanced on them. In some places the Flagellants seemed the harbingers of a deep social revolution, in which the bonds of social order would break apart as chaos reigned.

The Flagellants, and those who were excited by them, represented one pole of popular reactions to the Black Death. But other evidence suggests that many communities reacted with admirable calm and discipline. The government of Siena, far from collapsing in revolution, successfully raised taxes to pay its soldiers the wages they demanded, took part in a post-plague rebuilding of surrounding villages, and started attracting people who had fled back into the city. In many other communities (both large and small), legal routines may have suffered temporary breakdown at the height of the epidemic, but they were successfully resumed: people paid taxes, settled estates, and peacefully litigated disputes.

For the most part, the same calm seems to have been true of Muslim communities. Nor did the Mamlūk Egyptian government attempt to limit the free movement of peasants and others who sought a community with higher wages.

Some of the most serious social responses to the Black Death occurred in the decades that followed the epidemic. Popular revolts shook authorities, notably in France, England, and the Italian city-state of Florence. In each case, one of the issues was government attempts to intervene on behalf of landowners and large employers with such measures as the 1351 English law quoted earlier. In France, similar measures contributed to a series of peasants' rebellions in 1358 called the *Jacquerie*; in Florence, to the "Ciompi" rebellion in 1378; and in England, to the Peasants' Rebellion of 1381. The relation of these events to the Black Death, however, was more indirect (see the "Unresolved Historical Issues" section).

Later Phases of the Second Plague Pandemic

The different levels of response to the Black Death in some ways persisted through later stages of the Second Plague Pandemic, but important changes occurred as well.

Popular fears of plague remained powerful, and those fears still inspired pious invocations of God, religious processions, and prayer rituals. Religion (whether of Christians or of Muslims) continued to play an important role in both the explanation of the disease and response to it. But supernatural explanations of the disease fell away; God's primacy was still taken for granted, but often not dwelt on very much. Tracts about plague focused on immediate causes, not primary ones.

Some of the same medical advice persisted: avoid excitement, live moderately, and escape atmospheric corruption. The application of Galenic theory to plague underwent some modification, as the idea that the disease was a blood disorder gave way to emphasis on black bile as the offending humour. That in turn reduced the practice of bleeding as a medical response to plague and placed greater weight on the purging of the bowels. More important was the trial-and-error development, by physicians, apothecaries, and traditional empirical healers alike, of a variety of remedies and procedures that they at least claimed had some benefit. Healers, by the seventeenth century or earlier, *sounded* more confident in confronting plague. Whether they were is less clear, and the symptoms of plague often simply came on too rapidly and violently to allow any therapy to have meaningful effect.

The most important shift in responses came from European governments, which (in different places at different times) became increasingly active to countering what they argued was the *contagion* of plague. By the seventeenth century, northern Italian city-states had evolved elaborate public health mechanisms whose main focus was the prevention of plague; other European governments adopted some of the same measures with different degrees of success. Many of these actions involved a heavy-handed regulation of populations, especially of their movements; the motives might involve both countering contagion and controlling disorder and dissent.

Those actions of government illustrated that European society, at least, no longer felt helpless in the face of plague. It is also true, and an important contrasting development, that the hysteria generated (and represented) by the Flagellants did not recur, even in the epidemics of the later fourteenth century. Plague epidemics continued to occasion movements of social and political resistance, but they were stirred by opposition to government public health measures, not by millenarian expectations. For the significance and effectiveness of the evolving government responses, see the next section.

UNRESOLVED HISTORICAL ISSUES

The Black Death and subsequent Second Plague Pandemic have generated more historical writing and speculation than any other events in disease history, and many issues about them remain unresolved. Among those issues are the identity of the disease or diseases involved, the geographical origins of the pandemic, the actual extent of its mortality, its longer-range demographic effects, the relationship of both the Black Death and the later stages of the pandemic to a variety of political, social, economic, technological, and intellectual/cultural changes, and (for the pandemic as a whole) the causes and timing of its disappearance. These historical disputes have themselves related to larger questions of historical interpretation, especially of the character of the European Middle Ages and Renaissance.

The question of the identity of the disease has now been largely settled by the developing field of paleomicrobiology, using evidence from recombinant DNA obtained from the dental pulp of victims. That evidence has clearly established that *Yersinia pestis* was at least present in many victims of the First and Second

Plague Pandemics, and so may have been the primary cause of their catastrophic mortalities.

Yersinia pestis was therefore certainly a necessary cause of the Black Death, but was it a sufficient cause of those catastrophic mortalities? Some critics of the role of plague have proposed alternative great primary killers, but the geographical pattern of the Black Death characteristically illustrated an insect-borne bacterial infection, moving erratically, hitting some villages and cities while sparing others in the same season. An airborne viral infection such as smallpox, influenza, or any other such agent would spread much more uniformly across areas. But plague may have had affiliated assassins. Ann Carmichael (1986) suggested that the huge mortalities resulted from the workings of several diseases; typhus and malaria (both insect-borne) are possible accomplices. Plague may have initiated the Black Death, while other ailments multiplied its effects; for example, the social disruption caused by initial high mortality left many children without parental care and many of the otherwise vulnerable (such as lepers) without social support.

The relative importance of the different types of plague—bubonic, pneumonic, and septicemic—remains uncertain. Contemporary observers, especially the French surgeon Guy de Chauliac (Benedictow 2004, 236–238) whose writings are an important source, clearly described the symptoms and ravages of pneumonic plague in 1348. But did it persist in later plague outbreaks? Can rapidly spreading and fatal plague epidemics occur without it?

Where did the Black Death epidemic originate? For much of the twentieth century, historians placed its home in central Asia, or perhaps (less certainly) in China. The Mongol empire, founded in the early thirteenth century, opened the interior of Asia to overland trade routes across vast distances; perhaps plague, fleas, and rats made their way along such routes. Evidence for that belief is now weaker; the Mongol empire had broken into hostile pieces by the fourteenth century, so trade did not move as freely; other paths have been suggested, such as north from Kurdistan through the Caucasus. Benedictow (2004) simply argues that the southern Russian area identified as infected in 1346 was a focus of endemic plague anyway.

How great was the mortality from the Black Death, and from subsequent episodes of the pandemic? As stated earlier (see the "When and Where" section) estimates of mortality in the Black Death have varied. No clear and unambiguous censuses or population records were made in the fourteenth century, and so historians and demographers have exercised considerable ingenuity in reaching their estimates. Some general problems include the fact that contemporary documents did not record some proportion of any population, especially if, for example, they paid no taxes, or were not tied to any property, or escaped church records. And if a local record tells us that a population fell by one half, how many of those missing died, and how many fled elsewhere? Such issues (and many others) have dogged attempts at precision.

The longer-term demographic effects of the pandemic also remain controversial. Population levels in both Europe and the Near East were certainly reduced dramatically between 1347 and 1353, but at what point, and for what reason, did they begin to recover? What demographic role did the next plague epidemics (*pestis secunda* of the early 1360s, and *pestis tertia* of the 1370s) play? And what about the repeated plague visitations, at gradually lengthening intervals, throughout the fifteenth, sixteenth, and into the seventeenth centuries?

Some scholars have argued that Europe's population remained low until about 1380, under the pressure of the aftershocks (of the 1360s and 1370s) from the Black Death. Then, this argument goes, population stabilized; in the fifteenth century, some modest growth began. Others argue that the repeated pressure of high mortality in plague epidemics prevented any real recovery of population until sometime in the sixteenth century.

These arguments are intertwined with disagreements about the relative importance of mortality and fertility in population growth. Those who emphasize fertility also think that economic forces play a dominant role; in the case of plague epidemics, the relative prosperity of the survivors should lead to earlier marriages and higher fertility, and therefore economic forces lead to a rapid recovery of population after an epidemic. The countering view holds that plague epidemics, at intervals into the sixteenth or even seventeenth centuries, kept populations from recovering; epidemics served to hold population levels in a sink, and spurts of higher fertility were not enough for those levels to escape. To solve these issues, more reliable information about populations, especially in the fifteenth century, will be helpful.

Perhaps the overarching unresolved issue about the Black Death (and to a lesser extent the Second Plague Pandemic as a whole) might be stated thus: Was Western civilization changed so dramatically by the Black Death that it was no longer medieval, but on the road to being modern? Or were the changes that flowed from it simply reinforcements of trends that had begun long before 1347?

Those questions may be asked of demography. The Black Death certainly reduced populations sharply, but had population levels already begun to fall earlier in the fourteenth century or in the late thirteenth? Did the Black Death simply exaggerate trends that were already underway? If the latter was the case, was Europe already on the road (perhaps more gradually) to a different wage, rent, and price structure? Would slowing population growth have led to lower rents and prices, and higher wages, without the horrific intervention of an epidemic?

The same contrasting views—of continuity versus catastrophic change—may offer different interpretations of the development of more diverse consumer goods, of the emergence of new technologies, and of the breakup of the feudal economy. Did such new technologies as advanced clocks, watermills and windmills, improved mining techniques, and the printing press receive their great stimulus from a plague-created new situation, or were earlier medieval developments on the road to them anyway?

Positions taken on these issues—and on similar questions about art, thought, political administration, and mass psychology—may reflect underlying beliefs about the European (and Islamic) Middle Ages. Historians who contrast the Middle Ages with modernity may more likely emphasize the catastrophe of the Black Death as an event that forced change; they may also therefore lean toward high estimates of mortality, and argue that such disruptive episodes as the Flagellant processions are evidence of a society in crisis. Historians who emphasize the continuities between "medieval" and "modern" ages may be more prone to see the Black Death as a great shock, to be sure, but one whose effects either didn't last, or confirmed trends already underway. The histories of the Black Death, as Faye Getz (1991) has shown, have evolved together with more general opinions about the Middle Ages.

An important unresolved question about the Second Plague Pandemic as a whole asks: "What happened to it? Why did it come to an end?" It is not even clear *when* it came to an end (see the "When and Where" section). But between the seventeenth and the early nineteenth centuries, the Second Plague Pandemic, the one that had its origins in southern Russia and subsequently established colonies of plague-infested rodents throughout Europe, North Africa, and West Asia, lost its grip. In one country after another, its ravages ceased. Did that happen as a result of conscious human actions against the disease? Was it the inadvertent product of other human actions? Or did the pandemic die out as a result of changes in nature that occurred without people being conscious of them, what might be called *exogenous* changes? In short, how effective were human responses?

Since plague epidemics involve four different types of species (microorganisms, insects, rodents, and humans), the environments of any of them may affect the development of an epidemic. For that reason, many possibilities for an ecological exogenous explanation have been suggested. Fleas in particular are sensitive to temperature changes, so long-term changes in climate have been considered. Between the late sixteenth and early nineteenth centuries, Europe entered a "Little Ice Age," when average temperatures fell noticeably. Were fleas thus discouraged? Some rodents are more dangerous because they prefer living close to people; the black rat (*Rattus rattus*) was such a rodent, and so it has been argued that its displacement by the brown rat (*Rattus norvegicus*) in the seventeenth and eighteenth centuries had the effect of separating rats and people. But did that displacement occur in the right places at the right times? Black rats persisted in Britain, for instance, into the eighteenth century long after plague disappeared there; brown rats had long ousted black rats from Russia by the 1770s, when plague struck Moscow.

Another strong possibility is an evolutionary change in levels of immunity to the disease among rats. Plague spreads from rodents to people—at least initially—as a result of an epizootic outbreak that kills off the rat hosts, leaving the fleas no choice but to seek another warm (perhaps human) host. But if the immune systems of the rats can withstand the disease, the fleas stay put. This argument must, however, consider the continuing patchy appearance of plague between the late seventeenth and the early nineteenth centuries. Did the rats of England, for example, acquire greater levels of immunity before the rats of Egypt?

Other evolutionary changes may have occurred in *Yersinia pestis* itself. Did it become less lethal over time, either for rats or for people? For a time, its relation to a related microorganism (*Yersinia pseudotuberculosis*) was offered as an explanation for the Second Plague Pandemic's disappearance; in developing immunity to the latter, did rodents (or humans) also enjoy a cross-immunity to the former? More recently the molecular structure of *Yersinia pestis* has been understood; we now believe it to be a relatively recently evolved organism (perhaps within the period of human history), and that fact may strengthen the likelihood of such cross-immunities.

Human actions also affected the environment in which rats and fleas lived and moved. Changes in building materials might have separated people and rats. Sanitation campaigns might have had the same effect. The ideas of the eighteenth-century Enlightenment emphasized the general environmental causes of diseases and urged cleansing of cities and towns, although the great campaigns for better sewers only began later in the nineteenth century. Humans may have enjoyed improved nutrition, although whether they did so before the nineteenth century, and whether (in any case) nutritional status affects resistance to plague, remain unclear.

Deliberate human actions against plague had mixed results. Certainly, no effective understanding of the disease's epidemiology existed before the 1890s. Before that time not much notice was taken of rats; in fact, some cities in the Second Plague Pandemic blamed cats and dogs for spreading plague, ordered their deaths, and so allowed rats to flourish more than ever. While different trial-and-error therapies might have relieved some suffering, no effective cure existed before antibiotics of the mid-twentieth century. Isolating plague victims (or their families) in their own homes probably ensured that the whole family came in contact with infected rats and their fleas. That active measure may, therefore, have intensified an epidemic within a household at the same time that it slowed its outward spread. The imposition of quarantines, undertaken with increasing effectiveness in Italy (especially) in the sixteenth and seventeenth centuries and in place thereafter, was the conscious human action that might have most contributed to the end of the Second Plague Pandemic. Some historians (e.g., Cipolla 1976; Slack 1981) have made a strong case for their importance, especially in cutting the spread of plague from North Africa and West Asia to Mediterranean Europe.

This disappearance of plague in turn becomes part of another large (and important) historical puzzle: explaining the remarkable surge in the population of Western civilization that began in the middle of the eighteenth century and continued to the end of the nineteenth. That population surge coincided with the rise of Europe to unprecedented world prominence. Did the absence of the population brake (plague) lead to that growth in numbers?

The disappearance of plague did not last. A Third Plague Pandemic arose later in the nineteenth century, and its aftershocks still linger into the twenty-first century (see volume 2, chapter 31).

REFERENCES

Benedictow, Ole J. *The Black Death, 1346–1353: The Complete History.* Woodbridge, UK: Boydell, 2004.

Biraben, Jean-Noël. *Les Hommes et la peste en France et dans les pays européens et mediterranéens.* Paris: Mouton, 1975–1976.

Boccaccio, Giovanni. *The Decameron.* Translated by G. H. McWilliam. Harmondsworth: Penguin, 1972.

Campbell, Bruce M. S. *The Great Transition: Climate, Disease and Society in the Late-Medieval World.* Cambridge: Cambridge University Press, 2016.

Carmichael, Ann G. *Plague and the Poor in Renaissance Florence.* Cambridge: Cambridge University Press, 1986.

Cipolla, Carlo M. *Public Health and the Medical Profession in the Renaissance.* Cambridge: Cambridge University Press, 1976.

Dols, Michael W. *The Black Death in the Middle East.* Princeton, NJ: Princeton University Press, 1977.

Getz, Faye M. "Black Death and Silver Lining: Meaning, Continuity, and Revolutionary Change in Histories of Medieval Plague." *Journal of the History of Biology* 24 (1991): 265–289.

Horrox, Rosemary, ed. *The Black Death.* Manchester: Manchester University Press, 1994. *(A good collection of contemporary documents.)*

Slack, Paul. "The Disappearance of Plague: An Alternative View." *Economic History Review,* 2nd series, 34 (1981): 469–476.

Stephenson, Carl, and Frederick George Marcham, eds. *Sources of English Constitutional History: A Selection of Documents from A.D. 600 to the Present.* New York: Harper and Brothers, 1937.

SUGGESTED ADDITIONAL READING

Aberth, John. *The Black Death: The Great Mortality of 1346–1350, a Brief History with Documents.* Boston: Bedford/St. Martin's, 2005.

Appleby, Andrew B. "The Disappearance of Plague: A Continuing Puzzle." *Economic History Review,* 2nd series, 34 (1980): 161–173.

Benedictow, Ole J. *Plague in the Late Medieval Nordic Countries: Epidemiological Studies.* Oslo: Middelalderforlanet, 1992.

Bolton, J. L. "Looking for *Yersinia pestis:* Scientists, Historians and the Black Death." In *The Fifteenth Century XII: Society in an Age of Plague,* edited by Linda Clark and Carole Rawcliffe, 15–37. Woodbridge, UK: Boydell, 2013.

Bowsky, William M. "The Impact of the Black Death upon Sienese Government and Society." *Speculum* 39 (1964): 1–34.

Campbell, Anna M. *The Black Death and Men of Learning.* New York: Columbia University Press, 1931.

Carmichael, Ann G. "Plague Persistence in Western Europe: A Hypothesis." *The Medieval Globe* 1 (2014): 1–27.

Cohn, Norman. *The Pursuit of the Millennium: Revolutionary Millenarians and Mystical Anarchists of the Middle Ages.* New York: Oxford University Press, 1970.

Cohn, Samuel K., Jr. "The Black Death: End of a Paradigm." *American Historical Review* 107 (2002): 702–738.

Emery, Richard W. "The Black Death of 1348 in Perpignan." *Speculum* 42 (1967): 611–623.

Hatcher, John. *Rural Economy and Society in the Duchy of Cornwall, 1300–1500.* Cambridge: Cambridge University Press, 1970.

Hatcher, John. *Plague, Population and the English Economy, 1348–1530.* London: Macmillan, 1977.

Herlihy, David. *Medieval and Renaissance Pistoia: The Social History of an Italian Town, 1200–1430.* New Haven, CT: Yale University Press, 1967.

Ladurie, Emmanuel LeRoy. *The Peasants of Languedoc.* Translated by John Day. Urbana: University of Illinois Press, 1974.

Miskimin, Harry A. *The Economy of Early Renaissance Europe, 1300–1460.* Cambridge: Cambridge University Press, 1975.

Norris, John. "East or West? The Geographic Origin of the Black Death." *Bulletin of the History of Medicine* 51 (1977): 1–24.

Platt, Colin. *King Death: The Black Death and Its Aftermath in Late-Medieval England.* London: UCL Press, 1996.

Poos, L. R. *A Rural Society after the Black Death: Essex, 1350–1525.* Cambridge: Cambridge University Press, 1991.

Sallares, Robert. "Ecology, Evolution, and Epidemiology of Plague." In *Plague and the End of Antiquity: The Pandemic of 541–750*, edited by Lester K. Little, 231–289. New York: Cambridge University Press, 2007.

Sussman, George D. "Was the Black Death in India and China?" *Bulletin of the History of Medicine* 85 (2011): 319–355.

Williman, Daniel, ed. *The Black Death: The Impact of the Fourteenth-Century Plague.* Binghamton, NY: Center for Medieval and Early Renaissance Studies, 1982.

Ziegler, Philip. 1969. *The Black Death.* New York: Harper & Row, 1969.

6

Epidemics in Sixteenth-Century America

WHEN AND WHERE

Between 1493 and the end of the sixteenth century, the American continents suffered a repeated series of epidemics that had a catastrophic effect on their populations and civilizations. Those epidemics played a crucial role in the sudden and overwhelming conquests of the Americas by Europeans and also in the vast movement of Africans (as slaves) to the Americas. The sixteenth-century American epidemics therefore rank among the most decisive events of world disease history and indeed of world history generally.

Although many different epidemics—and diseases—occurred in sixteenth-century America, this chapter discusses them as a whole, regarding the American experience as one prolonged pandemic. The diseases involved were, for the most part, carried (although not deliberately) by people from Europe and Africa to the Americas where they spread among populations that had no previous experience with the responsible causative microorganisms (see the "Background" section). The "pandemic" might therefore be called "the diseases brought from the Old World to the New." The epidemics were an important aspect of what the historian Alfred Crosby (1972) called the "Columbian Exchange" and what others have styled the "Seeds of Change." This chapter's discussion concentrates on seven periods of epidemics in the late fifteenth and the entire sixteenth centuries, but it should become clear that the diseases set in motion then persisted in the Americas for a much longer period.

America: Late Fifteenth Century

Serious new epidemic disease first arrived in America in 1493, accompanying Christopher Columbus's second voyage. Unlike the famous 1492 trip, the second expedition was large (17 ships, over 1,000 men, and numerous domestic animals), for its intention was to found a settlement. The fleet reached the Caribbean in November, at a point when sickness (probably influenza) had badly weakened its

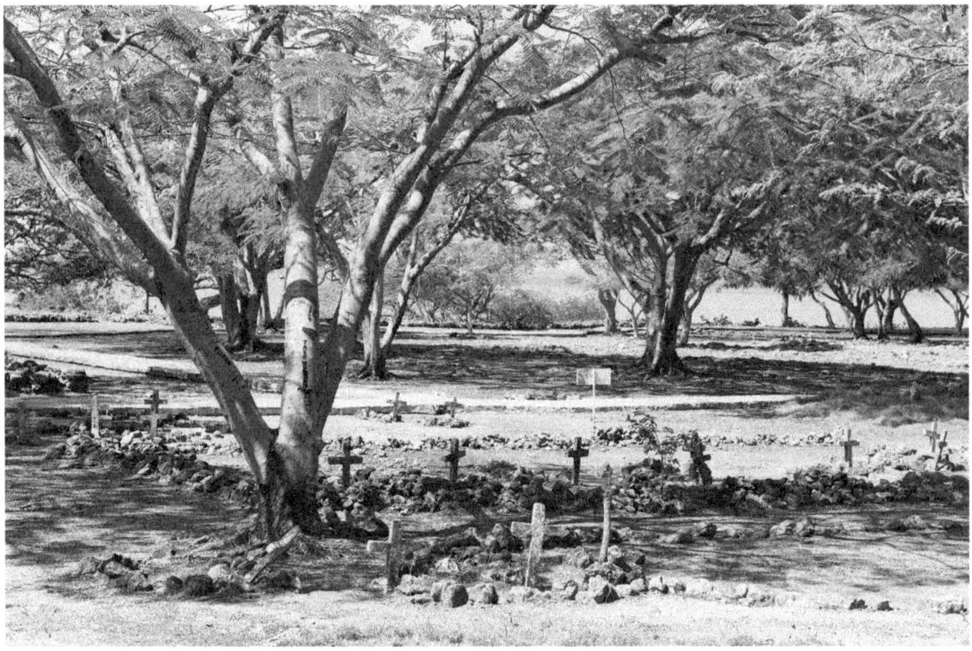

The site of the 1493 settlement of La Isabela, on Hispaniola, founded by Christopher Columbus. Epidemics had wiped out the population by 1496, as this ancient graveyard testifies. (Dmitry Chulov/Dreamstime.com)

personnel, and that illness then spread through the Native populations of the Caribbean Islands, especially Hispaniola where the Spaniards founded a settlement. The epidemic persisted through 1494, working simultaneously with hunger to reduce both European and American populations; one later Spanish writer claimed that two-thirds of the populations died between 1494 and 1496. When Columbus returned to Spain in 1496 only about half of his 1493 expedition was still living. In the next several decades, the combination of epidemic disease, social disruption, and economic tyranny dramatically reduced the Native population of the Caribbean Islands, as the Spanish conquerors exploited what little mineral wealth they could find and began agricultural plantations.

Smallpox in Mexico and the Caribbean, Early Sixteenth Century

Of all the epidemic diseases that assailed the American Indian peoples in the sixteenth century, smallpox—previously unknown in the Americas—was probably the foremost killer. (See the "Background" section for a discussion of smallpox's epidemiological effects.) Smallpox cases apparently first arrived in the Caribbean in late 1518, accompanying Spanish traffic, perhaps directly from Europe, perhaps through intermediary commerce in African slaves. Even before smallpox's arrival, the Native populations of the Caribbean had been dramatically reduced, perhaps to levels "nearing extinction" (Cook 1998, 60). Within a few weeks of the first outbreak of smallpox, about one-third of the surviving Natives on Hispaniola had succumbed to it, and it had spread to Puerto Rico as well. The outbreak of smallpox coincided with, and was worsened by, a new resettlement policy pursued by the Spanish overlords of Hispaniola. In the face of the precipitous decline of the Native workforce, the surviving Indians had been concentrated in fewer and more crowded settlements, which in effect spread the contagion more quickly.

Having jumped across the Atlantic Ocean, smallpox more easily moved from the Caribbean to the mainland of the Americas. Its eruption into Mexico played a role in one of the dramatic sagas of history: the overthrow of the Aztec Empire by the Spanish conquistador Hernán Cortés. Cortés, with several hundred soldiers, had set off from Cuba for Mexico in February 1519. In November 1519, he entered Tenochtitlan, the Aztec Empire's capital, seizing the ruler Moctezuma. His conquests exceeded his instructions, and another Spanish force was dispatched from Cuba to bring him under control. That military contingent, led by Pánfilo de Narváez, reportedly included at least one active case of smallpox, and when the expedition stopped at Cozumel on the Yucatan coast (in the spring of 1520), the disease apparently gained a foothold on the mainland.

In the summer of 1520, Cortés's hold on Tenochtitlan proved tenuous, so much so that in July he, his men, and his allies were forced out of the city by a revived Aztec military uprising. But between that event (the Noche Triste of Spanish historical legend) and September and October 1520, smallpox reached the Aztec lands. Both contemporaries and most later historical writers agreed that the ravages of the disease on a densely settled virgin soil population were catastrophic for both Aztec manpower and morale. By the summer of 1521, Cortés was able to reenter the city, and this time the Spanish conquerors (still remarkably few) completely mastered the large, populous, highly organized empire that had dominated central Mexico. The mortality of the Indians of Mexico in the years immediately following 1520 was enormous. Historical controversy persists about the actual death toll (see the "Unresolved Historical Issues" section for a further discussion), but much wider agreement exists about the crucial role of epidemic smallpox in the overthrow of the Aztec Empire.

Smallpox in Central and South America, Early Sixteenth Century

At about the same time that smallpox reached Mexico (1520, if not earlier), Spanish ships had also conveyed cases of the disease to the Isthmus of Panama. To and from that vital transit point men and goods moved, and with them moved pathogens. Diseases spread to Central American societies by 1520, perhaps from Mexico, perhaps from Panama. In the 1520s (the precise date is not clear from surviving evidence) smallpox began to infect the peoples of the Andes region, including the residents of the Inca Empire. Later testimony recounted how the Incan ruler, Huayna Capac, fell ill—apparently with smallpox—after he conquered the city of Quito (in modern Ecuador) sometime between 1524 and 1528. His death led to a struggle for power between different claimants for his throne, a struggle that broadened into a civil war. While the war progressed, the empire's population was simultaneously being weakened and reduced by smallpox, and the combination of epidemic and internal strife left the Incas vulnerable. When the ruthless Spanish conquistador Francisco Pizarro arrived in late 1532, the Inca realm quickly collapsed. Disease had done much of Pizarro's work for him.

Measles in Early Sixteenth-Century America

The sixteenth-century American population faced multiple diseases that were new to it, and that fact had especially serious consequences for any recovery of population levels. A devastating smallpox epidemic, such as that of the 1520s, might have killed many people, but it might also have left some survivors immune to the next smallpox visit. Any attempt to rebuild population numbers on that base, however, might be foiled if *another* virgin soil disease appeared among those survivors. That apparently happened in the Americas in the 1530s, when measles successfully made the voyage across the Atlantic and began infecting American populations. The measles epidemic that reached America may have originated in Seville, a large Spanish city that was the principal starting point for voyages across the Atlantic; measles more easily maintains a chain of infection in a large, dense population (see the "Background" section). Another group that may have been involved in the transmission of measles across the sea was the growing number of African slaves. In any case, measles first arrived through the islands of the Caribbean, the channel of most movement from Europe and Africa to the Americas.

By 1531 cases of measles were being described in Mexico; contemporaries saw a disease with a lighter skin rash than that of smallpox. In the next few years, measles reached the Pacific coasts of Mexico and Central America. To a virgin population measles can be lethal. Between 1531 and 1534, mortality in some American communities infected by measles may have reached 25% or 30%.

New Epidemics in the 1540s

A new wave of epidemics swept through middle America in the mid-1540s. Several diseases may have been involved in those years, including typhus, which had also become a very serious cause of death in Europe starting in the late fifteenth century. Especially suspicious was a badly infected Spanish fleet that arrived at Campeche Bay, Mexico, in December 1544. In 1545 a disease that killed its victims very quickly reached central Mexico and as far south as Guatemala. One contemporary claimed that mortality rates in this epidemic ranged from 60% to 90%; another reported 150,000 deaths in Tlaxcala (Mexico) alone. The suddenness and the extreme mortality of this epidemic suggests that pneumonic plague may have played a role, as well as typhus. One modern authority (McCaa 1995) claims that this epidemic inflicted the highest death rate in Mexico of any of the sixteenth century, although the total death toll from smallpox in the 1520s was higher because of the then much larger population.

Epidemics in the 1550s and 1560s

A panoply of diseases beset the Americas between 1557 and 1564. The late 1550s were years of an influenza pandemic across Europe, which spread across the Atlantic as well. Renewed infestations of smallpox began to assail the northern Andean region after 1558, perhaps conveyed from Hispaniola by infected slaves; between June 1559 and April 1560, the population of a province on the Colombia/Venezuela border fell by 35%. The Rio de la Plata region in southern South America was similarly struck by smallpox in the same years. And a serious plague epidemic in Lisbon in 1561 led (later that year) to the spread of the disease to Brazil, where it persisted through 1564.

Middle and South America, 1576–1591

Serious epidemics were widespread between 1576 and 1591. Mexico, in the midst of drought, crop failure, and famine between 1576 and 1579, suffered from repeated outbreaks of what was probably typhus; the Archbishop of Mexico claimed that half of the Indian population of his land had died in 1583; and between 1585 and 1591 a combination of typhus, smallpox, and measles (perhaps conveyed through the slave market at Cartagena in Colombia) swept through the Andean regions.

These seven epidemic periods should not be seen in isolation, but rather as relatively high points along a disastrous continuum. Once European (and African) disease pathogens reached the virgin soil of the Americas they took hold; different diseases interacted to dramatically reduce population levels and prevent the recovery of those levels. Disease was not the sole cause of the demographic collapse of the American Indians, but its role was very important (see the "Unresolved Historical Issues" section).

SIGNIFICANCE

Some of the significance of the sixteenth-century American epidemics is suggested by their awesome mortality figures. Modern scholars have argued about many of those numbers (see the "Unresolved Historical Issues" section), but widespread consensus holds that the population of the American continents may have fallen by 90% between the beginning and end of the sixteenth century, an unparalleled demographic catastrophe. Estimates about the pre-Columbian American population vary very widely, and so therefore do estimates of the actual number of deaths. But even the lowest estimates suggest a frightening loss. F. J. Brooks, whose population estimates are lower than those proposed by most other scholars, suggests that Mexican Indian numbers fell from five million to one million in the course of the century (Brooks 1993, 7): modest by comparison to Borah and Cook, who argued a Mexican decline from about 25 million to about 1.5 million, but still of obviously enormous significance.

To be sure, other forces worked in harness with these epidemics to reduce American numbers. Europeans subjected the American Indians to great violence and enslaved (or otherwise controlled) them in systems of brutal labor; economic and social changes led to weakening diets, and perhaps to social hopelessness. It is perhaps safest to say epidemic disease was a very important, perhaps necessary, component of the American demographic collapse, and that it played roles both in the initial cause of social changes and in the shape those changes took. (See the "Unresolved Historical Issues" section.)

Those changes in the social, economic, and political systems of the Americas occurred above all because of European conquest and settlement. The epidemic history of the century at least facilitated, and perhaps even made possible, the conquest, subjugation, and settlement of the Americas, by the Spaniards and Portuguese in the sixteenth century, and then by the French and English later.

The dramatic reduction of the Native American population also directly promoted the vast traffic in slaves from Africa to America. European conquerors demanded labor (in mines and plantations) to extract the riches they hoped to gain from their new possessions. When the Native Americans uncooperatively died of epidemic disease (or proved otherwise unsatisfactory), the Europeans turned to the west coast of Africa for an alternate (and less disease-prone; see the "Background" section) supply of forced labor.

BACKGROUND

The notion of virgin soil epidemics provides important background for the American sixteenth-century experience. Populations that have no previous experience with a particular disease and its causative pathogen often suffer much higher mortality and morbidity rates when such a disease appears. Several possible causes may explain virgin soil vulnerability: populations may lack inherited immunities, passed from mothers to fetuses through the placenta; populations may have undergone genetic modifications from an originally common type; or populations may have missed the winnowing effects of natural selection from previous epidemics.

The European exploratory voyages to America, beginning with those of Columbus in the 1490s, led to the most widespread illustration of this virgin soil theory. The American landmass and its inhabitants (both flora and fauna) had been long isolated from contact with Eurasia, Africa, and Australia; its human population had arrived from Asia (probably between Siberia and Alaska) perhaps 20,000 years ago. Between that time and the arrival of Europeans in 1492 those American populations (except for some few inhabitants of Greenland and Newfoundland between the eleventh and thirteenth centuries) had had no exposure to Eurasian or African pathogens. Francis Black has also suggested that the American populations had not mixed among themselves very much and so lacked genetic heterogeneity; diseases could "adapt to each population as a whole and cause unusual damage" (Black 1994, 301).

The Americas before Columbus certainly had a broad spectrum of diseases. Intestinal ailments—dysentery and diarrhea—were apparently common, as were fungal diseases. Streptococcal infections existed in America, and some form of tuberculosis (although perhaps not the pulmonary variety) was found as well. The pre-Columbian presence of malaria and yellow fever, both of which became especially important in Central America and the Caribbean, is very doubtful. Influenza's many subtypes and rapid mutation make tracing its past exceptionally difficult, so we can only speculate about its American existence. And American populations did harbor treponema pathogens, probably including that responsible for syphilis. America was therefore hardly a disease-free Eden when Columbus arrived.

But some important and very dangerous diseases were absent, including smallpox, measles, typhus, and plague. Some features of their epidemiologies may help our understanding of their effects when they arrived in America. Smallpox and measles both result from infection by viruses that spread from one person to another through the respiratory system; both, that is, are airborne infections and so can spread easily and quickly, especially in crowded settlements. An infected person may be a source of contagion when (in effect) he or she is actively sick; in the case of smallpox, "from just before the rash appeared until the last scab dropped off about three weeks later" (Hopkins 2002, 5). Generally, both diseases can only infect an individual once; a recovered smallpox victim is immune from another attack of smallpox, and a recovered measles victim won't again suffer from measles. That last characteristic means that both diseases persist by finding virgin subjects, and in most of their histories they have found such subjects in one generation of children after another.

The severity of smallpox and measles has varied at times and places. In recent times in the Western world, measles has been thought of as a relatively mild childhood disease, more serious than chicken pox but rarely a killer. At other times and places, measles has been very dangerous. In medieval Europe, smallpox may have been chiefly a childhood complaint, although evidence is mixed. The varying severity of smallpox stems in part from the fact that three different species of the causative virus exist, one of them (*Variola major*) much more serious than the others.

The transmission of smallpox and measles across the Atlantic Ocean in the early sixteenth century therefore depended on several chances, considering that the voyage might take four or six weeks. If a ship left Europe carrying one person ill with smallpox or measles, America would not be reached until after he had either died or recovered, and thus in either case ceased to be contagious. If the disease was to persist, it would have to spread from that person to others, and if all the other members of the crew had already contracted the disease the virus would not reach America. A swift crossing would increase the chances of the disease spreading, as would (obviously) a larger number of previously uninfected people on board. These circumstances may explain why smallpox did not reach America until about 1518, 26 years after Columbus's first voyage. Measles may have been marginally more difficult to transmit, perhaps because it was more likely that an entire crew had already been infected, perhaps because its period of infection in an individual is shorter, and perhaps because some smallpox virus may survive in scab material; in any case, measles apparently only reached the Americas in about 1530.

Influenza, which accompanied Columbus's second voyage, may occur repeatedly in the same individual, and so its rapid transmission across the Atlantic was much more likely. Plague and typhus, in contrast, spread differently. The spread of each depends on an insect vector (most often fleas for plague, lice for typhus) to carry their pathogens from one host (perhaps a human, perhaps another animal) to another.

The Native American population constituted a vast reservoir of virgin soil for smallpox and measles, the equivalent of a Europe populated only by newborn children, children who moreover lacked any inherited defenses. But did some characteristics of American societies also affect the spread of disease? Smallpox and measles both flourish in large and crowded human settlements, and such cities were relatively unusual in pre-Columbian America. They did, however, exist, especially in the highly centralized and powerful Aztec and Inca empires; Tenochtitlan and Cuzco were large cities by any sixteenth-century standard, and therefore airborne epidemics could spread rapidly and widely through them.

Some historians have also argued that central Mexico under the Aztecs had become dangerously overpopulated by 1500 and that the land could no longer produce adequate nutrition for its people. If so, the general health of the Indians may have been weak before the Spaniards (and their pathogens) even arrived. But this view, depending in part as it does on estimates of the total population, remains controversial; other scholars insist both that the Mexican population was smaller and that Native Mexican nutrition was adequate or better (see the "Unresolved Historical Issues" sections). The relative scarcity of domestic animals (especially large ones) in the Americas may also have increased Indian susceptibility to diseases. Many human ills originated among domestic animals, and human populations that long shared space with such creatures acquired resistance to such ailments. The Europeans brought not only pathogens, but cattle, horses, pigs, sheep, large dogs, and—inadvertently—rats.

Still another background factor that should be remembered is the strength of the European desire to control and settle the Americas. Many different forces motivated Europeans to cross the Atlantic, including greed, piety, and the extension of power; the European search for wealth quickly involved the enslavement of a Native labor force, and that enslavement meant extremely unhealthy living and working conditions. In those conditions, insect and rodent populations (perhaps carrying plague or typhus) might flourish. Disease was therefore even harder to resist, both for an individual body and for social networks of care and support. And because that search for wealth quickly led to the traffic in slaves brought by Europeans from the west coast of Africa, the background for epidemic disease included Africa as well as Europe and the Americas.

Smallpox, for example, might have reached the Americas from Africa as well as from Europe. For example, a clear link existed between Portuguese slave ports in west Africa and the spread of smallpox in Brazil. The first smallpox outbreak in Brazil, in 1562, probably originated in Europe, but later in the century most smallpox was borne to Brazil from Africa. Correlations have been shown (by Alden and Miller 1987) between periods of drought and famine in west Africa and subsequent Brazilian smallpox outbreaks. Such periods led to the movement of impoverished people from the African interior into coastal towns where they fell into the grip of slave traders; once enslaved, their overcrowded slave quarters (and slave ships) made the transmission of disease more likely.

HOW IT WAS UNDERSTOOD AT THE TIME

American Indian populations generally held holistic views of disease, seeing it as an outgrowth of a disordered cosmos. Gods had perhaps been angered or the order of the natural world had somehow been disturbed. Religion—and healing—relied heavily on shamans, people who mediated between humans and the divine order. The scale of the new epidemics of the sixteenth century, together with the fact that the symptoms of the diseases were often completely unfamiliar, led to despairing beliefs that the gods had turned against the people entirely.

For Europeans (and Africans) smallpox, measles, and plague had all become relatively familiar, although they still inspired varying degrees of fear. In addition to persistent beliefs that disease represented God's wrath, the prevailing general theory remained that of humoral imbalance, which should be rectified by bleedings and purgings. The contagious character of smallpox and measles was widely accepted; both had come to be seen as childhood diseases, and it may have been true that many or even most European adults had acquired immunity through childhood cases. In the course of the sixteenth century, however, a number of lethal smallpox epidemics occurred in European cities, and fears of it increased.

RESPONSES

American Indian responses to the sixteenth-century epidemics included both immediate attempts to cure disease (or to at least relieve its symptoms), and more shamanistic rituals to banish it. Americans had long had a body of various herbal medicines, which were employed against the new terrors without much effect. Some tried sweat baths, or rapid immersion in cold water, to relieve fevers and the itching from rashes. Flight was a common response (as it has been for many epidemics throughout world history), but—especially with smallpox—flight had important and unfortunate consequences. The flight of the healthy often left the sick helpless and hence more likely to succumb through lack of nourishment. And the fleeing healthy often were themselves infected, so that their flight became another mechanism for the epidemic's diffusion.

European responses to smallpox were not much more effective, however. Physicians attempted similar means to relieve symptoms. The prevailing medical theory called for corrections of the imbalance of humours; the rashes and pustules that accompanied smallpox and measles especially suggested that the body's blood was disordered, and therefore bleeding was often practiced. For several centuries, the "red treatment" for smallpox had been popular as well, in which the patient consumed red medications and liquids, and used red blankets and clothing.

It is also possible that some folk practitioners in both Europe and Africa had begun the practice of *variolation* or inoculation for smallpox. This procedure involved deliberately implanting pus from the scab of a sufferer into the veins of another, in the belief that a mild case could be thus induced that would prevent later, more serious, infection. European physicians took no notice of this practice until the early eighteenth century, when it suddenly became fashionable.

As the Spanish and Portuguese conquests advanced in the sixteenth century, the new rulers made determined attempts to stamp out Indian shamans, their beliefs, and the rituals they undertook in response to disease. They did so not because they wished disease to spread among the Indians (see the "Unresolved Historical Issues" section) but because they wished to convert the Indians to Roman Catholic Christianity. The result was a prolonged period of underground resistance on the part of the shamans and their followers, sometimes flaring into open rebellion. Native American responses to disease thus persisted despite the conquest.

UNRESOLVED HISTORICAL ISSUES

The dramatic collapse of important civilizations and cultures that occurred in sixteenth-century America has generated prolonged historical controversies, many of which raise questions about the role of epidemic disease in the process. It was really only in the twentieth century that historians seriously began to consider the place of disease in the story.

Before that time, European (and especially Spanish) cruelty most often explained the remarkable decline of the American populations and political systems. According to that view, the Spanish and Portuguese conquerors in the sixteenth century used their technological advantages (firearms, control of the oceans, and horses) to crush American Indian opposition. In the process, they murdered thousands of Americans and enslaved many thousands more, brutally punishing those who resisted, and forcing the slave population into inhuman living conditions. In those conditions, many of the surviving Americans lost their will to reproduce or even to live. This picture of colonial rule was supported, and in a sense begun by, the writings of such sixteenth-century Spaniards as Bartolomé de Las Casas, a Dominican missionary to America who denounced the Spanish colonial practices. This explanation of the decline of the American population fit nicely into the historical beliefs of much of Protestant Europe, which demonized Catholic Spain as the center of intolerant religious fanaticism.

But could a relatively small number of Europeans really have wreaked such havoc? American Indians often started dying in large numbers before Europeans actually came into physical contact with them; Indians died even in those places where European rule was benign. For those reasons, the role of disease began to be taken seriously (as indeed some contemporary Spaniards had noticed). Historians such as Alfred Crosby (1972) and William McNeill (1976) saw epidemics as the chief cause of the collapse of the American Indian societies.

Arguments continue about the respective importance of disease as opposed to political violence and economic exploitation. F. J. Brooks (1993) believes that the supposed death tolls from epidemics have been wildly overstated, that smallpox was not a very serious disease for anyone in the sixteenth century, and that in any case it could not have spread as rapidly as others have claimed that it did. Were epidemic diseases, then, a sufficient cause for the collapse of the American Indians? Were they even relevant? Or—as seems most likely—did epidemic disease work in tandem with wrenching political and economic change, both as cause and effect? A disastrous epidemic, for instance, might so disrupt social and economic routines that the production and distribution of food would slow or stop, malnutrition would increase, and the population would be more vulnerable to many causes of death.

These arguments also involve another set of unsettled questions, relating to the size of the pre-Columbian population of the Americas, and hence to the magnitude of the mortality of the sixteenth century. Population estimates have varied very widely; some historians have called the pre-Columbian population as many as 100 million, with up to 25 million in central Mexico alone (for instance, Borah and Cook 1963); others drastically reduce those numbers (for instance, Sanders 1992). Did 90 million die or did 9 million? Furthermore, high estimates of original population have been used to support the idea that some American places—notably central Mexico—were overpopulated in 1500, hence poorly nourished and more vulnerable to epidemic disease. A lower population estimate would deny that (e.g., Ortiz de Montellano 1990).

Such arguments in turn raise questions about the general level of pre-Columbian American civilization. Had its numbers outstripped its agricultural technology (and thus primitively regressed) or did its technology, well adapted to its environment, still provide adequate nutrition? How backward was it? And after the Europeans arrived, how successfully did the American Indians preserve parts of their cultures in the face of disaster, whether that of epidemic or of political violence? If the cultures were destroyed, with the total loss of their values, what role did disease play? Answers to such questions (largely outside the framework of this volume) may depend in part on political points of view. Did the Americans completely collapse? If so, the Europeans may be judged to have committed great crimes; are the Indians to be therefore pitied or scorned because of their weakness? Does evidence that American values and customs persisted speak to the brave persistence of Indian self-determination? Or is it simply evidence that the Europeans (and their diseases) were never as brutal as they've been made out to be?

Still another unresolved question relates to the possibility that the Europeans deliberately used disease as a weapon in their American conquests. There is little or no evidence that such a thing happened in the epidemics discussed in this chapter. In the sixteenth century, European notions of disease causation were very unsettled; while smallpox and measles were generally believed to be contagious, the precise mechanism of contagion was a mystery, and smallpox was coming to be feared by the Europeans themselves, suggesting that any use of it as a weapon might infect the Europeans too. And it is also important to remember that the sixteenth-century Spaniards and Portuguese had no economic motive for reducing their Indian populations, which they wished to preserve as a labor force. As the century went on, the Spanish authorities took increasing steps to provide care for some Indian communities, hoping to preserve them. So, while some Spanish and Portuguese colonists might praise God for sending diseases to smite the heathen Indians, no evidence exists that they tried to anticipate God's actions.

(The case of later English settlements in America is different. English settlers in seventeenth- and eighteenth-century North America hoped to drive the Natives out and settle the land themselves. They expressly urged the use of disease as a weapon, by, for example, proposing the distribution of blankets soaked with pus from smallpox scabs to the Indians.)

In the realm of the epidemiology of the diseases themselves, other questions remain, especially about smallpox. Was it a relatively mild disease for Europeans at the start of the sixteenth century, and if so, why did it become so suddenly dangerous, both to American Indians and to Europeans as well? Is the virgin soil character of the American population sufficient to explain high American mortality or did the European voyages to America coincide with a sudden increase in smallpox's virulence? If so, what caused that new virulence?

REFERENCES

Alden, Dauril, and Joseph C. Miller. "Out of Africa: The Slave Trade and the Transmission of Smallpox to Brazil, 1560–1831." *Journal of Interdisciplinary History* 18 (1987): 195–224.

Black, Francis L. "An Explanation of High Death Rates among New World Peoples When in Contact with Old World Diseases." *Perspectives in Biology and Medicine* 37 (1994): 292–307.

Borah, Woodrow, and Sherburne F. Cook. *The Aboriginal Population of Central Mexico on the Eve of the Spanish Conquest.* Berkeley: University of California Press, 1963.

Brooks, F. J. "Revising the Conquest of Mexico: Smallpox, Sources, and Populations." *Journal of Interdisciplinary History* 24 (1993): 1–29.

Cook, Noble David. *Born to Die: Disease and New World Conquest, 1492–1650.* Cambridge: Cambridge University Press, 1998.

Crosby, Alfred W. *The Columbian Exchange: Biological and Cultural Consequences of 1492.* Westport, CT: Greenwood, 1972.

Hopkins, Donald R. *The Greatest Killer: Smallpox in History.* Chicago: University of Chicago Press, 2002. (Orig. pub. 1983 as *Princes and Peasants: Smallpox in History.*)

McCaa, Robert. "Spanish and Nahuatl Views on Smallpox and Demographic Catastrophe in Mexico." *Journal of Interdisciplinary History* 25 (1995): 397–431.

McNeill, William H. *Plagues and Peoples.* Garden City, NY: Anchor/Doubleday, 1976.

Ortiz de Montellano, Bernard R. *Aztec Medicine, Health, and Nutrition.* New Brunswick, NJ: Rutgers University Press, 1990.

Sanders, William T. "The Population of the Central Mexican Symbiotic Region, the Basin of Mexico, and the Teotihuacán Valley in the Sixteenth Century." In *The Native Population of the Americas in 1492*, 2nd ed., edited by William M. Deneven, 85–150. Madison: University of Wisconsin Press, 1992.

SUGGESTED ADDITIONAL READING

Carmichael, Ann G., and Arthur M. Silverstein. "Smallpox in Europe before the Seventeenth Century: Virulent Killer or Benign Disease?" *Journal of the History of Medicine and Allied Sciences* 42 (1987): 147–168.

Cook, Noble David, and W. George Lovell, eds. *The Secret Judgments of God: Native Peoples and Old World Disease in Colonial Spanish America.* Norman: University of Oklahoma Press, 1992.

Crosby, Alfred W. *Ecological Imperialism: The Biological Expansion of Europe, 900–1900.* Cambridge: Cambridge University Press, 1986.

Crosby, Alfred W. "Virgin Soil Epidemics as a Factor in the Aboriginal Depopulation of America." *William and Mary Quarterly*, 3rd series, 33 (1976): 289–299.

Deneven, William M., ed. *The Native Population of the Americas in 1492.* 2nd ed. Madison: University of Wisconsin Press, 1992.

Guerra, Francisco. "The Earliest American Epidemic: The Influenza of 1493." *Social Science History* 12 (1988): 305–325.

Powell, Mary Lucas, and Della Collins Cook, eds. *The Myth of Syphilis: The Natural History of Treponematosis in North America.* Gainesville: University Press of Florida, 2005.

7

"French Disease" in Sixteenth-Century Europe

WHEN AND WHERE

In July 1495, a serious disease, apparently new, broke out among troops engaged in the battle of Fornovo, in northern Italy. War had begun in the Italian peninsula the previous year when the French king Charles VIII had invaded it to assert his claim to the Kingdom of Naples; alliances of other Italian states formed either to support or to resist the French claims. French troops associated the new disease with Naples, which they had earlier besieged, and so they called it the "Neapolitan disease." To Italians it became the Mal Francese, the "French disease," and that term became generally used by many others as well. It also acquired the name of the Great Pox, differentiating it from smallpox.

This disease spread through Europe with alarming speed. Armies carried it with them, both as they campaigned and then as they disbanded. In France, the ailment was reported in Lyons by March 1496, and in Paris by the fall. Lucerne, Switzerland, had infections by May 1496, Frankfurt, Germany, by the summer. England and Scotland recorded cases in 1497. All the countries of Europe experienced the disease, probably by 1500; by 1505, it had reached across Asia to China as well.

The new disease manifested itself in sharp pains in the joints, fever, sores, and swelling. Pustules formed on the body and cases then progressed to destruction of tissue, and the body seemed to rot. The victims gave off a powerful stench. These symptoms inspired particular horror. Alessandri Benedicti, an Italian physician, described it in 1497: "The entire body is so repulsive to look at and the suffering is so great, especially at night, that this sickness is even more horrifying than incurable leprosy or elephantiasis, and it can be fatal" (Quétel 1990, 10). The disease was, therefore, a very virulent one.

It also did not respect prominent people. Before 1500, it had already infected important figures in the court of Pope Alexander VI, including the pope's military adventurer son Cesare Borgia and Cardinal Giuliano della Rovere, the later Pope Julius II. (The powerful continued to be numbered among its victims throughout the sixteenth century, and at one point the humanist writer Erasmus claimed that if one hadn't experienced the disease one was evidently a naive rustic. King Francis I of France suffered from it.)

Its name remained a conflicted subject. The French blamed it on the Neapolitans, the Italians on the French, and other peoples blamed it on still other suspects. At some early point another idea took hold: that the disease had originated in America and had been brought back to Europe by the crews of Columbus and later explorers. The disease was *probably* venereal syphilis. The term "syphilis" was used in connection with the disease in the 1530 poem *Syphilis sive morbus gallicus,* by the Italian physician Girolamo Fracastoro, but that word did not come into general use for the disease until the eighteenth century. (See the "Unresolved Historical Issues" section.)

No reliable estimates of its sixteenth-century mortality and morbidity exist. Some evidence suggests that the disease became less virulent in the course of the sixteenth century, perhaps as the reservoir of the unexposed shrank. (See the "How It Was Understood at the Time" and "Unresolved Historical Issues" sections for the question of its newness.) It certainly became very widespread as the century went on, and syphilis has remained a well-entrenched and familiar ailment in the Western world ever since.

SIGNIFICANCE

The appearance of the "French disease" at the end of the fifteenth century contributed to reshaping European ideas about disease that had already begun with the Second Plague Pandemic. The nearly universal character of plague in the fourteenth century had forced thinkers to question the older assumption that explained disease as an individual aberration, a deviation from the desired mean of health. Plague affected so many people that it seemed to have an independent cause, acting outside the vagaries of individual bodies; the sudden explosion of the "French disease" likewise needed a more general explanation. Both diseases, therefore, led thinkers to begin regarding diseases as autonomous, separate entities apart from the balances (such as those of the "humours") of the human frame. And the "French disease," again like the plague, encouraged thinkers to believe that contagion was an important aspect of disease.

If the disease really was new, what did that say about the wisdom of the ancient Greeks and Romans who had remained the authorities for medieval opinion? Was it possible that the ancients did not know everything? (The nearly simultaneous geographical discoveries of Vasco da Gama and Columbus had something of the same effect.)

In modern historical writing, the sudden appearance of the "French disease" has been bracketed with the contemporary spread to the Americas of several massive new epidemics. They have all been seen as virgin soil epidemics, the results of new human contacts between different, previously isolated, continents. But the newness of the "French disease" to Europe remains controversial (see the "Unresolved Historical Issues" section).

The history of this disease also marks the first time in Western history when a remedy for a disease was prepared and actively promoted by commercial interests.

The "French disease" therefore stands as a forerunner to many important later Western responses, and as a curious early example of the growth of market economies in Western history (see the "Responses" section).

BACKGROUND

Columbus returned from his first voyage to America at the end of 1492; Vasco da Gama completed his voyage around Africa to India in 1498 and returned in 1499. Diseases from three great land masses—the Americas, Eurasia, and Africa—might thereafter be spread by ocean voyagers.

The prevalence of warfare in sixteenth-century Europe, and the character of the armies of the time, both contributed to the diffusion of disease. The sixteenth century, the age of the Protestant Reformation and its Catholic counterpart, was a time of frequent armed conflict that had both new religious and old dynastic motives. Armies were usually poorly paid, ill-disciplined, dirty, recruited from many places, and frequently disbanded and reassembled; they were therefore ideal diffusers of epidemic diseases.

The appearance of the "French disease" in Italy occurred at a particular time of crisis (widely seen as such at the time). The French invasion of 1494–1495 touched off a period of political turmoil in Italian states, which coincided with widespread floods and famines to which the new epidemic was added. Millenarian prophecies (as the year 1500 approached) were common. Girolamo Savonarola, the charismatic Dominican, rose to political ascendancy in Florence in 1494, an extreme example of the highly strung public mood when the "French disease" appeared.

HOW IT WAS UNDERSTOOD AT THE TIME

As with the Black Death in the fourteenth century, some of the first reactions to the new disease looked to God's anger as the cause. Were sinners being punished? Some such thought persisted through the sixteenth century. In Fracastoro's allegorical poem (1530) the shepherd Syphilis offends the "Sun God" by worshipping at other altars and so is stricken with the disease.

And as in the fourteenth century, some thinkers saw God's will being worked through the movements of the heavens. If anything, convictions about astrology had strengthened by the late fifteenth century, as an aspect of Renaissance Neoplatonism. For some, the new disease resulted from an unfortunate conjunction of the planets.

Most physicians, however, were not convinced that the disease was new, and their writings paid less attention to either God's wrath or planetary conjunctions. In their training, the ideas and writings of classical antiquity loomed large; for them, the knowledge of the ancients surpassed that of the moderns, and if so, could a disease *exist* that had been unknown to the ancients? This new disease, therefore, could only be understood within the categories of disease found in the Hippocratic writings, in Galen, and in Arab commentators such as Avicenna.

Using categories from Galen and Avicenna, doctors concluded that the new disease was in fact a humoral disorder, especially an excess of phlegm. This view of the disease at least suggested that doctors could do something active about it: remove the phlegm (see the "Responses" section). Opinions about the newness of the disease, then, in part related to the possibility of curing it. Doctors might be helpless in the face of a "new" disease.

Opinions differed about ways in which individuals contracted the disease. Some ideas did not become more specific than a simple assertion that the atmosphere was disturbed by the planetary conjunctions, but humoral theories usually saw disease as resulting from an alteration in what were sometimes called the nonnaturals, meaning air, food and drink, sleep, exercise, excretion, and emotion. That is, did the disease stem from something one ate or drank? Or was the disease a *contagion*, which spread from one person to another? If so, how? That line led to an early emphasis by many authorities (although not all) on sexual activity as the mode of contagion for the Great Pox. And as the sixteenth century progressed, that view—that the disease was venereal—gained strength.

It was also quickly understood that the "French disease" differed from plague in an important respect: it was *chronic*. Its symptoms, while changing, could linger for years. Its social effects, therefore, were more akin to those of leprosy; it did not cause plague's sudden drop in populations, but rather created populations set apart by their grotesque symptoms and suffering.

RESPONSES

The major medical response to the new disease appeared fairly quickly: promoting either sweating or spitting were attempts to expel excess phlegm from the body. Descriptions of a "dry stove" date from as early as 1497; the device simply consisted of a closed box containing a stove or some other fire, and the patient would be placed in the box to sweat.

At some point in the early sixteenth century another element entered into this heat treatment: the hard American wood called *guaiacum*. Especially for those who believed that the disease was both new and had its origins in America, the idea of an American cure was appealing; God would surely provide a corresponding American cure for an American ailment. Guaiacum was ground into a powder, and either eaten or spread in a salve on the sores of the sick. These remedies accompanied such sweating treatments as the dry stove.

Guaiacum owed its popularity, in part, to the writings of a young German humanist, Ulrich von Hutten, whose 1519 book *De guaiaci medicina et morbo gallico* ("On the guaiac medicine and the French disease") became one of the standard and most widely read early treatises. (Von Hutten himself had suffered from the disease, and so his writing carried particular conviction.) But the popularity of guaiacum also owed something to commercial advertising. The important German banking and merchant house of the Fuggers imported it and promoted its sale.

There existed a rival remedy to guaiacum, one that had in fact been used almost from the disease's first appearance: compounds of mercury. Mercuric ointments had been prescribed for various skin ailments for several centuries, especially by Arabic physicians. Their use promoted profuse spitting (which medical science,

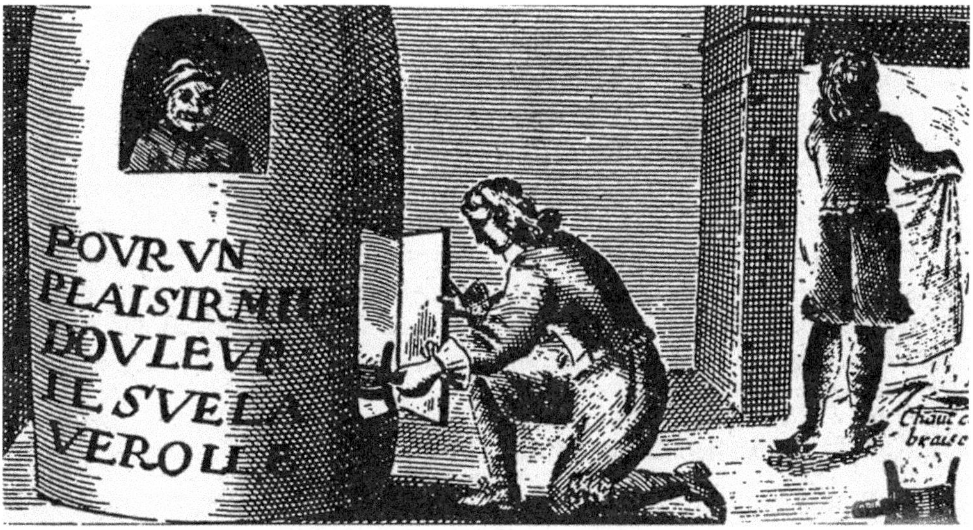

Acting on the belief that syphilis, the "French disease," was caused by an excess of the bodily humor phlegm, treatment consisted of promoting profuse sweating to right the humoral imbalance. From a French engraving, c. 1659–1663. (Science History Images/ Alamy Stock Photo)

much later, would identify as a symptom of mercury poisoning), and that effect seemed the desired expulsion of offensive phlegm. Mercury found a particularly vigorous exponent in the radical Swiss healer Paracelsus (1493–1541), for whom the mercuric treatment was part of a much larger and more systematic attack on Galenic and Aristotelian traditions. In practice, many healers combined the use of heat, guaiacum, and mercury, in different proportions.

Other medical treatments existed as well, as healers wrestled with a loathsome and dangerous disease. They included bleeding the patient, especially if you believed that the offending humor was blood, not phlegm; cauterization of the pustules of the sick; and baths, taken with herbs or perhaps with a powder of guaiacum. And for those who maintained that astrological influences caused the disease, the best advice was to avoid exposure to heaven-sent atmospheric disturbance: stay indoors, avoid the exertion and emotion that would mean rapid breathing.

These different medical responses applied to the treatment of ailing individuals. Other responses were social and political. Governments were only slowly (and in some places) developing public health responses to plague (see volume 2, chapter 5); this new disease ultimately reinforced the fear of contagion that plague had begun to inspire, but many of the early collective responses were those of voluntary organizations such as religious confraternities and privately supported hospitals. Specialized hospitals (called Incurabili hospitals in Italy, where they were widespread), or at least separate isolation wards for victims, received the backing of the papacy by 1515. In some places more extreme isolation was proposed or even carried out, as in Edinburgh, where "French disease" victims were banished to an island. In some ways these early communal reactions to the Great Pox mirrored long-standing approaches to another chronic, loathsome disease, leprosy. As the sixteenth century progressed, however, the belief that the "French disease" might be curable strengthened, and the Incurabili hospitals became, in fact, places where cure was the goal.

The association of the disease with sexual contacts suggested another official response: the control of prostitutes. Such measures were urged as early as 1500 by a papal physician, Gaspar Torrella: "Leaders like the Pope, the Emperor, kings and other lords should send matrons to investigate the disease, especially among prostitutes who, if they be found to be infected, should be confined to a place designated for this purpose by the community or the lord, and treated by a physician or surgeon paid to do so" (Arrizabalaga et al. 1997, 34). Such proposals were often voiced, but were not implemented on any significant scale until the nineteenth century.

UNRESOLVED HISTORICAL ISSUES

The origins of the "French disease" in Europe began to be disputed almost since it was first noticed, and they have remained so. Two main theories emerged early: that it had been in Europe all along or that it had been imported from America in the wake of Columbus. Those theories persist, now called (respectively) the *unitary treponema* theory and the *Columbian* theory.

The unitary treponema theory holds that venereal syphilis is just one of a family of related diseases caused by the class of closely related microorganisms called *treponematoses.* Those diseases include the tropical diseases pinta (in Central America) and yaws (in Africa), and the Near Eastern disease bejel (or endemic syphilis). The theory (and there have been several variants of it proposed) holds that *treponematoses* have existed in all human populations for thousands of years and their diseases have taken different forms at different times, slowly evolving from one manifestation to another. What was suddenly noticed in 1495 Europe was not really new, but the suddenly visible outcrop of disease states that had earlier been called something else (perhaps leprosy) or even simply ignored.

The Columbian theory maintains that the 1495 epidemic *was* new to Europe and that the form of *treponema* responsible for venereal syphilis had evolved separately in the New World. The American Indians, in this view, had long suffered from it, and the peoples of Asia, Africa, and Europe had not. Columbus's 1492 voyage changed all that and began a very important period of disease exchange in which new microbes invaded virgin soil populations with devastating results. The "French disease" epidemic in Europe was one such.

Some strong circumstances have bolstered the Columbian theory. Many people in the years around 1500 *thought* the disease was new, even though physicians wanted very much to be able to fit it into the established Galenic framework. The apparent slow decline of the disease's virulence in the sixteenth century also argues that it may have been new in 1500; as the previously virgin population of Europe acquired resistant experience with the microorganism, its effects lessened. Paleopathological evidence from the remains of American Indian dead have been less certain, and controversy persists. But the prospect of increasingly precise paleopathology promises an eventual settlement of the Columbian versus unitary treponema dispute.)

While strong, the Columbian theory did not hold the field unanimously in the early modern period. West Africans transported as slaves to the Caribbean region brought with them beliefs and preventive practices about yaws. Those ideas particularly informed British opinion about the origins of syphilis in the seventeenth and eighteenth centuries, more so as opposition to the slave trade arose in popular and political opinion.

The evolution of medical understanding, from the "French disease" of the sixteenth century to the venereal syphilis of the late nineteenth, also illustrates the continuing unresolved issues that surround past epidemics. The causative organism of syphilis was not identified until the early twentieth century. Shortly thereafter a compound (a "magic bullet") was developed that specifically attacked that microorganism in the body and opened a whole new world of curative possibilities. Until that point, mercury compounds continued to be used, with some effect on the symptoms of syphilis; guaiacum also remained listed as a remedy, although its effects could only have been psychological.

REFERENCES

Arrizabalaga, Jon, John Henderson, and Roger French. *The Great Pox: The French Disease in Renaissance Europe.* New Haven, CT: Yale University Press, 1997.

Quétel, Claude. *History of Syphilis.* Baltimore: Johns Hopkins University Press, 1990.

SUGGESTED ADDITIONAL READING

Crosby, Alfred W., Jr. *The Columbian Exchange: Biological and Cultural Consequences of 1492.* Westport, CT: Greenwood, 1972.

Munger, Robert S. "Guaiacum, the Holy Wood from the New World." *Journal of the History of Medicine and Allied Sciences* 4 (1949): 196–227.

Paugh, Katherine. "Yaws, Syphilis, Sexuality, and the Circulation of Medical Knowledge in the British Caribbean and the Atlantic World." *Bulletin of the History of Medicine* 88 (2014): 225–252.

This article summarizes some different opinions about the geographical origin of syphilis:

Guerra, Francisco. "The Dispute over Syphilis: Europe versus America." *Clio Medica* 13 (1978): 39–61.

8

Epidemics and the Thirty Years' War, 1618–1648

WHEN AND WHERE

The complex series of wars that occurred in Europe between 1618 and 1648 have been called the Thirty Years' War, although that term specifically refers to events in and near Germany. Most of the fighting took place in the German areas of central Europe, although the war drew in nearly all the states of the continent, as other wars (marked by different dates) interacted with German events. The conflict stemmed from multiple causes, including religious struggles between Catholic and Protestant states in central Europe, increasingly overlaid by dynastic and state power issues.

The circumstances of the war were particularly favorable for the spread of epidemic diseases. The most consistent and dangerous epidemic disease that accompanied the war was typhus, which all through the early modern period was often endemic in the armies of the time and was spread by them. Especially in the early 1630s, plague joined typhus as a major killer in the zones affected by war and may have been responsible for the single episodes with the highest mortalities. But other diseases were important as well, including dysentery, typhoid fever, and (probably) relapsing fever.

Within the German states wide regional variations existed in the war-related disease toll. The immediate cause of the war was a revolt in Bohemia that ousted the Hapsburg (Catholic) dynasty and chose Frederick, the (Protestant) Elector of the Palatinate, as the new king. The Hapsburg heir presumptive, Ferdinand, responded with military force, and thus Bohemia, the diverse lands of the Palatinate, and adjoining regions such as Württemberg became and remained zones of high mortality from both disease and warfare. Another region of high disease mortality was northeastern Germany, including Mecklenburg and Pomerania. Northwestern Germany, which saw relatively little fighting, suffered little. While the most vivid and best-documented examples of epidemics occurred in cities and towns, villages may have suffered proportionately more because they had little or no defense against marauding armies and did not enjoy the reserves of food that cities might accumulate.

The complex events of the Thirty Years' War, occurring as they did at a time of climate change involving bitter cold and storms that meant crop failures and famine, compounded the ravages of epidemics with their violence and social disorder. The panoply of disasters perhaps explains the difficulty in sorting out the relative importance of disease in the total figures of mortality and morbidity and have thus frustrated simple general narratives of diseases in the war. Some specific examples may illustrate themes of the relations between war and epidemics.

1. The revolt in Bohemia, where Protestants ousted the Catholic Hapsburg claimant to the throne, touched off the war in 1618. Catholic forces responded by mustering an army of about 50,000, but by the end of 1620 about half of them had been lost to some combination of disease, battle deaths, and desertion. As that army moved through Bavaria, Austria, and Württemberg, it spread diseases through those regions. Meanwhile a countering Protestant army under the soldier of fortune Ernst von Mansfeld campaigned in Franconia and the Palatinate, carrying more typhus with it; when Mansfeld reached Strasbourg in 1622, that city suffered over 4,300 deaths, many of them from typhus. Over 1,700 died in Frankfurt, where the usual annual death toll was only about 600. The first campaigns of the war, then, introduced the theme of disease diffusion by lice-infested armies. (Mansfeld himself died in 1626, apparently suffering from both typhus and tuberculosis.)
2. In the years between 1618 and 1624, the Hapsburg imperial authorities raised a total of 69 regiments of troops. By 1625 the manpower for only 15 regiments survived (Wilson 2009, 397).
3. In 1627 and 1628, the army of Count Wallenstein, in the service of the Hapsburg emperor Ferdinand II, carried the war into northeastern Germany. His troops repeatedly ravaged Pomerania between 1628 and 1631. The city of Kolberg had 3,000 deaths in six months in that period.
4. In 1630 the Swedish king Gustavus II Adolphus entered the war and thus intensified the fighting in Germany. His army occupied the city of Augsburg between 1632 and 1635. Between September 1634 and March 1635, an opposing Imperial army besieged the Swedes in Augsburg. In the period of the Swedish occupation and the Imperial siege, the population of the city was reduced from about 48,000 to about 16,000, with typhus and plague playing major roles. Disease and death struck other towns in the Augsburg area as well; in Memmingen, southwest of Augsburg, 3,000 died in 1635, while in Füssen 1,200 people—one-fourth of the population—died in the same year.
5. Some examples chosen from a single year, 1633, illustrate the deepening disease crisis that accompanied the continuing war in Germany. Altenburg, in central Germany, lost 2,100 people to disease in the wake of its occupation by the Swedes in January. Breslau, in Silesia, suffered 18,000 deaths; in the area of Schweidnitz, near camps of both the Swedes and Wallenstein, perhaps 16,000 people died, more than two-thirds the population.

6. After the crucial battle of Nördlingen in 1634, the Swedes and their Protestant allies retreated across Württemberg with the Imperial forces in pursuit, and the resulting movements of armies meant disaster for that section of Germany. The city of Stuttgart, with about 8,300 people in 1631, suffered nearly 1,000 deaths in 1634, and then in 1635 (when the town was filled with filled with fugitives from the surrounding countryside) a further 4,300. When an Imperial army left the city in 1638, it left behind about 6,000 wounded or diseased soldiers. Adjoining communities were stricken as well: Cannstatt, 1,300 deaths in 1635; Goppingen, occupied by the Imperialists after Nördlingen, 600 pestilence deaths in three months in 1634; Gmünd, 30–40 deaths daily in 1636, and the town could only dispose of bodies in mass graves; Weinsberg, over 600 deaths in a total population of 1,400 in 1635; Vaihingen, 1,800 deaths in 1635 where only 48 had died in 1631; Tübingen, where the famous university's faculty fled the city in 1635 to escape an army-spread plague; and the Ulm region, which may have lost as many as 15,000 in eight months in 1635, many from plague.

   One estimate holds that the population of the Duchy of Württemberg fell by 57% between 1634 and 1655, and that it did not regain its 1618 numbers until after 1710. These figures are very uncertain, and some number of the losses may been accounted for by flight or disappearance rather than death.

Modern historians believe that the years of the Thirty Years' War resulted in a population loss of 15% or 20% in the German states as a whole. (See the "Significance" and "Unresolved Historical Issues" sections.)

SIGNIFICANCE

The Thirty Years' War stands as the most vivid example of the interconnection of warfare and epidemic disease in early modern European history. Other wars of the sixteenth, seventeenth, and eighteenth centuries shared many of its characteristics and were also accompanied by epidemic disease. But the Thirty Years' War became in both historical writing and popular folk culture the most extreme such case.

Earlier historical opinion, especially that which developed in the nineteenth century, pictured the war, and its death tolls from disease and violence alike, as a catastrophic interruption of the course of German history. The subsequent misfortunes of Germany (e.g., the perceived lack of economic progress compared with that of Britain and France or the dominance of a land-holding military class) were traced to that disaster. According to this older interpretation, perhaps half of the German population perished in the war, and the country could not recover for more than a century.

Modern historians now reject such a dramatic view and believe that the total population loss of the German states was between 15% and 20%. That still represents a serious demographic blow, but it was one from which the society may have recovered relatively quickly.

BACKGROUND

Armies in early modern Europe were in many ways ideal diffusers of epidemic disease. The states of the period were only gradually moving toward control of full-time armies and that control only became generally effective in the eighteenth century. Many sixteenth- and seventeenth-century armies were mercenary, recruited by states for a campaign and then disbanded. Even when war continued, armies often broke up during the winter months, to be reassembled in the spring. These armies were therefore poorly paid, often badly disciplined if at all, and drawn largely from the most unfortunate classes of society. Many of their commanders tried to compensate them by allowing them license to loot, pillage, and rape. At times such an army could be an unpaid, itinerant, unwashed, promiscuous mob, living in close quarters among themselves and in close proximity to unwilling others. And the army moved from place to place both during campaigns and when it disbanded and scattered, carrying its diseases with it.

Many different diseases might flourish in such a body of men, but typhus seemed particularly favored. Epidemic typhus is passed from one human to another by lice. The louse ingests the microorganism that causes the disease when it feeds on the blood of an infected person. The louse then moves to another person, and the microorganism reaches the new victim when the feces of the louse enters his circulatory system either through the skin or by inhalation of dust containing dried louse feces. A group of unwashed people, infested by lice, living in close contact with one another, therefore form a pool in which typhus infection can easily and rapidly spread. Other diseases could run riot as well in a situation such as that illustrated by the makeup of Wallenstein's army in 1632: 55,000 troops, 50,000 camp followers, 45,000 horses, four tons of human excrement per day, and an untold swarm of accompanying rats and flies (Wilson 2009, 501–502).

As the following sections show, the disruptions of war played havoc with the public health responses to epidemic disease that existed in the seventeenth century. War therefore not just assembled the masses of poorly fed and unwashed people to initiate and sustain an epidemic; it also made any effective response to the epidemic much more difficult, and so guaranteed its persistence.

HOW IT WAS UNDERSTOOD AT THE TIME

Seventeenth-century understanding of diseases did not clearly differentiate many ailments that would later be considered separate entities. The term "pestilence" included many different possibilities. Fevers were often placed on a continuum, in which one fever differed from another only in degree.

The diseases that were rife during the Thirty Years' War were sometimes collectively and indiscriminately called "war plague," "head disease," "soldiers' disease," or "Hungarian fever." Most often those terms described typhus or an outbreak that involved typhoid fever and influenza as well as typhus. (The identification of the causative microorganism of typhus and the role of lice in its transmission was only made in the early twentieth century.)

Plague was more clearly recognized as a separate ailment. By the seventeenth century, if not before, an elaborate public health response to plague had evolved. That response was based on the growing conviction that plague was a contagious disease, and that conviction was sometimes extended to the "fevers" of wartime as well. (See volume 2, chapters 5 and 9.)

RESPONSES

The public health measures deployed against plague were designed to interrupt contagion. These included isolation facilities for the sick, quarantines, sanitary cordons, the issuance of health passes allowing travelers to proceed, and the destruction (often by burning) of the possessions of the sick or the dead. Attempts were made to implement such responses, whether against plague or the fevers of war.

The circumstances of the war, however, meant that such responses never had a chance. Marauding armies would not respect quarantines or sanitary cordons; the thousands of people whom the war uprooted overwhelmed any attempt at population control. Wherever the war went, the political and social institutions responsible for public health often simply collapsed. The tragedy of the Thirty Years' War's epidemics, therefore, grew from both the diseases themselves and the war's disruption of human responses to them.

UNRESOLVED HISTORICAL ISSUES

Questions remain about the actual extent of the epidemics in the Thirty Years' War, about the mortality they extracted, and about the long-term effects of that mortality on the German states and their people. It is clear, however, that earlier accounts claiming 50% or higher mortality were exaggerations. Places where populations may have fallen by half or more between 1618 and 1648 lost an unknown number not to death but to flight; many population losses were in fact transfers from one place to another.

The precise identification of the diseases responsible for the epidemics of the time also remains unsettled and will probably never be solved. Typhus, plague, and influenza remain the chief suspects.

SUGGESTED ADDITIONAL READING

Friedrichs, Christopher J. "The War and German Society." In *The Thirty Years' War*, 2nd ed., edited by Geoffrey Parker, 186–192. London: Routledge, 1997.

Parker, Geoffrey. *Global Crisis: War, Climate Change and Catastrophe in the Seventeenth Century*. New Haven, CT: Yale University Press, 2013.

Prinzing, Friedrich. *Epidemics Resulting from Wars*. Oxford: Clarendon, 1916.

Wilson, Peter H. *The Thirty Years War: Europe's Tragedy*. Cambridge, MA: Belknap Press of Harvard University, 2009.

Zinsser, Hans. *Rats, Lice and History*. Boston: Little, Brown, 1935. (Paperback ed., New York: Bantam, 1960.)

9

Plague in Italian Cities, 1630s

WHERE AND WHEN

Italian cities had suffered periodic plague epidemics since the Second Plague Pandemic first reached there in 1347. (See volume 2, chapter 5.) For many of the important Italian cities, the last surge of these plague epidemics occurred between 1629 and 1633. At that point plague had not visited the cities for several generations: not since 1531 in Florence and 1577 in Venice, for example. In all, at least 34 Italian cities experienced plague in 1630, and 21 in 1631.

Plague claimed high mortalities in all the major cities of northern Italy in those years, although some places were more seriously hit than others. In Verona, an estimated 33,000 people (of a total of 54,000) died in 1630–1631, a frightening 61% of the population. Of the larger cities in those years, Venice lost 46,000 (of 140,000), Milan 60,000 (of 130,000), and Florence 9,000 (of 76,000). Surrounding rural communities were affected as well, although wide variations apparently existed. Plague missed some villages in Tuscany entirely, while exacting mortalities near 50% in others. Over northern Italy as a whole perhaps one million people, of a population of about four million, died. Morbidity—the rate of illness—was high as well. Although morbidity has been difficult to estimate precisely, the total number of those who fell ill with plague may have reached as high as 50% of the population.

No one could have predicted that these would be the last plague years for some northern Italian cities, but they were. At least in western Europe, the Second Plague Pandemic was coming to an end.

SIGNIFICANCE

This set of epidemics in 1630s Italy is one of the best-documented episodes of the Second Plague Pandemic, and one that has inspired considerable modern historical writing. The epidemics clearly illustrated the changing conceptions of plague that had evolved since the pandemic began in the fourteenth century, particularly the growing conviction that plague was a contagious disease (although it was still thought to have originated in miasmatic causes). Since the fourteenth century, the city-states of northern Italy had developed complex and sophisticated government mechanisms specifically in response to the threat of plague, and the story of the epidemics of the 1630s clearly demonstrates the measures that city governments took in the face of a disastrous disease.

Those measures possibly contributed to bringing the Second Plague Pandemic to an end. For most of the cities of northern Italy, the long period of plague years ended in the 1630s. The last plague year for Bologna and Mantua was 1630; for Padua, Pistoia, and Venice, 1631; for Parma, Pisa, and Turin, 1632; for Florence, 1633; and for Milan, 1637. The anti-contagion policies illustrated in the 1630s, therefore, may be part of the answer to the large historical problem of why the Second Plague Pandemic disappeared from the West when it did.

The measures undertaken by the Italian cities in the 1630s also served as an early model for comprehensive public health regulations, and in so doing raised questions that persist into the twenty-first century: How far may the needs of a community's public health encroach on individual freedoms and traditional social customs?

BACKGROUND

The Second Plague Pandemic, which reached Europe in 1347, persisted into the eighteenth century. After the great Black Death epidemic of 1347–1350, Europe suffered several centuries of repeated plague visitations, aftershocks that came (at first) every 10 or 15 years, then at gradually lengthening intervals. For the cities of northern Italy, for example, serious plague epidemics occurred in 1360–1363, 1373–1374, 1382–1383, 1400, 1456–1457, 1478, 1484–1486, 1522–1529, and 1575–1577, before the 1630s epidemics began. Plague had, in some sense, become endemic in Europe; some plague was reported *somewhere* in Europe every year between 1356 and 1670. In the years between the Black Death of 1348 and the 1630s epidemics, plague was found in Italy about two years (on average) out of every three. But an unusually long interval separated the epidemics of the 1570s from those of the 1630s, and so without previous exposure the Italian population may have been especially vulnerable.

The cities of northern Italy—Venice, Genoa, Milan, Florence, Bologna, and others—had long been the major urban concentration of Europe. As they had been in the fourteenth century, they could still be regarded in the seventeenth century as city-states, each controlling the territories that surrounded them. (Their forms of government differed, for some were ruled by hereditary princes while others were republics.) Repeated experience with plague epidemics had led them to adopt pioneering public health systems, with standing boards of health charged with directing the city-state's response to epidemics. Venice made such a board permanent in 1486, Florence in 1527, and Milan in 1534. These boards were more administrative than medical in their compositions and functions. While physicians would serve on some of them, they were dominated by men of political standing and prestige, for they needed to overawe their populations into obedience of often-unpopular measures (see the "Responses" section).

Although the boards of health had evolved a set of beliefs about where plague came from—it was a contagious disease that was carried from somewhere else—they had no accepted notion of what the mechanism of contagion was.

HOW IT WAS UNDERSTOOD AT THE TIME

By the early seventeenth century, a widespread consensus had been reached among Italian physicians and public authorities that plague was above all a contagious disease, which spread from one person to another, and which was carried from one place to another by the movements of people. Plague originated in environmental miasmas, sometimes pictured as "venomous atoms" given off from some source of infection, including those already sick. The task of the public authority was to limit the disease's spread from one person to another. While it would be generally agreed that ultimately God caused all natural phenomena, the immediate hand of the Almighty received less attention in seventeenth-century plague thinking than it had in the fourteenth century.

This belief in contagion dictated the measures that city governments undertook in response to threatened (and actual) plague epidemics, above all the imposition of quarantines to prevent the disease from reaching their territories, and the isolation of plague victims to prevent its spread to others. But since ultimately plague began with fatal miasmas, those had to be guarded against as well, and church authorities still insisted on the importance of religious responses. On a popular level, many resisted the theory of contagion, perhaps because it led to great hardship for them, and perhaps because they did not see *how* contagion worked.

No clear notion of the mechanism of contagion existed. If plague originated with the effusions from some infected source, what was that source? Numerous possibilities were considered, including the already-sick and their possessions, domestic animals (believed by some to be carriers of plague), and any other possible corruption of the air, including garbage. The fact that plague was most common in summer months (when smelly corruptions were more obvious) seemed to confirm that point. Experience also connected greater risk of plague with contact with textiles, especially wool.

A variety of different ailments may have been lumped together as plague, for plague's main sign was the *bubo,* or ulcerated swelling in the groin, armpit, or neck; undoubtedly some other diseases that included swellings or rashes might have been called plague. (See also volume 2, chapter 5, especially "Unresolved Historical Issues" section.)

RESPONSES

When a city-state government learned that plaguc had broken out in another city or region, it declared a quarantine on people and goods coming from that place. (It would learn about such an outbreak from its own ambassadors, from the infected place itself, or from a report from a third city.) Quarantines had differing degrees of severity. In some cases, the quarantine simply forbade the entry of people or goods from the infected place into the city proclaiming the quarantine. In others, the travelers and their goods would be isolated in a location (perhaps an island if it were available) within the territory of the city-state imposing the quarantine, perhaps for a period of 40 days.

A city determined to keep plague out could also impose a *cordon sanitaire* (sanitary cordon) around its borders. Entrance to the city-state would depend on a traveler's possession of a health pass from an authority certifying freedom from disease; border police turned those without such a pass away. City authorities therefore especially suspected a wide variety of transients: shepherds, day laborers, peddlers, vagrants, beggars, and soldiers (and army deserters). Such groups received extra (and unwelcome) attention from city-state authorities in plague years.

By such measures, city-state governments hoped to keep plague from reaching their territory. Once plague broke out within that territory, the health boards attempted to isolate its victims from others. Authorities ordered the sick into a *pesthouse* (perhaps a permanent installation, perhaps a building commandeered for the epidemic) and held them there for a specified time (again, perhaps 40 days). Pesthouses would house the sick, those recuperating from illness, and even those suspected of illness. The families of those bundled off to a pesthouse would be confined in their houses, whose doors and first-floor windows would be sealed; they would be supplied with food, perhaps through open windows on upper floors. Suspect possessions of the sick, especially clothes and bedding, would be seized and burnt. Contagion from the dead victims of plague was also greatly feared, and so health boards provided for the rapid, unceremonious disposal of corpses, avoiding the established cemetery grounds.

These responses to a plague epidemic meant considerable expense for a city-state government. Border guards, house inspectors, physicians and surgeons, and gravediggers had to be paid; supplies for isolated families had to be bought; and property for a pesthouse had to be acquired. And because the health boards also had to act against the underlying miasmas that were thought to exist, still other expenses arose. Thus, in 1630, the Florentine health board recommended that "all cities of the Grand Duchy [of Tuscany] keep their streets as clean as possible" (Cipolla 1981, 52).

The sweeping measures against plague that city-state health boards had evolved by the seventeenth century gave rise to many and serious grievances among their people. Quarantines obviously could devastate trade between cities, and isolation of victims and their families could likewise suspend business within the city. Artisans, many of whom worked in home shops, could lose their business, and perhaps also their materials when they were seized and burned. Textile materials were particularly subject to seizure, for they were feared as likely producers of venomous particles; for example, the physicians of Pistoia urged the prohibition of silkworms and an end of silk production there. The seizure of private property by health authorities was therefore widely resented.

The people of the cities feared pesthouses and regarded isolation in them as equivalent to a death sentence. The isolation routine disrupted family life. The rapid disposal of the bodies of plague victims deeply offended traditional funeral customs, interfered with mourning routines, and perhaps denied victims burial in consecrated ground. In many ways, then, the actions of health boards seemed both to interfere with individual behavior and to menace long-standing and important social customs.

And by the seventeenth century, the decrees of health boards also came into conflict with religious authorities. Fearing contagion, health authorities banned religious processions and assemblies, moves that angered church leaders and many other people for whom a prayer service and procession asking for the intercession of a saint were important defenses against the epidemic. Monastic or other church property would be claimed for a pesthouse; churchmen, accustomed to traveling freely, found their paths blocked by quarantines and sanitary cordons.

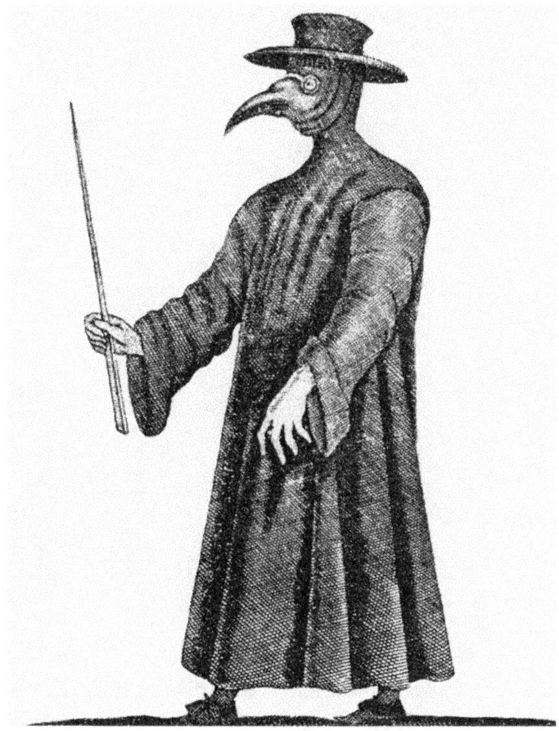

Illustration from a seventeenth-century manuscript, depicting a "plague doctor." The distinctive attire is intended as protection against contagion through airborne exposure and physical contact. Typically, such gowns were made from heavy fabric or leather and were usually waxed. The beak contained pungent substances such as herbs or perfumes, thought at the time to purify the air and helpful in relieving the stench. The person also carried a pointer or rod to keep patients at a distance. (Wellcome Collection)

Both increased taxation and brutal police power accompanied these assertions of state power in the name of public health. Both led to complaints; resistance to public health measures would call down a very heavy state response, which (in Florence, for example) routinely included inflicting torture on suspects.

Popular grievances against health boards and their measures occasionally expressed themselves violently. In Milan in 1630 a crowd cursed and threw stones at two members of the health board as they moved through a busy street; in Florence in 1633 hundreds of women had angry confrontations with barber-surgeons that led to the official (if temporary) closure of pesthouses. In the village of Monte Lupo, in Florentine territory, a 1630 religious procession took place in defiance of health board rules, and in the ensuing uproar the village stockade was destroyed. Probably more common, however, was quiet resistance to the rules and unofficial easing of

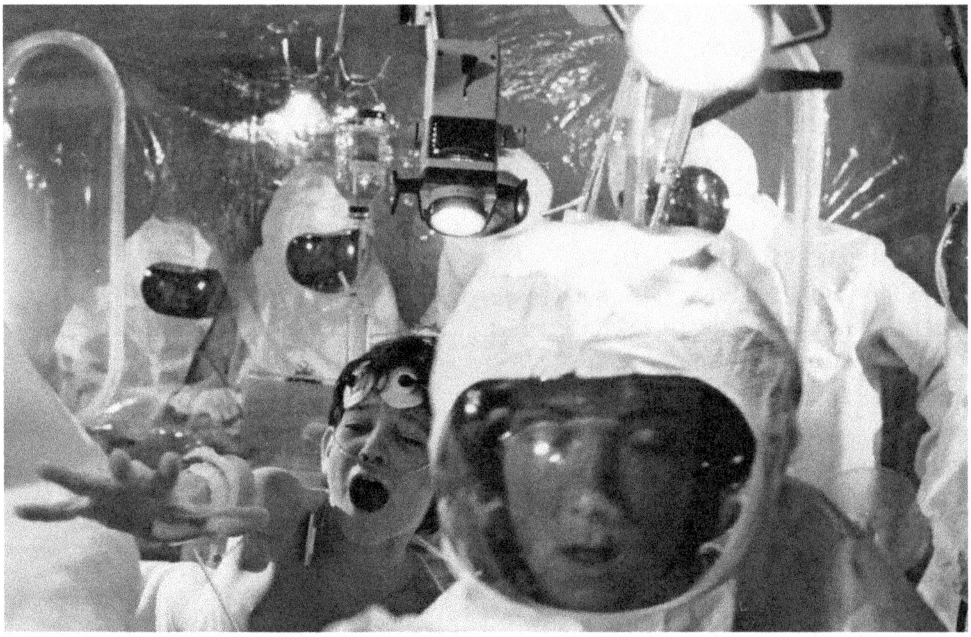

A late twentieth-century version of a costume to ward off possible disease, scene from *E.T. the Extra-Terrestrial* (1982), directed by Steven Spielberg. When compared to the seventeenth-century garb, it illustrates that little has changed. (Collection Christophel/ Alamy)

them, often through corruption. Surgeons and inspectors could be bribed to turn their backs on suspected plague cases or to desist in the seizure and destruction of property; and grave diggers could be bribed to bury victims in church cemeteries. The same officials would extort favors from those in their power, in effect compelling payment of a bribe. In those ways, the traditional community and the aggressive health bureaucracy reached some mutual accommodation.

Physicians and surgeons had a number of techniques that at least tried to combat the disease, although most were in fact of little use. By the seventeenth century, a plague-fighting costume for physicians and surgeons had been developed, an ominous robe with the head encased in a sort of beak. The beak contained perfumes to ward off the plague's venom. The physicians could prescribe a variety of remedies of which some were herbal mixtures and some were chemical in character. The chemically prepared substances, especially arsenic compounds, represented a more modern approach that began to be used in the sixteenth century. Such substances would be placed on the spots of infection, especially on the buboes that identified plague. Physicians also engaged in the long-standing attempt to correct humoral imbalances, through bleeding and purging the bowels. Some healers recommended lancing the buboes to expel the poison from the body.

UNRESOLVED HISTORICAL ISSUES

These epidemics undoubtedly crippled the Italian city-states, and to some extent (this is a subject of debate) contributed to the economic decline that eroded their long-dominant position in European society. Their dominance had been shaken by a series of causes in the early sixteenth century (including their plague epidemics in the 1520s), but the position of Milan, Florence, Venice, and their sister cities as centers of trade, manufacture, and finance had revived after 1550. Then in the early seventeenth century, long-term problems again built up; Italian manufacturers had trouble meeting the increased competition from France, England, and the Netherlands for international markets, while troubles beset traditional Italian customers in Germany (see volume 2, chapter 8). In that situation, writes Carlo Cipolla, "a drastic and rapid fall in population like that caused by the plague of 1630 had the effect of raising wages and putting Italian exports in an even more difficult position" (1994, 248–249). By the end of the seventeenth century, Italy had ceased to be an important manufacturing center.

These 1630s plague epidemics were among the last suffered by northern Italian cities, although plague lingered in southern Italy into the eighteenth century. The disappearance of plague from such densely settled targets as Florence and Venice is an important part of a historical puzzle: Why did the Second Plague Pandemic disappear? While the policies of quarantine and isolation certainly generated controversy in their time, some modern historians have credited them with a role in the larger question of the pandemic's disappearance. Others disagree, noting that while the isolation and confinement of people may have prevented plague from spreading from one place to another, the same policies may have increased local mortalities by confining the still-healthy in areas infected by plague-bearing rodents and fleas. See volume 2, chapter 5 for a more complete discussion of the issue.

REFERENCES

Cipolla, Carlo M. *Before the Industrial Revolution: European Society and Economy, 1000–1700*. 3rd ed. New York: W. W. Norton, 1994.

Cipolla, Carlo M. *Fighting the Plague in Seventeenth-Century Italy*. Madison: University of Wisconsin Press, 1981.

SUGGESTED ADDITIONAL READING

Benedictow, O. J. "Morbidity in Historical Plague Epidemics." *Population Studies* 41 (1987): 401–431.

Calvi, Guilia. *Histories of a Plague Year: The Social and the Imaginary in Baroque Florence*. Berkeley: University of California Press, 1989.

Cipolla, Carlo M. *Faith, Reason, and the Plague in Seventeenth-Century Tuscany*. Ithaca, NY: Cornell University Press, 1979.

Cipolla, Carlo M. *Public Health and the Medical Profession in the Renaissance*. Cambridge: Cambridge University Press, 1976.

10

Epidemics in China, 1635–1644

WHEN AND WHERE

In the period between about 1635 and 1644, a series of natural and human disasters struck China, including famines, floods, civil unrest and rebellion, and (especially in the years from 1640) devastating epidemic diseases. Those epidemics affected most of the country; of the densely settled areas only the provinces of Guangdong in the south and Sichuan in the southwest were spared.

Epidemics had apparently become more serious in the 1630s, in the wake of severely cold weather, prolonged droughts, and famine. The regions then affected ranged from Shanxi (southwest of Beijing) to the Mongolian border regions. By 1639 diseases reached the Yangzi valley. The cascade of epidemics peaked in 1641, when (according to one modern authority) the local gazetteers of 103 different locales reported epidemics, a great majority of them called "big" epidemics. The entire eastern half of the Ming Empire was stricken, and whole villages were "completely exterminated" (Brook 2010, 251).

We can only guess at the total mortality in these epidemics. It is likely that between 20% and 40% of the population died in many places in 1641. In Chekiang, 80–90% of the households were reported affected by disease; other statements of about 80–90% mortality may refer to mortality of those who fell ill, not of the entire population. Contemporary Chinese sources used such terms as "countless deaths" or "deaths beyond reckoning" (Elvin 1973, 311).

The identity of the diseases involved in these deadly episodes also remains uncertain. It is likely that several different epidemic diseases worked in tandem in those years; the fact that epidemics raged throughout all seasons of the year makes such combinations seem more likely, for many possible single diseases (such as malaria and bubonic plague) are largely seasonal. From contemporary descriptions, bubonic plague does seem to have been present, perhaps as early as the 1630s. The social conditions of China in the 1640s made typhus, typhoid fever, malaria, and dysentery all likely participants in the disasters of the decade. The descriptions of one disease ("sheep's wool fever") suggest a fungus ailment, or perhaps anthrax. Smallpox was endemic as well (Dunstan 1975, 19–28).

A few reports from specific places may illustrate the gravity of the epidemics. In Wuxian in 1641, what was likely an epidemic of dysentery killed perhaps 70% of its victims; "tens of thousands" of bodies were collected *daily*, in the worst epidemic since the twelfth century (Leung 1987, 142). In Nanjing in the same year, the same phrase—"tens of thousands"—described the toll. In Wuxian in 1644, entire families died, and the people begged the gods for mercy. And in Shanxi province in 1644, plague struck, resulting in 80–90% mortalities. The descriptions of that episode suggest that both bubonic and pneumonic forms of plague had appeared; those descriptions mention the characteristic buboes in the armpits, coughing up blood, and rapid death of pneumonic plague. (The descriptions of buboes are not found in accounts from the earlier 1640s.)

SIGNIFICANCE

The effects of these epidemics were certainly very great, but those effects should be seen in the context of a panoply of disasters that struck Ming China in what has been called the "Chongzhen Slough," a period of drought (punctuated by floods), frigid temperatures, locust infestations, crop failures and resulting famine, in which reports circulated of desperate people eating dirt and digging up corpses for food. The ravages of epidemic disease certainly contributed to the weakening and eventual collapse of the Ming dynasty that led to the assumption to power by the Manchu-based Ch'ing dynasty in 1644, but to what degree? Did high mortality ease the pressure of population on the land, and thus open the way for dramatic social and economic change? (See the "Unresolved Historical Issues" section.)

BACKGROUND

China, with its large and densely settled population, had a long history of serious epidemics. Crowd diseases flourished there; Chinese sources from as early as the thirteenth century describe what was probably typhus. Chinese chronicles often grouped epidemics with other natural catastrophes, such as famines and floods. Before the 1640s, another very serious epidemic period had occurred in 1586–1587.

China also had a long and active medical tradition that responded to epidemics. Chinese medicine placed particular emphasis on pharmaceutical remedies. In the period of the Ming dynasty (between the fourteenth and seventeenth centuries), the state provided for medical bureaus throughout the country, although by the time of the epidemics of the 1640s those offices had become ineffective (as will be seen later). But the imperial government regarded epidemics as crises. It took vigorous direct action in its capital, Beijing (see the "Responses" section), and expected local officials elsewhere to distribute medicines and money. In the 1587 epidemic in Beijing, the state distributed medicines to 100,000 people.

The social and economic situation of China in the 1640s contributed to the severity of the epidemics in the decade. The overall population of the country had risen steadily from the late fourteenth century to the late sixteenth, and while it had then begun falling, cities in the 1640s were still overcrowded. The streets overflowed with excrement and other filth, flies abounded, and flooding was frequent. The dense, unwashed crowds made typhus infections likely; the flies could spread typhoid fever, and mosquitoes (breeding in the flooded streets) spread malaria.

Dietary deficiencies were common, and malnourished people were more likely to succumb to some epidemics.

HOW IT WAS UNDERSTOOD AT THE TIME

Chinese medical traditions emphasized the role of the environment as the general underlying cause of disease, and the disorders in the internal balance of the body as the immediate manifestation of it. Disease, perhaps generated by an environmental miasma, invaded the body from without. The result, perhaps made more likely by prior weaknesses of an individual, was a systemic breakdown of internal balances, analogous to but different from the humoral theory of Western medicine. Those balances might be expressed in terms of "twelve pulses" or of "five phases"; another, more general, set of balances existed between the underlying principles of "yin" and "yang" (Elvin 1973, 189–191). Diseases, then, were often seen along a continuum, one of greater or lesser imbalance, rather than as a number of separate ailments.

In the 1640s an important medical thinker, Wu Yu-hsing, found explanations that depended on an individual's weakness being inadequate in a time of widespread or even universal sickness. He therefore emphasized the role of general environmental forces, especially heat and cold, in the generation of what he regarded as a more specific, separate disease (Dunstan 1975, 38–43; Elvin 1973, 190).

These Chinese medical understandings of epidemics overlapped with the persistent belief in the role of "unpacified spirits" that caused disease. By the late Ming period belief in such demons had revived, and the society also strongly stressed the relation between morality (of the individual, but especially of the society as a whole) and the spread of epidemics.

RESPONSES

State machinery to deal with epidemics included providing medicines to the population, staffing medical bureaus, distributing money to the poor, and arranging burials (including providing coffins). By the 1630s, in the chaos of the time, the state bureaucracy was largely ineffective.

It may be, however, that the magnitude of the epidemics simply overwhelmed what any government could have done, whether its bureaucracy was efficient or not. A revealing account (Leung 1987, 142) suggests that even though the imperial government heavily subsidized the Academy of Medicine of Beijing, its expenses for collecting dead bodies and for their burial exceeded that sum by *20* times. Official response may have been practically limited to the disposal of the dead.

Medical responses concentrated on the prescription of remedies whose goal was restoring the proper balances in the body's system. Wu Yu-hsing's prescriptions enjoyed some success in the 1640s, which gave his more general ideas of the cause of epidemics some influence. In general, if people recovered from an epidemic, they would credit the medicines they had taken. The frequent failure of medicines inspired a general fatalism, however.

For a variety of reasons, Chinese ideas about disease had little concept of contagion, and so the anti-contagion responses common in Western places in the seventeenth century were not pursued. The dominance of theories of environmental cause discouraged belief in contagion, and the moral ethos of the community placed great value on care of its sick members; quarantine might be seen as abandoning them. An exception to the general neglect of the concept of contagion did exist, however: to some uncertain extent Chinese medicine had adopted the practice of variolation—inoculation—to prevent a full-blown smallpox infection. The adjoining Mongols, however, had not adopted the practice and clearly feared the contagion of smallpox, which (despite the efforts of variolators) was endemic in crowded China and not in more thinly settled Mongol lands. Mongol armies that attacked China in the 1630s deliberately placed in the lead detachments of soldiers who already had contracted smallpox.

In addition to medical responses, the Chinese—both officials and the public—appealed to the supernatural in their confrontation with epidemics. Rituals were performed, propitiatory dramas were staged, and prisoners were released in a gesture of clemency in the hope that the gods would similarly show mercy. In 1643 the emperor "issued an edict commanding all his subjects, from the highest official to the lowest day laborer, to purge the evil thoughts lurking in his heart so that Heaven might be persuaded to end the punishment of drought and bring back the rain" (Brook 2010, 250). It was widely believed that the epidemic resulted from the failure of the society's moral foundations, and perhaps charity would inspire a moral renewal.

UNRESOLVED HISTORICAL ISSUES

The 1640s were certainly a time of great crisis in China. The Ming dynasty collapsed, to be succeeded by the Manchu-based Ch'ing, in 1644. A series of rebellions and peasant unrests had occurred prior to that collapse, as well as famines, crop failures, and the epidemics discussed here. Questions remain about the relative place of each of those calamities in the cause of the political changes. Mark Elvin (1973) has argued that the 1640s epidemics led to a shortage of military manpower that weakened the dynasty's ability to defend itself.

Other questions have been raised about the role of the epidemics in demographic change, and (in turn) about the extent and permanence of that demographic change. Lack of evidence makes a convincing quantitative argument difficult. Elvin believes that, as a result of the epidemics in the 1640s, population pressure on the land eased significantly, while the area of cultivation continued to expand. The result was a burst of food production that laid the foundation for a long-term dramatic *increase* in the Chinese population, one that condemned the country to a perpetual cycle of low individual incomes. But Elvin's argument remains highly speculative.

China's difficulties have been seen (by Geoffrey Parker) as part of a worldwide "Global Crisis" in the seventeenth century, a crisis in which climate change played a decisive role. This sweeping argument may also be applied to this volume's chapters 8 and 9.

Remaining unsettled is the identity of the diseases that struck China in the 1630s and 1640s.

REFERENCES

Brook, Timothy. *The Troubled Empire: China in the Yuan and Ming Dynasties.* Cambridge, MA: Belknap Press of Harvard University Press, 2010.

Dunstan, Helen. "The Late Ming Epidemics: A Preliminary Survey." *Ch'ing-Shih wen-t'i* 3 (1975): 1–59. (*This work, which may be relatively difficult for some readers to find, remains the best source of information on the subject.*)

Elvin, Mark. *The Pattern of the Chinese Past.* Palo Alto, CA: Stanford University Press, 1973.

Leung, Angela Ki Che. "Organized Medicine in Ming-Qing China: State and Private Medical Institutions in the Lower Yangzi Region." *Late Imperial China* 8 (1987): 134–166.

SUGGESTED ADDITIONAL READING

Parker, Geoffrey. *Global Crisis: War, Climate Change & Catastrophe in the Seventeenth Century.* New Haven, CT: Yale University Press, 2013.

Parsons, James B. *The Peasant Rebellions of the Late Ming Dynasty.* Tucson: University of Arizona Press, 1970.

Serruys, Henry. "Smallpox in Mongolia during the Ming and Ch'ing Dynasties." *Zentralasiatische Studien* 14 (1980): 41–63.

Twitchett, Denis. "Population and Pestilence in T'ang China." In *Studia Sino-Mongolica: Festschrift für Herbert Franke*, edited by Wolfgang Bauer, 35–68. Wiesbaden: Franz Steiner Verlag, 1979.

Unscheld, Paul U. *Medicine in China: A History of Ideas.* Berkeley: University of California Press, 1985.

11

Plague in London, 1665

WHEN AND WHERE

Between April 1665 and January 1666, London suffered a major epidemic of bubonic plague. While the total toll of the epidemic cannot be known precisely, modern estimates place the number of deaths at about 75,000, and perhaps as many as 100,000. (About 56,000 plague burials were officially recorded, but many plague deaths almost certainly went unrecorded.) The population of the city, including its suburbs, was then about 460,000.

An outbreak of plague in the Netherlands in 1663 alarmed the English government, which decreed a quarantine on traffic from the United Provinces. Comets in the skies in December 1664 and March 1665 frightened the population, and astrologers forecast a coming plague (see the "Background" section to understand that such a prediction was neither unusual nor risky). By April 1665, a few plague deaths were reported in the parish of St. Giles-in-the-Fields, which adjoined London to the west; the central government's Privy Council (a body of royal advisers) began ordering that households containing plague cases be shut up and their inhabitants forbidden to leave. In May, although the number of reported plague cases remained low and continued to be centered in the St. Giles-in-the-Fields district, popular fears mounted and some Londoners began fleeing the city. By June, the government was attempting to control movements of people and goods to and from the affected parish, while more Londoners left the city. In the second and third weeks of June, the number of reported plague deaths began to rise, and the epidemic began to have a noticeable effect on London life. The Inns of Court (the centers of the English legal profession) were deserted, as was the College of Physicians. In a telling illustration of plague's disruption of routine, the delivery of prisoners to jail in London stopped in June, not to resume until 1666.

In July, the epidemic's death toll began rising dramatically, reaching over 1,000 per week in the third week. While St. Giles-in-the-Fields remained the epicenter of plague, the infection now spread significantly to other parishes, especially others in the poor suburban fringes of the City of London proper. Deaths in

St. Martin's-in-the-Fields (adjoining the royal palace at Whitehall) alarmed the court, which on July 9 moved to the palace at Hampton Court, a few miles west of London. On July 6, the government proclaimed that days of prayer and fasting would be observed on July 12 and at stated intervals thereafter until the plague abated. Churches throughout the country began collections for the relief of London.

August and September saw the epidemic peak. Recorded deaths from plague exceeded 6,000 in the third week of August and remained at that level through the third week of September. Other poor fringe parishes, such as Cripplegate to the north (in August) and Stepney to the east (in September), now felt the full force of the disease. King Charles II and his court left the London area altogether, moving to Salisbury on August 1 and later to Oxford. Most of the governing Privy Council was no longer resident in the capital.

In October the epidemic was clearly on the wane. Although plague mortalities remained high, reported plague deaths fell from over 4,000 in the second week of the month to less than 2,000 in the third week. By the third week of November the toll was less than 1,000, and it continued to decline as winter came on. By the end of the year, London life was beginning to return to normal. London was to have no further plague epidemic, but some cases of the disease continued to be reported there until 1679.

The epidemic struck London very unevenly. Generally, the worst-affected areas were the poor parishes in the suburban fringes of London, beginning in the west, then spreading to the north, east, and across the Thames to the south. The City of London, especially the well-off areas in its center, suffered less, but some plague could be found everywhere in metropolitan London in 1665.

While London's experience was dramatic, bubonic plague also ravaged other English cities and towns in 1665 and 1666. Especially serious epidemics struck East Anglia, to the northeast of London. In Norwich over 2,200 people succumbed to plague between October 1665 and October 1666, a loss proportional to London's; in Colchester plague carried off the frightening number of about 5,000 (perhaps half the total population) between August 1665 and the end of 1666; and in Cambridge, the university dispersed for nearly two years from the summer of 1665 until the summer of 1667.

SIGNIFICANCE

While the plague epidemic that struck London in 1665 inflicted very heavy mortality on the city, its significance derives more from its subsequent position in literary culture. In the words of the modern historian Paul Slack, the epidemic has become "part of the common currency of historical knowledge," certainly in Great Britain, and perhaps more widely (Slack 1985, 144). Two classics of English letters have contributed to that reputation: Samuel Pepys's *Diary*, which provides eyewitness testimony about the epidemic, and Daniel Defoe's *A Journal of the Plague Year*, published in 1722. The latter is a work of historical fiction, not an eyewitness account. While Defoe drew on some contemporary records, the readers of his *A Journal of the Plague Year* should remember that it is not a history of

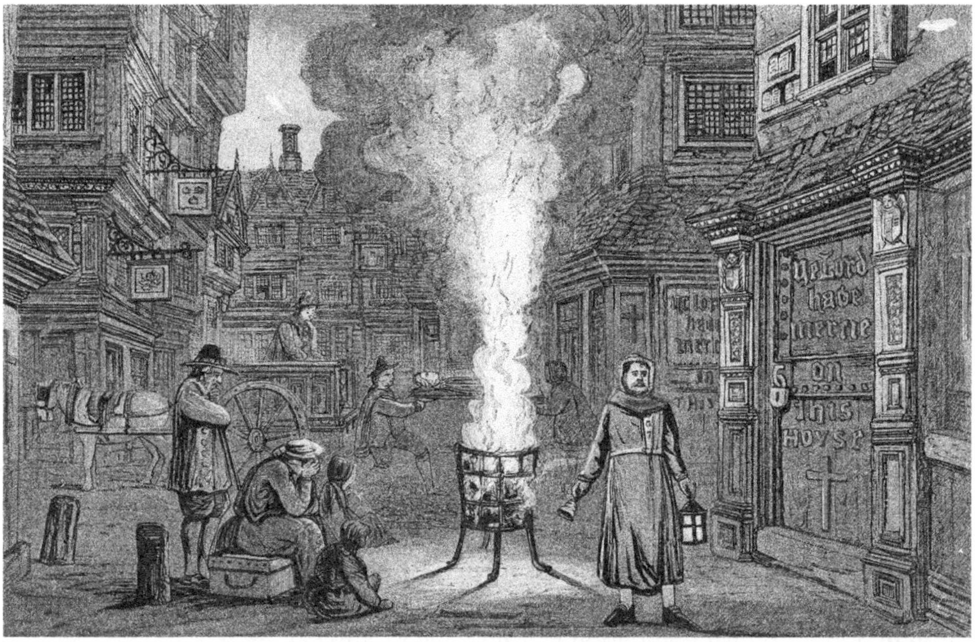

An engraving of a London street scene during the 1665 plague. The town crier calls, "Bring out your dead," while corpses are placed on a horse-drawn cart. The accompanying fire was thought to dispel plague "vapors." (Wellcome Library)

the event. Many subsequent literary allusions to the Great Plague of 1665 exist, as well as another classic fictional account, William Harrison Ainsworth's *Old Saint Paul's*, published in 1841. Also contributing to the 1665 epidemic's position in collective memory was the near-coincidence of the epidemic with the Great Fire of London in 1666; the great city suffered two hammer blows within a few months.

The 1665 plague in London was certainly an important event in its own right, but of London's sixteenth- and seventeenth-century plagues, it did not in fact inflict the highest mortality rate. Epidemics in 1563, 1603, and perhaps 1625 all killed a greater proportion of Londoners than did that of 1665, although the total death toll in 1665 was higher. That said, the 1665 epidemic had numerous short-run effects on social, political, and economic life. For a time, trade throughout England was disrupted, both by quarantines and by the reduced production of goods because of workshop closures. London was a major center of manufactured items for the country and was also the entrepôt through which both domestic and international trade moved. The coincidence of a major epidemic in 1665, a disastrous fire in 1666, and a war with the United Provinces of the Netherlands between 1665 and 1667 strained the English government's finances.

The 1665 epidemic resulted in an important shift in public health policy by the English government. At the time that the epidemic struck, the government was still following guidelines laid down in 1578 for its response to plague. The 1665 experience catalyzed a new set of regulations (see the "Responses" section). It also contributed to an evolution in conceptions about the disease's nature and cause (see the "How It Was Understood at the Time" section).

Although some cases of plague continued into the 1670s in the British Isles, the events of 1665 (and 1666 in some other English towns) represented the last plague epidemic there. It was therefore one of the final western European events of the Second Plague Pandemic, and so its history enters into the complex issue of why that pandemic died out.

BACKGROUND

Between the beginning of the Second Plague Pandemic (which reached England in 1348) and the London epidemic of 1665, bubonic plague had a nearly continuous history both in the British Isles in general and in London. Serious plague epidemics continued into the sixteenth and seventeenth centuries, although at gradually lengthening intervals. Slack has documented 17 periods of national "crisis mortality" between 1500 and 1670, and has argued that plague was almost always present somewhere in England in that period (although, perhaps significantly for the impact of the 1665 epidemic, not between 1654 and 1664). While plague was therefore a major cause of death, and an even more important source of terror for the population, its epidemic intervals had widened enough that the long-term growth of the English population was no longer regulated by it.

London's place in the history of these recurring plague epidemics varied. On some occasions (e.g., 1592–1593), the city bore a disproportionately heavy share of the country's plague deaths. That was decidedly true in 1665. In other years, other cities and regions suffered more than London did. Before the 1665 epidemic, the London plague visitations of 1563 and 1603 had each, in their times, been called the Great Plague, a term that would be appropriated for 1665. And indeed, about 20% of the 1563 London population died of plague, compared with about 18% in 1603 and about 12% in 1665. (The percentages reflect the official plague death count, which in each case was probably an underestimate.)

Certainly by the sixteenth century, far larger than any other city in the kingdom, London had a reputation as an unhealthy and dirty place. By the end of the century, the word *wen* (an unsightly and congested city) was being applied to it. As London relied increasingly on "sea coal" (coal brought by sea from Newcastle) for fuel, its air became choked with smoke and its surfaces coated with soot. (That fact in itself did not worry those who feared plague, for it was widely believed that fires and smoke might prevent the disease.) London was also remarkably congested, and in the seventeenth century the area of dense settlement expanded beyond the walls of the city to take in suburbs. That circumstance was reflected in the 1665 epidemic. The earlier Great Plagues, such as 1563 and 1603, had begun in the eastern part of the city along the river and its docks, and then moved west. By 1665 some of the most densely settled areas of London were now suburban: Southwark, Stepney, Clerkenwell, Westminster—these were all outside the old walls. In those areas crowded tenements housed masses of poor people, and there were also markets and granaries, where rats gathered and where commerce and goods moved from many places. The London fringe areas had become ideal nurseries for bubonic plague. In 1665 (see the "When and Where" section), the epidemic spread into the old city from outside the walls.

But the high plague mortalities in 1665–1666 in Norwich, Colchester, and other places suggest that the environment of London, while favorable to plague, was evidently not uniquely so.

HOW IT WAS UNDERSTOOD AT THE TIME

By the mid-seventeenth century, the Second Plague Pandemic had affected the West for about 300 years, and understanding of the disease had undergone some changes since its first appearance. Natural explanations had, by then, gained favor over supernatural and religious ones, but the natural and supernatural still coexisted in the thinking of most of those affected by bubonic plague. That tension had long characterized English thought, which understood the disease as a manifestation of divine providence and power, as a product of an environmental miasma, and as an infectious contagion that moved from one person to another. Seventeenth-century English policies reflected beliefs in all three of those explanations (see the "Responses" section).

Part of those natural environmental arguments now also related plague to social conditions, attributing the disease to the filth of poor, dirty, and crowded living conditions. Those who lived in those conditions were therefore thought to be at greater risk (as were those who cared for plague victims). The circumstances of the London epidemic of 1665 confirmed and strengthened those beliefs (see the "When and Where" and "Background" sections).

Many still emphasized the power of Providence in addition to, or instead of, natural and social factors. Prayers were regularly (and fervently) offered, and a variety of omens and charms were consulted. Astrologers claimed to have forecast the 1665 epidemic's appearance (as well as the 1666 fire), and Londoners consulted them.

Orthodox medicine had, by the seventeenth century, agreed on many of the symptoms that it interpreted as evidence of bubonic plague. Above all, the telltale symptoms were first the buboes, the ugly dark swellings in the groin, armpit, neck, or other glandular sites, and second the *petechiae*, the black spots elsewhere on the body. The course of the disease from first infection to crisis and (likely) death was also symptomatic. The buboes and the petechiae stemmed from, and illustrated, an imbalance of the body's humours. While many physicians admitted their relative powerlessness in the face of plague, they tried a wide range of medical responses (see the "Responses" section), and by the seventeenth century some tensions existed between traditional Galenic responses and those of the newer Paracelsian medical beliefs.

RESPONSES

The English government's responses to seventeenth-century plague epidemics shared some common features with those that had been developed in Italian city-states, but the English state on the whole was less active and intervened less in its society than did the Italian cities. At the time of the 1665 London epidemic, the guiding government document was still a set of orders laid down by the Privy Council in 1578 and subsequently embodied in statute law in 1604. The orders placed the greatest emphasis on avoiding contagion by requiring—at least in theory—the isolation of households where plague was found. The inhabitants of such houses were to be shut up within them for six weeks. Responsibility for enforcing this policy was laid on justices of the peace, the particular English local officials who combined administrative and judicial functions. Local governments—parishes in particular—bore the costs of anti-plague measures by imposing local taxes. Local authorities, therefore, both isolated households in their dwellings for six weeks and raised local taxes to supply them with food. The central government laid down policy and left its implementation to localities. The local, unpaid officials on whom the system relied would be beholden to their constituents, fearful of or angry at them, perhaps amenable to bribery, or—because they lived among them—dead or dying themselves.

In contrast to the Italian city-states, the 1578 English government's orders made little effort to provide pesthouses within which the sick could be segregated, and they did not provide for boards of health that had long been standard in Italy. The central government could and did proclaim quarantines in times of epidemic, but left local authorities to collect information on morbidity and mortality, burn the clothing and bedding of the plague-stricken, and attempt to control burials to minimize contagion. (London authorities, for example, had begun publishing statistics of mortality in the sixteenth century, and these evolved, by the early seventeenth, into the weekly London "Bills of Mortality," a source of great interest to historians.) For a wide variety of local reasons, significant gaps often existed between the intentions of the 1578 orders and their actual implementation.

When plague broke out in the Netherlands in 1663, the Privy Council imposed a quarantine (at first 30 days, then 40) on traffic from the Low Countries. Plague reached London regardless (see the "When and Where" section), and by March 1665 the relevance of quarantine declined in any case, owing to the war declared that month between England and the United Provinces, a war that largely canceled trade between the two countries.

The major initial official response was to isolate households. Inhabitants of plague-infected buildings were shut in, while a vivid red cross was placed on the door, together with a sign that read "Lord Have Mercy on Us." These sequestrations faced some real, and more potential, resistance. As early as April 1665, some householders in St. Giles-in-the-Fields removed the red cross and sign from the door of one of their neighbors, allowing those within to escape. Official responses did not, therefore, always meet with popular support. The Privy Council soon authorized harsh punishments for those who violated rules, especially those who resisted isolation; throughout the epidemic authorities feared the linkage of plague and social disorder. And by August 1665, the death toll, the number of households that had to be isolated, and the shortage of available bodies to enforce the rules meant that the isolation policy was gradually (but perhaps inevitably) abandoned in parts of London.

The Privy Council also urged a wide variety of measures intended to clean the environment and remove the contingencies that furthered contagion. Stray animals—especially dogs, but also pigs—were feared as sources of contagion, and so their destruction (or at least confinement) was ordered. (Since the rat-flea connections of bubonic plague's epidemiology were advanced in the late nineteenth century, historians have been especially critical of those moves, which seemingly allowed rats to proliferate.) Local authorities were urged to remove heaps of rubbish from the streets and to clear obstructions from ditches so that water could rinse them. On the other hand, fires and smoke were thought to be deterrents of plague and so positively beneficial. The same authorities that fumigated houses and removed rubbish also lit fires in the streets, ordered the discharge of guns, and encouraged the use of smoking tobacco.

Funeral processions and customs particularly worried authorities combating plague. The corpses themselves would be a source of contagion; the crowds that gathered to follow the deceased to the grave might be another. Efforts were made to limit attendance at funeral processions, but such measures flew in the face of deeply held social customs and proved difficult to enforce. The rising death toll in the epidemic badly strained the supply of coffins and the available burial grounds, and so mass graves of bodies wrapped only in shrouds replaced more traditional burials. As was true in contemporary Italy, regulation of burials became a particular point of dispute between official policy and popular culture.

Authorities also regulated some commerce and trades, especially those that involved materials thought to give rise to dangerous miasmas. Those who dealt in fish, meat, fruit, and grain had their sales controlled (at least in theory); bread could not be taken from bakeries until it cooled; and street vendors were forbidden from selling old clothing. Many alehouses were closed in the hope of reducing contagious crowding.

Official fears of contagion mirrored popular reactions. Across England, people traveling from stricken London were suspect. Samuel Pepys found people in Romford fearful of Londoners: "But Lord, to see, among other things, how all these great people here are afeared of London, being doubtful of anything that comes from thence or that hath lately been there, that I was forced to say that I lived wholly at Woolwich [which he did not]" (Pepys 1972, 161). Objects from London, as well as people, were feared. For a time, Pepys hesitated to wear a new wig "because the plague was in Westminster when I bought it" (Pepys 1972, 210). Excise collectors reported that they had difficulty collecting because people feared to frequent those taverns and inns that remained open. That fear of contagion led to very widespread flight away from the city, noticeable in May followed by a rush in June. Those who fled were, of course, predominantly those who could afford to do so and who had someplace else to go. The flight of the well-to-do contributed to the disproportionate toll the epidemic took on the poor, those who had little choice but to remain behind. King Charles II and the court moved first to Hampton Court Palace (to the west of London), and then on August 1 left the area entirely, going first to Salisbury and then to Oxford. When Parliament reconvened in October, it did so in Oxford.

Some important men remained in London. Among them was the Lord Mayor, Sir John Lawrence; two others who assumed positions of importance in the struggle against the plague were General George Monck (the Duke of Albemarle) and

William, Lord Craven. Craven's 1665 experiences led him to propose major modifications in the 1578 Privy Council plague orders, and in response to his urging, new orders were issued in 1666. Those new orders placed greater emphasis on the importance of pesthouses where the sick could be isolated from the healthy. At the start of the 1665 epidemic, only five such pesthouses existed in London, and while more were begun during the year, their capacity proved grossly inadequate.

Popular responses to the threat of plague varied very widely. A great number of omens were consulted and charms were employed; people sought hope, or solace, in churches and from informal preachers in the streets. A broad range of healers, on a continuum from orthodox physicians through surgeons and apothecaries to folk practitioners and enterprising quacks, offered their remedies. Among the most common were some version of *theriac* (also called *treacle*) or *mithridatium* (varying mixtures of opium and viper's flesh believed to be poison antidotes), and herbs such as rue. Within the community of orthodox physicians, two opposing camps—the Galenists and the Paracelsians—proposed somewhat different remedies, but their treatments differed little in practice. Physicians and surgeons also attempted to lance buboes and bleed petechiae, in the belief that errant humours could thus be expelled.

UNRESOLVED HISTORICAL ISSUES

The 1665 London epidemic was not the last episode of the Second Plague Pandemic, but it was part of the last major plague visitation in the British Isles, and one of the last dramatic ones anywhere in western Europe. Its story therefore has entered the broader discussion of what caused the Second Plague Pandemic to recede. Did human actions, illustrated by those of 1665 London, help speed the pandemic's departure? In the light of more modern understandings of the cause and epidemiology of plague, were the responses effective?

Some historians now argue that, indeed, some of the 1665 actions may have dampened the spread of plague. Quarantines, by cutting down on traffic that rats and fleas might accompany, may have made movements of plague across distances less likely. The English practice of isolating households in shut-in dwellings was more dubious and may have put more people at risk than removing the plague victims to a separate pesthouse would have done. But in that connection, it is interesting that multiple infections within the same household were less common in 1665 London than was once supposed or than one would assume based on the practice of sequestering household inhabitants together with plague victims. Perhaps the sequestration rules were not effectively enforced. Historians agree that the elimination of dogs and cats was a mistake, for it allowed rats to flourish.

In the 1665 London epidemic, the mortality rate for women was significantly higher than that for men, a fact that has only recently been realized, and one that invites theories about why that was so. J. A. I. Champion (1995) has suggested several possibilities: in wealthy households, the masters left women domestics in London when they fled to the country; domestic servants generally were at greater risk because they were sent out to obtain provisions, and women were generally weakened by poverty and poor nutrition. The gender issues of the epidemic have only begun to be considered.

A tantalizing, if unresolvable, issue is the relation between the 1665 epidemic and the creative thought of Isaac Newton, the great scientific figure of the seventeenth century. With the University of Cambridge closed because of the epidemic, Newton returned to his home in rural Lincolnshire between June 1665 and April 1667. In that period, Newton later claimed, he had developed the calculus, realized that white light contained the colors of the spectrum, and conceived of his theory of universal gravitation. "All this," he said, "was in the two plague years 1665–1666. For in those days I was in the prime of my age for invention & minded Mathematicks & Philosophy more then at any time since" (quoted in Westfall 1980, 143). Did the plague-enforced isolation lead to an astonishing burst of creativity, an *annus mirabilis* in Newton's life? Newton's recollections encouraged (perhaps deliberately) such a dramatic interpretation. R. S. Westfall (among other modern scholars) argues, however, that excessive attention to the plague years "disregards the continuity of [Newton's] development" (Westfall 1980, 143).

REFERENCES

Champion, J. A. I. *London's Dreaded Visitation: The Social Geography of the Great Plague in 1665.* Historical Geography Research Series, no 31. London: Center for Metropolitan History, 1995.

Pepys, Samuel. *The Diary of Samuel Pepys.* Vol. 6, *1665.* Edited by Robert Latham and William Matthews. Berkeley: University of California Press, 1972.

Slack, Paul. *The Impact of Plague in Tudor and Stuart England.* London: Routledge & Kegan Paul, 1985.

Westfall, Richard S. *Never at Rest: A Biography of Isaac Newton.* Cambridge: Cambridge University Press, 1980.

SUGGESTED ADDITIONAL READING

Bucholz, Robert O., and Joseph P. Ward. *London: A Social and Cultural History, 1550–1750.* Cambridge: Cambridge University Press, 2012.

Moote, A. Lloyd, and Dorothy C. Moote. *The Great Plague: The Story of London's Most Deadly Year.* Baltimore, MD: Johns Hopkins University Press, 2003.

Porter, Stephen. *The Great Plague.* Stroud: Sutton, 1999.

12

Plague in Marseille, 1720–1722

WHEN AND WHERE

On May 25, 1720, a ship docked at the French Mediterranean port of Marseille. The vessel's voyage began at Sidon, in Syria; when it arrived at Marseille, its crew included men suffering from bubonic plague. Marseille authorities impounded the cargo and ordered the crew quarantined for 15 days. Those restrictions were lifted on June 14, when some goods were sold in the city and some of the crew disappeared. When some of the customers who had bought goods from the ship fell ill, the authorities re-impounded the suspect merchandise (and subsequently burned it), and again isolated the crew.

Those measures came too late, for the goods already sold and distributed in the city apparently carried fleas infected by bubonic plague. In late June, illness and deaths began in one street in the poor section of the city, a district where there were no physicians. When doctors were called to the street, on July 9, they warned the city authorities of an epidemic. For the next two weeks (although the illnesses spread to another, adjoining, street) the epidemic seemed contained, and physicians and authorities debated whether the disease was truly plague or some "malignant fevers, possibly caused by intestinal worms" (Biraben 1972, 234).

But then in the last week of July, the epidemic exploded. Fourteen deaths were reported on July 23, and the number rapidly grew thereafter. On August 1, the parliament at Aix, the presiding judicial authority for the province, decreed the isolation of Marseille and began establishing a cordon around the city that would prevent traffic moving in or out. Some difficulties arose in implementing the cordon, however; for one thing the city needed to gather provisions to feed itself if it were to be isolated, and for another the soldiers needed to man the cordon could not be assembled overnight. Only on August 20 did the cordon become effective. By that time about 10,000 people had already fled Marseille and infected goods had escaped as well. On the same day that the parliament acted (August 1), cases of plague appeared in Aix itself, and by August 20, the disease had appeared in Toulon, about 35 miles east of Marseille.

In August, Marseille was experiencing a major epidemic. The number of dead bodies threatened to overwhelm the city's ability to dispose of them; first beggars were enlisted to haul bodies, and then the convicts in the galleys were employed in the grim task. Throughout August, mortality in the city rose at a frightening rate. It peaked in early September, then began falling rapidly by mid-October. Deaths (although few) continued through the year and into 1721. Authorities imposed two final periods of quarantine from August through November 1721, at the conclusion of which the epidemic was declared to be over. It was, however, not over; another flare-up of plague occurred in early 1722, with 260 cases resulting in 194 deaths in the city. Meanwhile plague had also spread throughout Provence and the northern and eastern portions of adjoining Languedoc.

The epidemic's toll was remarkably high. The population of Marseille in 1720 was about 90,000. About 39,300 of those people died in the epidemic, 43.7% of the population; of the 80,000 who remained in the city, 49.1%. Certain groups of the population suffered devastating losses: 543 galley convicts in a population of 784; 350 cobblers in a population of 400; all but 3 of the millers of the city; all but 3 of the meat-cutters; 32 of 35 surgeons.

Across Provence as a whole, 94,000 deaths were officially recorded; a modern historian (Biraben 1972) thinks the actual total was probably about 105,000. The other cities of Provence suffered mortalities comparable to those of Marseille: 50.6% of the population of Toulon, 42.7% of Arles, 31.4% of Aix, and 31.3% of nearby Avignon. Some small villages also suffered grievously. Forcalqueyret began the epidemic with 230 people, of whom 174 died.

SIGNIFICANCE

The Marseille (and Provence) epidemic of 1720–1722 was "the last important epidemic of the plague in Western Europe" (Biraben 1972, 233). For western Europe, therefore, it marked the end of the great Second Plague Pandemic. Among the individual epidemic episodes of that pandemic, 1720–1722 gains special significance because of the rich documentation that exists about it. This epidemic has therefore been subjected to close historical study. Some findings about the 1720–1722 epidemic have been projected backward in time in an attempt to generalize about the earlier phases of the Second Plague Pandemic or even about plague epidemics in general. (See the "Unresolved Historical Issues" section; see also volume 2, chapter 5.)

BACKGROUND

France suffered from recurrent plague epidemics during the Second Plague Pandemic, as did most of Europe. By the second half of the seventeenth century, however, the interval between those epidemics lengthened. After a prolonged string of bad plague years between 1622 and 1640 (especially in 1628–1631), more epidemics occurred in 1650 and 1652–1653. The next years of widespread French plague were 1668–1669, and only the northern part of the country was affected.

No plague was found in the country at all between 1689 and the Marseille outbreak of 1720. Marseille itself had last been infected by plague in 1664. Two generations, and perhaps three, of its people therefore had had no exposure to plague in 1720.

In the course of the seventeenth century, French governmental machinery for responding to the threat of plague improved. Some aspects of the official response to the epidemic in Marseille in 1720 revealed an administration out of practice (see the "Responses" section).

Marseille was a city with long traditions of Mediterranean trade and of close associations with Italian cities. Its leaders were therefore familiar with the long-established northern Italian urban public health measures. But as a Mediterranean port, it also had regular contact with places in western Asia where plague still flourished, as the 1720 epidemic illustrated.

HOW IT WAS UNDERSTOOD AT THE TIME

Despite the long history of experience with plague and the widespread consensus that had developed by the seventeenth century about its contagious character, some uncertainties still remained. A period of denial, or at least alternative diagnoses, occurred in the early weeks of the 1720 epidemic (see the "When and Where" section); religious beliefs still heavily conditioned popular understanding of the disease (see also volume 2, chapter 5).

RESPONSES

Initial official responses to the plague epidemic focused on halting its potential for contagion. A maritime quarantine that would isolate the suspect ship, its crew, and its cargo was quickly imposed. When the city itself seemed infected, the provincial parliament responded with a cordon around it. The determination to dispose of the rapidly growing number of bodies, the extraordinary efforts to obtain assistance to do so, and the recognized danger of that task, all demonstrated serious fears of contagion and an official wish to stop it.

For other measures, the city seemed less prepared, and the measures long familiar in northern Italy had to be improvised. Only after the epidemic began did physicians urge the creation of a standing board of health, or at least an ad hoc one. There was no pesthouse, and when some physicians advocated the creation of one, arguments raged about where it would be put. Only in mid-August 1720 was a pesthouse finally opened; only in October did more plague hospitals and centers join the first.

Physicians remained conflicted about possible medical treatments for the disease, as they had been for much of the Second Plague Pandemic. Some advocated vigorous bleeding and purging, others lanced buboes, and still others offered a variety of gentler herbal remedies. In 1720 Marseille, as at other times and places in response to different diseases, some physicians advocated cleansing the air of dangerous miasmas by lighting fires and setting off explosions. The city authorities agreed to try it.

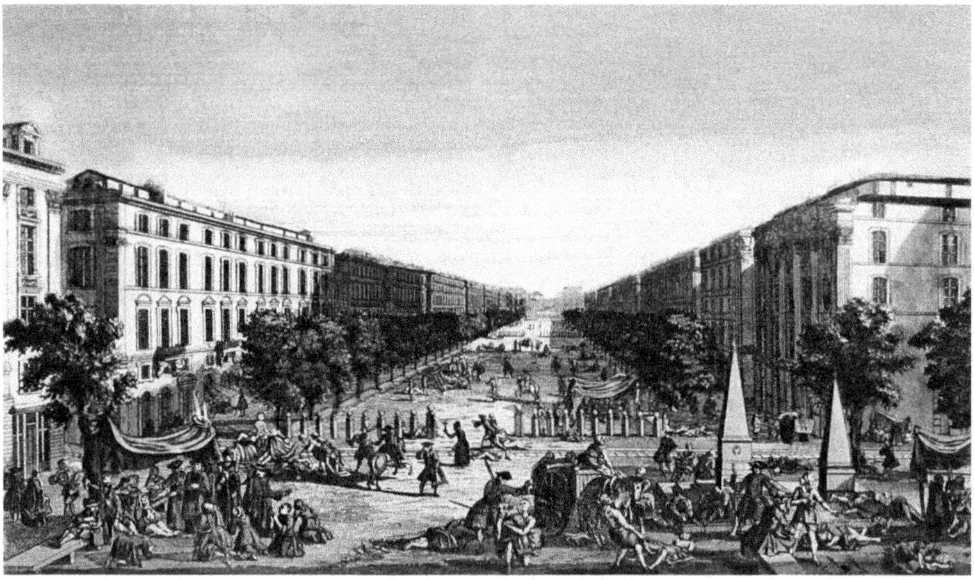

View of a main boulevard in Marseille in 1720, with plague victims in the foreground and lining the street, an illustration of the city's great difficulty in removing bodies. (National Library of Medicine)

Some of the official responses sparked popular resentment, as (again) had happened in earlier plague epidemics. Especially unpopular were the effects of the cordon on the supply and hence the price of food in the city. All through the eighteenth century, the price of grain was a flash point for popular disturbances in France, and 1720 Marseille illustrated that.

Official policy also stood in the way of another popular response (one that could have been an effective way of avoiding the disease): flight. About 10,000 people fled the city in the early weeks of the epidemic, before the cordon became effective in late August.

And religion remained an important element in popular and official responses. An incident involving a vision and a proposed procession illustrated its importance. A girl, "distinguished for her piety," related to her confessor a vision she had received as she lay mortally stricken with plague. She said that the Virgin Mary had appeared to her and assured her that "the present scourge which afflicted Marseille would not cease, until the two churches of the cathedral and St. Victor, united in a general procession, should expose all their reliques to the view of the faithful" (Bertrand 1805, 213–214). The confessor relayed this revelation to the bishop, who, impressed, agreed to such a procession. St. Victor, an abbey church, evidently had a prickly relationship with the cathedral; the abbot was sensitive about his precedence as opposed to the bishop's. The abbey, citing doubts about the trustworthiness of the revelation, also argued that processions flew in the face of good public health practice. The procession "could not be put in practice without the utmost danger, not only to the ministers of the Lord, but equally to that of the people at large, in mingling all kinds of persons indiscriminately together; for it must reasonably be supposed, that among these would be many tainted with the infection, which would thus be communicated to numbers of their fellow-citizens who might otherwise escape it" (Bertrand 1805, 219–220). The joint procession was not held, but the bishop erected an altar in a prominent public place, approached it barefoot, and celebrated mass in great pomp.

UNRESOLVED HISTORICAL ISSUES

This epidemic, because many of the facts about it are well documented, has allowed unsettled questions about the plague's history to be put with unusual sharpness. A summary of the differing views of J.-N. Biraben and O. J. Benedictow illustrates the issues at stake.

Biraben, a thorough student of the 1720 Marseille epidemic, was impressed by several facts about it. As he mapped its spread from Marseille into outlying parts of Provence, he became convinced that it seemed to follow human communication routes and that it was more likely to affect places with a larger concentration of people. All the places in Provence of a certain size were badly hit by the epidemic; many smaller villages escaped, and those that were affected were found on major communication routes. Biraben concluded that humans living in some density were at greater risk and that humans on the move carried plague with them. To explain these facts, he argued that the 1720 epidemic—and by implication other, earlier, stages of the Second Plague Pandemic—was at least to some extent spread directly from one person to another by *human* fleas. Depending on the accidental meeting between *rat* fleas and humans could not adequately account for the evident importance of human density and human traffic.

Benedictow (1987) raised several objections to these arguments. He showed cases (from other plague epidemics) where plague mortalities were very high in small villages completely isolated from lines of communication. He suggested that while human density was important for plague epidemics, so too were the densities of fleas and rodents, and that those densities might be higher in rural areas with fewer people. He therefore downplayed the role of human fleas in plague epidemics, emphasizing instead the vital (or fatal) interconnection between humans, rodents, and fleas.

As the last major plague epidemic in western Europe, the 1720 Marseille plague has entered into the larger historical questions surrounding the Second Plague Pandemic. (See the "Unresolved Historical Issues" section in volume 2, chapter 5)

REFERENCES

Bertrand, J.-B. *A Historical Relation of the Plague at Marseilles in the Year 1720.* Translated by Anne Plumptre. London: Joseph Mawman, 1805. Reprint, Farnborough, UK: Gregg International, 1973.

Biraben, Jean-Noël. "Certain Demographic Characteristics of the Plague Epidemic in France, 1720–1722." In *Population and Social Change*, edited by D. V. Glass and Roger Revelle, 233–241. London: Edward Arnold, 1972.

SUGGESTED ADDITIONAL READING

Benedictow, O. J. "Morbidity in Historical Plague Epidemics." *Population Studies* 41 (1987): 401–431.

This chapter summarizes material found in more detail in:

Biraben, Jean-Noël. *Les Hommes et la peste en France et dans les pays européens et mediterranéens.* Vol. 1, *La Peste dans l'histoire.* Paris: Mouton, 1975.

Refer to volume 2, chapter 5 "The Black Death Begins: The Second Plague Pandemic, 1346–1352," for additional reading suggestions.

13

Smallpox in Boston, 1721

WHEN AND WHERE

In 1721 a major smallpox epidemic struck the still-small city of Boston, in the British colony of Massachusetts. More than half of the people of Boston fell ill, and over 800 of them died in the epidemic.

Two merchant ships that entered Boston harbor in April carried people who were ill with smallpox, and although the two known cases were immediately isolated, others apparently had reached that brief stage in which they were infected and contagious but the telling rash had not yet appeared. Those people came ashore without hindrance, and so the disease began to spread through the town. At first the spread was slow, but by June, the number of cases had grown to the point where the city government could no longer find the resources to post a guard over every infected house. On June 26, Zabdiel Boylston, a doctor (although one with informal medical qualifications), performed the first of what would become very controversial inoculations for smallpox (see the "Responses" section). The city government designated the next day, June 27, as one of public fasting and humiliation in the hope of appeasing the wrath of God.

But the death toll only became really serious late in the summer and into the fall months. Through the end of August, 46 people in Boston had died of smallpox since the epidemic began. In September, deaths numbered 101, and then came the worst time, October, with 411 deaths. November's toll was still high: 249. Only in December did smallpox in Boston abate. In those peak months, the public life of Boston nearly came to a halt, as stores closed and streets were deserted. The authorities even placed limits on tolling funeral church bells, if only so the population could get some sleep.

By the end of the year, smallpox deaths in Boston numbered 842, nearly 8% of the total population (about 10,700) of the town. Smallpox accounted for 76% of all deaths in 1721 Boston. More striking even than the death count was the number of Bostonians who had fallen ill with smallpox: the official number was 5,759, nearly 54% of the population. Since an unknown number of residents fled the city during the epidemic, the proportion of smallpox sufferers among those who remained must have been even higher.

Although both mortality and morbidity in Boston were therefore very high, the epidemic remained largely confined to the city itself. While a few adjoining towns reported smallpox cases, a wider-ranging regional epidemic did not occur. A few cases of the disease appeared in 1722 (as well as further inoculations by Boylston), but the next Boston epidemic did not occur until 1730.

SIGNIFICANCE

Simply from the numbers of sick and dead, the 1721 Boston smallpox epidemic was evidently unusually severe. But its significance was broader than its immediate impact on human suffering. The 1721 Boston experience was the first epidemic in the Western world that inspired a deliberate campaign of inoculation, urged and practiced by the community's educated elite.

That inoculation campaign led to a major controversy, one in which the first widespread airing of the pros and cons of the inoculation procedure occurred. The arguments about the wisdom (and morality) of deliberately administering a case of a potentially fatal disease to prevent a more serious case began in Boston in 1721 and persisted into the twentieth century.

That controversy also became an important example of the conflicting and ambiguous claims of religious and scientific authority that have characterized many world responses to epidemics.

BACKGROUND

Smallpox epidemics had begun among the English settlers of Massachusetts as early as the 1640s. Before the 1721 epidemic, the most recent one had occurred in 1702 and 1703, when over 200 Bostonians died of the disease. The 18-year interval between that outbreak and 1721 meant that a substantial population of young people in the town had not been exposed to smallpox.

Reflecting the widespread conviction that smallpox was above all a contagious disease, the principal defenses that had been erected in the past were quarantine and isolation, and Boston employed them. By 1717 a quarantine hospital had been established for such eventualities.

Although Massachusetts (and British North America generally) lay on the fringes of European civilization, the medical beliefs and practices of its people followed European models. In 1721 only one physician in Boston (William Douglass) had received a European medical degree, but the community included a number of widely educated healers regarded as physicians. European scientific ideas did reach the population of Boston; for example (as will be shown later), the educated Boston elite sometimes read the Royal Society of London's journal, *Philosophical Transactions.*

The colony of Massachusetts, founded in the seventeenth century by English Puritans, remained in 1721 a community in which religious leaders played an important role in public life. Its founders had planned a Godly commonwealth. The colony's town meetings in some ways represented an early manifestation of democracy but often in practice enforced religious conformity. Trials for witchcraft had been important events. Pastors remained the most important figures in most Massachusetts communities, and the colony gave up religious qualifications for citizenship only late in the seventeenth century.

HOW IT WAS UNDERSTOOD AT THE TIME

The contagious nature of smallpox was well understood, although the mechanism of contagion remained in dispute. A few years prior to 1721, the authorities of Boston had provided a quarantine hospital to isolate cases. Many of the responses to the 1721 epidemic (discussed later) illustrated the fears of contagion. Those fears persisted after the 1721 epidemic as well; in 1731 a law required that all cases be reported so that a red flag of warning could be placed in front of the stricken house.

As might be expected in a community with such deep religious roots, many people in Massachusetts saw smallpox as a product of the will of God. Increase Mather, the influential Congregationalist pastor, warned in 1720 that God was preparing to scourge the sinful city, and when smallpox arrived the next year his prophecy seemed borne out.

RESPONSES

Boston moved as quickly as it could to throttle the contagion of smallpox, but not all the active cases were isolated in time. By May 1721, the suspected ships had been moved to a quarantine island, and guards had been posted to keep people living in infected houses locked up there. Streets were ordered to be cleaned, reflecting one of the competing beliefs about the mechanism of contagion: that it moved through a polluted environment. On June 21, Harvard College barred the public from its annual commencement ceremonies, again demonstrating fears of contagion.

But by June another response was underway: the inoculation of individuals with live smallpox before they developed a natural case. The arguments in favor of this procedure came initially from Cotton Mather (1663–1728), who, like his father Increase, was a leading Congregationalist pastor. Cotton Mather had apparently heard about inoculation as early as 1706, when he was told of it by an African-born slave who recalled the common folk practice of inserting (by incision or by scarification) the pus from a smallpox scab into the skin of a healthy person. What resulted would be—it was hoped—a slight case of the disease, one that would confer subsequent immunity. (This technique was apparently of great antiquity in several different folk traditions of Asia and Africa.) About 10 years later, several accounts of inoculation began appearing in European scientific literature, and Mather read two such accounts (by physicians based in Constantinople, Emanuel Timoni and Giacomo Pylarini) in the *Philosophical Transactions* of

London's Royal Society in 1714 and 1716. In 1721 Mather emerged as an enthusiastic proponent of inoculation.

In early June 1721, Cotton Mather urged Boston's healers to adopt the method of inoculation to protect the people of the town. One such healer Zabdiel Boylston agreed, and on June 26 performed the procedure on his six-year-old son and two African slaves. The successful results (all survived) inspired more trials by Boylston in July. By the end of that month, a raging controversy had begun. William Douglass, the sole physician with a European medical education, denounced Boylston (and Mather), claiming that inoculation was a very dangerous and untried procedure. It was simply very unwise to spread a highly contagious (and often lethal) disease deliberately. Boston's newspapers warred with each other over the merits and demerits of inoculation.

Most of official Boston opinion agreed with Douglass. The Board of Selectmen severely reprimanded Boylston, and later Boston voters specified that anyone coming into Boston from outside for the purpose of being inoculated should be put into a pesthouse. Nevertheless, the number of the inoculated grew. Boylston performed 17 inoculations in August, 31 in September, 18 in October, and (in the wake of the very high mortality of October) no less than 104 in November. By the spring of 1722, 280 Bostonians had been inoculated, most of them by Boylston.

Douglass's arguments against inoculation were first and foremost medical ones: the procedure was dangerous and untried. (And, in fact, six of those inoculated by Boylston developed fatal cases of smallpox.) Inoculation threatened to spread the epidemic even more widely by giving smallpox to healthy people who otherwise might have remained so. (Boylston made no effort to isolate the people he inoculated.) Other arguments against inoculation gathered around those points. Should matters be left in God's hands, if He were responsible for the epidemic in the first place? Only repentance would succeed; Mather presumed to speak for the Almighty.

Mather, Boylston, and their allies countered that the procedure was not dangerous and that it had been long-established in other societies. (And while it may have been true that six of Boylston's patients died, that represented only about 2% of those inoculated. Of those Bostonians who caught natural smallpox in 1721, nearly 15% died.) Mather countered the religious objection by arguing that God wants us to use the means that He has provided to us to better our health.

Behind the arguments of Douglass and Mather lay other issues, one of which was countering assertions of authority in the Boston community. Both, in different ways, claimed to speak for both science and religion; both had contentious personalities.

UNRESOLVED HISTORICAL ISSUES

Was the Douglass-Mather controversy a simple science versus religion, enlightenment versus superstition, quarrel? Clearly not, although in the light of later beliefs about the virtues of inoculation it might seem so. But the pastor (Mather) who had earlier in his career endorsed the Salem witch trials was the defender of Enlightenment (as later opinion might have seen it), while the physician (Douglass) seemed to speak for reactionary conservatism. Both, however, claimed to speak for God's will. Both invoked arguments of reason, disagreeing largely over whether the procedure was dangerous (Douglass) or safe (Mather). Perry Miller (1953) argued convincingly that the issue between them really concerned their respective power and authority in the Boston community, not a clear conflict between science and superstition. According to John Blake, Mather believed that he should "control the life of the community," while Douglass felt that he was "defending the integrity of the medical profession . . . against credulous laymen" (Blake 1959, 69, 70).

Did inoculation subsequently become well established in Boston? Its merits were certainly not settled by the 1721 experience. When Boylston resumed inoculations in 1722, the controversy boiled over again immediately. His patients were isolated on an island. Called before a town meeting, Boylston promised to cease inoculating until the town gave him official permission. A new smallpox epidemic in 1730 meant reviving the argument, although Douglass now agreed that inoculation, if done carefully, might provide protection. At least compared to the enthusiastic reception of inoculation in some other American colonial cities (such as Philadelphia and Charleston), the popularity of the technique in Boston remained uncertain. Its application in times of epidemic, such as 1752 and 1754, grew larger; in the 1764 epidemic Boston electors voted to allow it, and about 3,000 people were inoculated within a few weeks. But its acceptance in nonepidemic times remained uncertain, as Boston continued to emphasize measures against contagion (guards on infected houses, notification, isolation) rather than the preventive approach that inoculation represented.

REFERENCES

Blake, John B. *Public Health in the Town of Boston, 1630–1822.* Cambridge, MA: Harvard University Press, 1959.

Mather, Cotton. *An Account of the Method and Success of Inoculating the Small-pox, in Boston in New-England.* London: J. Peels, 1722. Reprinted in I. Bernard Cohen, ed. *Cotton Mather and American Science and Medicine*, 2:8–10 (orig. 1722 pagination). New York: Arno, 1980.

Miller, Perry. *The New England Mind from Colony to Province.* Cambridge, MA: Harvard University Press, 1953.

SUGGESTED ADDITIONAL READING

Coss, Stephen. *The Fever of 1721: The Epidemic that Revolutionized Medicine and American Politics.* New York: Simon & Schuster, 2016.

Hopkins, Donald R. *The Greatest Killer: Smallpox in History.* Chicago: University of Chicago Press, 2002. (Orig. pub. 1983 as *Princes and Peasants: Smallpox in History.*)

Winslow, Ola E. *A Destroying Angel.* Boston: Houghton Mifflin, 1974.

14

Smallpox in Eighteenth-Century Europe

WHEN AND WHERE

In the eighteenth century, smallpox succeeded plague as the great epidemic disease of Europe. Waves of epidemic smallpox repeatedly assailed the entire continent; in the larger cities, the disease was a nearly constant presence that flared in periods of higher mortality and morbidity, while less densely settled areas had periods of relative health interrupted by violent outbreaks of smallpox. No reliable estimate of the disease's complete eighteenth-century toll exists, but the deaths certainly numbered in the millions. One modern estimate claims that by the end of the century smallpox was claiming 400,000 European lives a year, at a time when the population of the continent numbered less than 200 million.

Cities were especially vulnerable to a disease such as smallpox, which spreads by contagion from one person to another and which depends on finding previously unexposed people for its continuance. It was therefore particularly a scourge of children, but those cities that grew in the eighteenth century did so largely by attracting migrants from rural areas where longer intervals separated smallpox epidemics. Those migrants accordingly represented another vulnerable population, and their constant city-bound flows helped sustain urban epidemics. London is a prime example of a large and growing city where smallpox was both a constant presence and a periodic epidemic. That city averaged perhaps 2,000 smallpox deaths a year through the century, or about 300 deaths per 100,000 population per year, a serious epidemic disease death rate. In some years, however (e.g., 1710, 1719, 1723, 1736, 1746, 1752, 1763, 1779, 1781, and 1796), the toll of Londoners was considerably higher than that. London was not unique. The mortality rate in Copenhagen exceeded that in London, reaching about 350 per 100,000 people per year in the second half of the century. In Paris in 1719, smallpox may have killed as many as 14,000.

Young children and infants everywhere were especially susceptible. Through the century smallpox resulted in the deaths of perhaps 10% of all the infants of Sweden every year, and the death rate of infants in Russia may have been even higher. In Berlin about 6,700 people died of smallpox between 1758 and 1774, and nearly all of them were children.

Epidemic smallpox in the eighteenth century generally resulted in death for about 25% of those infected by it. The experience of the illness was particularly unpleasant; an initial headache and fever progressed to a painful rash that swelled to pustules, while the skin seemed to be on fire. Skin and glands might be destroyed and an overpowering odor surrounded the victim. The survivors were most often badly scarred for the rest of their lives, especially on their faces. In some cases, permanent blindness resulted, in others, infertility.

SIGNIFICANCE

The incidence and severity of smallpox made it the great epidemic disease of the eighteenth century in the West. Plague, although still a widely feared menace, made its last important western appearance in the 1720s; cholera, the later shock disease for the West, only arrived in western Europe in the 1830s. Smallpox made a particular impact by attacking all segments of the population indiscriminately; the rich suffered as well as the poor, which was not the case in earlier plague epidemics and would not be true in later cholera visitations. Donald Hopkins, a modern smallpox authority, had reason to call his 1983 book on the disease's history *Princes and Peasants*. As Hopkins noted, smallpox in the eighteenth century ravaged the royal houses of Europe, claiming the lives of the Hapsburg Emperor Joseph I in 1711, King Luis of Spain in 1724, Czar Peter II of Russia in 1730, Queen Ulrika of Sweden in 1741, and King Louis XV of France in 1774. Other members of royal families were stricken as well, altering the succession paths in dynasties such as the Austrian Hapsburgs and the British Stuarts.

Smallpox was feared in part because of its disfiguring and disabling effects on its surviving victims. Young beauty spoiled by the scars of smallpox became a theme of eighteenth-century literature:

> Lo, the smallpox with horrid glare
> Levelled its terrors at the fair;
> And rifling every youthful grace,
> Left but the remnant of a face.
>
> (Goldsmith 1966, 370–371)

Widespread blindness in some European populations (notably that of Poland) also had a social impact. And apart from the immediate impact on government from the death of a king, smallpox epidemics occasionally intruded on larger political events. France, at war with Britain, prepared a powerful invasion fleet in 1779. Before it could land its troops in southern England, however, smallpox spread through the ships, resulting in over 8,000 deaths and the abandonment of the invasion.

The eighteenth-century smallpox epidemics also led to very significant responses, perhaps the first clearly successful deliberate steps to prevent a specific disease. No cases of smallpox have occurred in the world since 1977, in large measure the result of the application of techniques developed during, and in response to, the eighteenth-century smallpox epidemics (see the "Responses" section).

BACKGROUND

Smallpox had clearly infected Europeans for many centuries before the eighteenth; it had probably been responsible for some of the important epidemics of classical antiquity (such as the so-called "Plague of Thucydides" that struck Athens in 430 BCE). Such Muslim authors as Rhazes (of the ninth century) and Averroes (of the twelfth century) had described it and distinguished it from other diseases. European Christian authors of the thirteenth century, relying on the earlier Muslim writers, described it as well. Its effects on Europeans throughout the sixteenth century remain in dispute; some evidence suggests that for many it was in that period a relatively mild childhood disease that could at times become more serious; this at a time when European contacts with others resulted in catastrophic mortalities in the Americas, with smallpox likely the most responsible. But smallpox had, without doubt, also become a major killer of Europeans by the seventeenth century, if not before.

Its spread in seventeenth- and eighteenth-century Europe was certainly assisted by the growth of such cities as London, Amsterdam, Madrid, and Vienna. Smallpox can best establish itself in crowded populations of a certain minimum size, one that provides a large enough number of susceptible people who have not yet been exposed to it.

HOW IT WAS UNDERSTOOD AT THE TIME

By the eighteenth century, smallpox was becoming familiar enough to be understood as a specific disease, although some continued to see various *poxes* on a continuum that might have included syphilis (the *great pox*), measles, and chicken pox.

Very widespread agreement existed on one point: smallpox was highly contagious. The extraordinary precautions taken with the body of King Louis XV of France in 1774 illustrated that conviction. The corpses of deceased monarchs usually lay in state for the public, but no such ceremony surrounded Louis XV's remains. The modern historian Claude Manceron described the scene:

> Louis XV had already been bundled off to the crypt at Saint-Denis. Panic gripped the witnesses of his final agony the moment he was pronounced dead. No one would come near them. "The body was so putrefied that it had to be placed immediately in a lead casket. The commonest laborers were summoned to perform this task. The casket was first enclosed in an aromatized packing case, but all this could not prevent the odor from seeping through." . . . Indeed Versailles was acting as if the plague had hit. Absolute chaos. A flock of courtiers had rushed off to a remote wing of the palace where the dauphin and Marie Antoinette, now king and queen, were quarantined. At a distance, without kissing hands, they paid their respects to the painfully young and awkward couple standing there, eyes brimming with tears, looking scared to death. . . . Mesdames had been bundled off in a coach like a colony of lepers, while the steady clatter of departing carriages bespoke everyone's impatience to escape the palace's befouled air. (Manceron 1977, 58–59)

But if agreement existed on the contagiousness of smallpox, controversy still surrounded many other ideas about it, especially those relating to its origins. Did it spring from an "innate seed" in the body, before spreading contagiously to others? Or was it the product of some contamination of the environment? Did a microscopic organism cause it? Those arguments went on through the century, reflecting more general Enlightenment uncertainties about the etiology of diseases.

Overshadowing all thoughts about smallpox was the frequently acknowledged role of God's Providence. The strength of beliefs in the role of God would show themselves in the histories of inoculation and vaccination (see the "Responses" section).

RESPONSES

The fear of contagion led many eighteenth-century governments to erect quarantines against smallpox and to insist on isolating its victims. After the death of Czar Peter II from smallpox in 1730, the Russian government became increasingly insistent that cases of smallpox be reported so that its progress through the country could be traced. In many places, the fear of contagion led to the careful and swift disposal of bodies, as the foreshortened rites for Louis XV illustrated. And some therapies that had evolved over the preceding centuries continued to be applied, although their effectiveness was never clearly shown. Some physicians continued to bleed smallpox patients. Others argued about the wisdom of opening skin pustules to drain the "matter" of smallpox away, as opposed to letting scabs fall off of their own accord. Some favored applying heat to patients, while others, urging the reverse, cooled them. An old, traditional, and nearly worldwide treatment involved covering the patient with red cloth and bathing the sickroom in red light.

The most important set of responses to smallpox in the eighteenth century were, however, in the realm of prevention, not cure—the techniques of inoculation and vaccination (the first an ancient folk practice, as well as a formal method of older Chinese and African medicine adopted and made official by Western medical practitioners, the second a triumph of eighteenth-century experimental science).

Inoculation for smallpox involved the deliberate introduction of the matter of smallpox into a healthy person's body. The matter of the disease might be found (it was thought) in the scabs left on the skin of smallpox sufferers, or perhaps in fluid drained from the pustules that formed on their skin. Different techniques of inoculation had evolved in different traditions; in China, for example, dried scabs were blown into the nasal passages of the person being inoculated, while in other places (including sub-Saharan Africa) fluid was inserted into scratches or incisions in the skin. Those who performed the procedure hoped that a mild case of smallpox conferring immunity on the person inoculated would occur. Occasionally a serious or even fatal case did result.

This procedure was of unknown antiquity, certainly practiced in many parts of Asia and Africa, and perhaps in some rural areas of Europe as well. It was, however, unknown to (or at least unrecognized by) the formally educated physicians of Europe until the early eighteenth century. Among several such physicians were Emanuel Timoni and Giacomo Pylarini, practicing in Constantinople, who between 1714 and 1718 published separate accounts of inoculation in the *Philosophical Transactions* of the Royal Society of London. Shortly afterward two prominent nonmedical figures began to press for the general adoption of the practice: Cotton Mather, a prominent Massachusetts divine, and Lady Mary Wortley Montagu, a fashionable young Englishwoman.

Montagu, the wife of the British ambassador to Ottoman Turkey, had earlier suffered from a case of smallpox that marred her celebrated beauty. Aware of the inoculations performed by Constantinople folk practitioners and determined to spare her children the ravages of smallpox, she had her son inoculated in 1718. She then publicized the successful results in a series of letters to her English friends. In the next several years, her efforts were seconded by Charles Maitland, an English surgeon, and Sir Hans Sloane, a prominent English physician. Between them, they convinced Caroline, Princess of Wales, of the merits of inoculation. After some experiments on convicts succeeded, Caroline agreed to have her children (who included the heir to the British throne) inoculated. By the 1720s, inoculation thus became fashionable in Great Britain, beyond the isolated rural settlements where it had traditionally been practiced.

The fashion did not entirely take hold, however. Some deaths followed some inoculations; doubts about the wisdom of deliberately spreading a highly contagious disease persisted. Religious objections arose as well: Was not inoculation an attempt to thwart the will of God? And many physicians, sensitive about their professional dignity, were reluctant to perform a procedure that had originated with unlettered folk practitioners. For some combination of all these reasons, inoculation spread only haltingly until the 1760s. For some of the leading spokesmen of the Enlightenment, it became a cause—a symbol of the march of scientific progress opposed by ignorant superstition; thus, the great French *Encyclopédie* praised it, as did Voltaire. But resistance to inoculation proved especially strong in France.

Further refinements in the procedure, combined with more enthusiastic support from the crowned heads of Europe, led to new levels of acceptance of inoculation from the 1760s onward. Those physicians and surgeons who had become inoculators had insisted on lengthy (and costly) periods of preparation before the actual incision. In the 1760s, Robert Sutton and his son Daniel, a pair of English inoculators, developed methods that involved shallower incisions in the skin, which may have reduced not only mortality rates among the inoculated and rates of contagion from them but also time and expense of the procedure. The Suttons—especially Daniel—were very enthusiastic proponents of their method; Daniel claimed to have inoculated thousands of people within a few years. The popularity of inoculation grew in Great Britain as its costs fell.

The acceptance of inoculation in continental Europe was furthered by the example of three monarchs: Catherine II of Russia (1762–1796), Frederick II of Prussia (1740–1786), and Maria Theresa of Hapsburg Austria (1740–1780). Catherine II summoned one of Sutton's competitors, the English physician Thomas Dimsdale, to St. Petersburg in 1768. His successful inoculation of the empress established the credibility of the procedure in Russian society. In the same year Maria Theresa, in whose court smallpox had been especially deadly in the 1760s, imported the Dutch physician Jan Ingenhousz to inoculate her family and founded an inoculation infirmary in Vienna. Hoping to spread the practice to Prussia, Frederick II employed English inoculators in 1775.

By the last quarter of the eighteenth century, therefore, inoculation had become an accepted medical technique in much of Europe. How widespread the practice became in those years remains a subject of historical debate (see the "Unresolved Historical Issues" section), but its application may have had a real effect on morbidity and mortality rates from smallpox.

Inoculation may also be seen as a stepping stone toward a related response: the technique that was called vaccination. While inoculation had a very old history in folk practices, vaccination emerged in the 1790s as a result of deliberate experiment by a medical professional, the surgeon Edward Jenner. Jenner's practice in rural western England led him to observe the curious fact (which others had noticed as well) that people who had contracted the mild disease called *cowpox*—especially common among those who worked with cows, such as milkmaids—rarely suffered from smallpox. By 1791 he had begun a file of cases of people whose cowpox had led to apparent smallpox immunity. In 1796 he began experiments in which he first transferred cowpox to new subjects (using the techniques of inoculation), and then attempted to inoculate the same people with smallpox "matter." When not even the slightest symptoms of smallpox appeared, Jenner was convinced that his cowpox had resulted in immunity.

In 1798 Jenner published the results of his findings in a work entitled *Inquiry into the Causes and Effects of the Variolae Vaccinae, or Cow-Pox.* The term "vaccine" (derived from the Latin *vacca*, cow) was later generally applied to all preparations of disease agents administered to prevent cases of the disease (e.g., Salk vaccine for poliomyelitis), but it initially referred to Jenner's cowpox used to prevent smallpox. Cowpox, a mild disease that left no scars, apparently prevented later cases of smallpox. Although not everyone was immediately convinced by Jenner's arguments (see the "Unresolved Historical Issues" section), many were, and demand for the vaccine soared in different European states. Within a few years, Jenner had been hailed as a benefactor of the human race, a symbol of the progress that came from science and enlightenment. Napoleon admired him; the British Parliament lavished gifts of money on him. In Britain, 100,000 people had been vaccinated by 1801; in France, 1.7 million by 1811; in Russia, 2 million by 1814.

UNRESOLVED HISTORICAL ISSUES

Jenner's introduction of a vaccination, while a dramatic event in human responses to epidemics, did not abruptly end the menace of smallpox. Contemporary questions about the effectiveness and use of vaccination persisted throughout the nineteenth century, as did smallpox itself. And some important questions about the eighteenth-century smallpox epidemic are still debated by historians.

While many of his contemporaries hailed Jenner and his vaccine, many others remained dubious or openly critical. The older technique of inoculation conferred lifetime immunity from smallpox, since it resulted in an actual (although mild) case of that disease. Could vaccination make the same claim? Jenner, at least initially, said that it could. Doubts persisted, however, and by the 1820s (if not earlier) enough evidence had amassed that the vaccination's immunity eventually wore off, leaving the vaccinated vulnerable to smallpox. Revaccination was therefore necessary, but, in the meantime, some people understandably lost faith in the procedure that seemed not to work as advertised. And even if vaccination worked, questions remained about its safety or about the comparative safety of vaccination and inoculation. Would introducing an animal disease into a human disturb essential humanity, thus "animalize" one? And by the time Jenner announced his vaccine, a substantial number of European health practitioners (including both physicians and unofficial rural healers) had established themselves as inoculators, and they formed a formidable body of opposition to vaccination. Perhaps they distrusted the new method's safety; perhaps their professional positions were threatened by it.

Another unresolved question revolved around the role and powers of the state. Could the state compel the vaccination of its population? Even if it wished to, did it have the means to do so? Those questions loomed large in later smallpox epidemics.

Many features of the history of eighteenth-century smallpox remain in dispute. What accounts for the apparently greater virulence of the disease in Europe by the seventeenth and eighteenth centuries? We now know that the virus responsible for the disease occurs in several subtypes, especially those called *Variola major* and *Variola minor*, the latter much less virulent than the former. Was *Variola minor* more common in earlier centuries, and was it being replaced by *Variola major* during this epidemic period? In the eighteenth century, smallpox may have simultaneously become more lethal in Africa and India as well; could that increase be related to social or economic change, akin to European urban growth? Or did the pattern of European (or African or Indian) immunities change for some reason? Did urban population densities increase with rural migrants providing a steady stream of people without immunity?

The importance of eighteenth-century inoculation has been the subject of particular debate. Peter Razzell (1977) has claimed that inoculation (especially in England) became such a widespread practice that it actually resulted in an important reduction of overall mortality rates. Inoculation might therefore have been one of the first active medical measures to contribute to increasing life expectancy for a whole population. As early as 1756, some English parishes—the local government unit responsible for care of the poor—began inoculating their entire populations in the belief that preventing an epidemic would save public money, and the Sutton method reinforced that cost argument.

While no one doubts that inoculation (and the later vaccination) represented important medical interventions against a specific disease, other scholars (notably Thomas McKeown 1978) have questioned both whether inoculation was carried on to the extent that Razzell and others have argued and whether it was efficacious. How many people died of smallpox as the *result* of an inoculation?

Finally, doubts also persist about just what Jenner did and specifically about the composition of his vaccine. Was it cowpox, as he asserted? Or was it (as his contemporary opponents asserted) simply a contaminated form of the "matter" of smallpox itself? Derrick Baxby (1981) has argued that Jenner's vaccine was most likely a variety of yet another disease of animals, horsepox, or perhaps an indeterminant mixture of different benign animal "poxes."

REFERENCES

Goldsmith, Oliver. "The Double Transformation: A Tale." In *Collected Works of Oliver Goldsmith*, edited by Arthur Friedman, 370–371. Oxford: Clarendon, 1966.

Jenner, Edward. "The Three Original Publications on Vaccination against Smallpox." In *The Harvard Classics: Scientific Papers: Physiology, Medicine, Surgery, and Geology*, 164–165. New York: P. F. Collier & Son, 1910. (Orig. pub. 1798 as *Inquiry into the Causes and Effects of the Variolae Vaccinae, or Cow-Pox.*)

Manceron, Claude. *Twilight of the Old Order, 1774–1778*. In *Age of the French Revolution*, translated by Patricia Wolf, 1:58–59. New York: Knopf, 1977.

SUGGESTED ADDITIONAL READING

Baxby, Derrick. *Jenner's Smallpox Vaccine: The Riddle of Vaccina Virus and Its Origins.* London: Heinemann, 1981.

Carmichael, Ann G., and Arthur Silverstein. "Smallpox in Europe before the Seventeenth Century: Virulent Killer or Benign Disease?" *Journal of the History of Medicine and Allied Sciences* 42 (1987): 147–168.

Glynn, Ian, and Jenifer Glynn. *The Life and Death of Smallpox.* Cambridge: Cambridge University Press, 2004.

Herbert, Eugenia W. "Smallpox Inoculation in Africa." *Journal of African History* 16 (1975): 539–559.

Hopkins, Donald R. *The Greatest Killer: Smallpox in History.* Chicago: University of Chicago Press, 2002. (Orig. pub. 1983 as *Princes and Peasants: Smallpox in History.*)

May, Maisie. "Inoculating the Urban Poor in the Late Eighteenth Century." *British Journal for the History of Science* 30 (1997): 291–305.

McKeown, Thomas. "Fertility, Mortality and Causes of Death: An Examination of Issues Related to the Modern Rise of Population." *Population Studies* 32 (1978): 535–542.

Miller, Genevieve. *The Adoption of Inoculation for Smallpox in England and France.* Philadelphia: University of Pennsylvania Press, 1957.

Patterson, A. T. *The Other Armada.* Manchester: Manchester University Press, 1960.

Razzell, Peter. *The Conquest of Smallpox: The Impact of Inoculation on Smallpox Mortality in Eighteenth Century Britain.* Firle: Caliban, 1977.

15

Plague in Moscow, 1771

WHEN AND WHERE

In 1771 the most serious epidemic of plague in Russian history occurred. The epidemic especially affected the city of Moscow, the old capital of the country that stood in Russia's heartland. The disease apparently arrived in the environs of Moscow in late 1770. After a period of alarms and apparent containments of plague, the epidemic rapidly reached a peak late in the summer of 1771. With the onset of cold weather in October and November, mortality declined, and the epidemic had passed by the end of the year.

This epidemic reached Moscow from the southwest. In 1768 a war began between Russia and Ottoman Turkey. By early 1770, Russian forces had occupied the Danubian provinces of Wallachia and Moldavia, and plague apparently spread from those territories into the Russian Empire itself. In the summer months of 1770, Kiev was struck by plague, which killed perhaps 3,200 of its 20,000 people. By November, mysterious deaths (or at least thought to be mysterious) were occurring in a suburban area of Moscow that included both textile manufacturing and a military hospital; in December, the alarm about plague was raised there, only to die down by year's end. On January 15, authorities declared the end of the emergency.

But plague had apparently never left, and by February mortality started to rise, especially in a very large woolen textile factory in Moscow called the "Big Woolen Court." Officials ordered that establishment be quarantined and then evacuated in March, and the imperial government in St. Petersburg prepared to isolate the entire city of Moscow. In early April, the epidemic waned again, and by May the precautions had been dropped. By late June, however, plague mortality again began to rise, especially in families connected with textile manufacturing. Sudden further surges in deaths occurred in late July and mid-August. In the latter month over 7,200 plague deaths were reported in Moscow and corpses accumulated in the streets. The terrible toll rose to over 21,000 in September.

At the height of the epidemic, on September 15 (a day when 920 plague deaths were reported in Moscow), a major riot began in the city, in the course of which a crowd battered Archbishop Amvrosii to death. The Czarina Catherine II had already dispatched a special official, Grigori Orlov, to Moscow to take charge of the struggle against the disease; Orlov was now empowered to restore order as well as health (see the "Responses" section). Mortality from plague began to decline in late September and continued to do so in the next month (although another 17,500 plague deaths occurred then, and daily mortality remained above 600 until October 19). By December, the epidemic had abated.

Several estimates were made of total mortality. The Plague Commission, organized by Orlov, put the deaths at about 56,900; other contemporaries suggested as many as 100,000. The modern historian John Alexander estimates that 50,000 died in the city itself and another 50,000 in the central region of Russia that immediately surrounded it. These numbers may have represented 20–30% of Moscow's population, estimates of which range from 150,000 to 300,000; probably no more than 150,000 had remained in the city in the peak months of the epidemic.

SIGNIFICANCE

The 1771 Moscow epidemic was the worst plague visitation in Russian history. Its death toll almost certainly exceeded that suffered by the then-thinly-populated Russia during the fourteenth-century Black Death (see volume 2, chapter 5), as well as those of the earlier serious epidemics of 1570 and 1654.

The experience of the epidemic had a number of immediate effects on the Russian economy, government, and medical system. It stimulated a surge in medical literature in the Russian language and underlined the need felt by Russians for contacts with the medical thinking and practices of western Europe. The experiences of 1771 strengthened convictions among the Russian medical and political establishments that disease was most often borne by contagion, and in subsequent decades Russian policies against epidemics were strongly anti-contagion.

The epidemic immediately and seriously disturbed the economy of Moscow, for those possessing hard-to-replace mercantile and artisanal skills suffered high mortalities. It struck perhaps two-thirds of the city's industrial establishments. The particularly high toll in such large manufactories as the Big Woolen Court, an industrial structure that employed and housed several thousand, led to a determined decentralization of Moscow industry after 1771. Smaller workshops replaced such large textile factories, and other industries transferred out of the city altogether.

Political effects were serious as well, although perhaps more diffuse. The Russian ruler, the Czarina Catherine II, disliked Moscow anyway, and the epidemic (and the riot that accompanied it) made her even more determined to reform and modernize the city (see the "Responses" section). It may have contributed to a Muscovite sense of martyrdom and separateness from the Westernized capital city, St. Petersburg. And in some larger way, the Moscow epidemic of 1771 entered into a larger pattern of events that made the years 1768–1774 a period of crisis in Catherine II's rule (see the "Unresolved Historical Issues" section).

BACKGROUND

In Russia, as in western Europe, plague had regularly recurred from the fourteenth century through the seventeenth, with increasingly long intervals between epidemics. Illustrating the persistence of the Second Plague Pandemic, particularly serious epidemics occurred in Moscow in 1570 and 1654; on the latter occasion, civil authority briefly collapsed in violence and looting. Periodic plague outbreaks continued to affect different areas of the Russian Empire (e.g., in 1690 and 1738), but Moscow remained free of plague between 1654 and the 1771 epidemic.

In the light of much later understanding of plague, we can now see that Moscow was especially vulnerable to the disease in the middle and late eighteenth century. It was a large, crowded city built largely of wood; water channels and rivers honeycombed it. Moscow had become an important textile manufacturing center, where large stocks of such imported raw materials as wool and silk accumulated; it was also a major grain market. The wooden dwellings and the water channels provided ideal environments for rats to live and move, the wool and silk could harbor fleas, and the granaries drew rats. The city contained very crowded working and living quarters and also had a large transient population of beggars, soldiers (and their followers), convicts, and clerics without pastoral responsibilities. The movement of people in and out of Moscow made the spread of disease from elsewhere more likely.

In the immediate background of the 1771 epidemic was a war between Russia and Ottoman Turkey, which began in October 1768. Russians had long connected plague epidemics with contacts with Turkey, and Russian conquest of the Turkish Danubian provinces in 1770 led to the rapid progress of the epidemic from the southwest toward Moscow. To commercial traffic was added the movement of military personnel and supplies between the Russian heartland and the war zones.

HOW IT WAS UNDERSTOOD AT THE TIME

By the eighteenth century, Russian opinion about plague largely mirrored that found elsewhere in Europe. Plague was explained in terms that combined beliefs in contagion and miasma. If anything, Russian authorities (medical and political) emphasized contagion more than others did, but the differences were of degree. Plague, it was thought, had its origins in some locally based miasma or local corruption of the atmosphere; it then spread from its point of origin by contagion, passing from person to person. Russians were convinced that this disease came from outside their homeland, especially from Ottoman Turkey. Some opinion also recognized that the poorest quarters of cities were more vulnerable, but no agreement existed about why that was so. Did the poor lead a life that engendered dangerous miasmas? Were they simply heedless of precautions? Or did crowded conditions ease the path of contagion?

Many Russians—perhaps more in proportion to population than elsewhere in Europe—remained convinced that plague stemmed from divine displeasure, human sin, and/or malignant magic. Medical interpretations, especially those of western Europe, had only begun to enter Russian society. Only in the reign of Czar Peter I (1689–1725) did the Russian state begin to take medical opinion into account in its formulation of policy during epidemics. The population as a whole had not absorbed much sense that physicians held the keys to disease; on the eve of the 1771 Moscow plague, physicians in the entire Russian Empire numbered about 100. As recently as 1738, a woman had been tortured into confessing that she had transformed herself into a goat and infected others with evil spirits (Alexander 1980, 30). In the 1771 epidemic, such religious views of disease were frequently expressed and dramatically acted on.

One additional understanding of the disease was important in the 1771 epidemic: For a variety of medical and political reasons, Moscow (and imperial) authorities remained uncertain about the identification of the disease against which they bent their efforts. Was it plague? If it was, then certain draconian measures were called for, which would both disrupt society and commerce and give rise to dangerous outbreaks of mass emotion. Many motives existed for states of denial.

RESPONSES

In line with the dominant theory of plague's cause, over a long period Russian authorities evolved a set of responses to a disease thought to be carried from elsewhere by contagion: quarantines and cordons to keep the disease away and isolation of those infected if the quarantines failed to stop plague. Those measures dominated the responses to the 1771 Moscow epidemic, but that event also illustrates the ways in which they might not be thoroughly applied, even though the state, in theory, could use ferocious punishments to enforce them.

The 1771 epidemic appeared (or seemed to appear) in three phases, and the responses to them had an on-again, off-again character. Measures were decreed and perhaps put in place; then they would be lifted; then reinstated more comprehensively; and then the same cycle repeated itself. Plague first appeared in the Moscow suburbs in November 1770, but it was only when the death toll became truly catastrophic in September 1771 that arguments about the identity of the disease ceased. And even then, the measures taken against it were vigorously contested, for the isolation of the city by quarantines and cordons coincided with a serious crisis in the food supply.

By the time plague made its November appearance in the Moscow suburbs, the government had been implementing cordons and quarantines in response to the disease's spread to the northeast from the conquered Danubian provinces since early 1770. But doubt and perhaps concealment marked its arrival in Moscow. The affected sites—a textile factory and a military hospital—were isolated, but no general quarantine was imposed for Moscow. The central government in St. Petersburg blamed Turkey for the epidemic and prohibited the importation of cloth from the Danubian provinces, but by the end of December the epidemic had apparently ceased and in practice the measures were abandoned.

The epidemic's second appearance, by February 1771, was concentrated in the so-called Big Woolen Court. That structure was isolated, a pesthouse was established to separate victims from the healthy, and the healthy population of the factory was evacuated. Other factories were fumigated, public baths were closed, and burials within the city were forbidden. An imperial official, Peter Eropkin, was empowered to control measures against the epidemic. But throughout this phase (March and April) no public admission of plague appeared, and the owners of factories were urged not to alarm their workforces with strict anti-plague discipline. As the danger passed (by late April), the public baths were reopened, sequestered factory workers were released, and cloth shipments to and from the Big Woolen Court resumed.

By July plague mortality had reached a new peak, and with that came a renewal of official measures. In the next several weeks, public baths were again closed, burials within the city were again forbidden, the healthy workers of infected factories were again sequestered, buildings were again fumigated. Inspectors now moved through the city, registering deaths, tracing the sick, and ordering property be burned. And on August 20 (in a month when the official plague toll exceeded 7,000), Czarina Catherine II ordered that Moscow be isolated from outside contacts.

Opposition mounted to these more active government policies. One source of resistance originated in religious belief and practices. Processions through the streets, in which icons were borne by the faithful, had begun in late July. Believing that the disease was contagious, authorities had attempted to discourage these crowds, and that action further disturbed the pious, who found their traditional funeral customs (washing and kissing the dead, and following coffins in funeral processions) similarly restricted. Catherine II's dislike of the backward city of Moscow was countered by Muscovite suspicion of the Western, "foreign," St. Petersburg court. Most of the physicians in Moscow (and indeed in Russia) were in some way foreign, in training at least, and popular resentments increasingly focused on them. Crowds threatened doctors and inspectors of goods. The Moscow city authorities, fearing the likely violent reaction to the isolation of the city in a time of serious food shortages, resisted Catherine's quarantine proclamation. On September 20, Catherine ordered a new imperial official—her favorite Grigori Orlov—to Moscow to assume supreme command of the city.

But by then the accumulated grievances against the government plague policies had exploded in a serious riot. Word spread that miracles were occurring at an icon hanging from one of the city's gates, and a crowd gathered there, which included priests resentful of government interference with their funeral practices. Eropkin, the imperial official, and the archbishop of Moscow, Amvrosii, hoped to calm the situation by summoning the angry priests to a meeting, but their messengers to the scene (six soldiers, an official, and a priest) were resisted by the crowd, as a rumor spread that the archbishop and his soldiers intended to seize the icon. (Amvrosii had for some time been worried by the behavior of clergy who seemed out of his control and who, he believed, fed popular superstitions about plague.) By the evening of September 15, thousands of Muscovites were in the streets and a full-scale riot was underway. The rioters broke into the palace precinct of the Kremlin and looted the archbishop's lodgings. The next day attempts to coax the looters out of the Kremlin failed; some of the crowd, now inflamed by the Kremlin's wine cellars, found the archbishop in a monastery, battered him for two hours, and finally killed him. Late in the day on September 16, Eropkin assembled troops and regained control of the Kremlin, but crowds in the streets continued the fighting through the night. When the violence finally ended, an unknown number of people lay dead; the official tally was 78, but other estimates ranged much higher.

In response to this collapse of authority, Eropkin decided to (once again) ease the plague policies, modifying the insistence on sequestering the healthy. But those orders were promptly countermanded by Orlov, who arrived with Catherine's direct authority to restore order on September 26. Orlov began a thorough anti-contagion program, reintroducing compulsory isolation for all those infected and sequestering others. A commission was appointed to oversee more active policies, which included supervising medical providers. New pesthouses were created, medical staff was conscripted, those who concealed facts—as well as looters—were punished. Dogs and cats from infected places were killed.

Medical responses to plague in 1771 Moscow resembled many of the practices in other plague epidemics late in the Second Plague Pandemic, although Moscow's population of physicians was small and relatively recently established. Physicians bled and purged the sick, attempted to lance plague buboes, and prescribed a wide variety of herbal and chemical concoctions. For a time, the *cool regimen*, in which patients were placed in cool rooms, bathed in cold water, and rubbed with ice, enjoyed some favor. Far more common were the ministrations of irregular and folk healers, and the performance of symbolic religious gestures.

UNRESOLVED HISTORICAL ISSUES

The 1771 Moscow epidemic was one of the last events of the Second Plague Pandemic in the Western world. Its story, therefore, enters into the larger unresolved questions about that pandemic, especially any explanation of the pandemic's disappearance. It was the last visitation of epidemic plague in the Russian interior. John Alexander, the modern authority on this epidemic, argues that it occurred as a result of a unique combination of circumstances. Weather conditions played a role: a warm late fall allowed plague to reach Moscow in November; a short winter allowed it to survive and reappear; a suddenly cold late spring apparently drove it away; but then a warm summer brought it back again in all its fury. The war between Russia and Ottoman Turkey opened paths of human contagion. The simultaneous crisis in food supply contributed to both a high death toll and to escalating social tensions. The development of industries in Moscow had created congested working and living places, where materials (wool, silk) harboring fleas were brought. Moscow, an overwhelmingly wooden city, provided ideal conditions for rats.

If Alexander is correct, were all urban epidemics toward the end of the Second Plague Pandemic the products of local circumstances? If so, could the disappearance of the second pandemic be explained by changes in those circumstances? Did the conditions of Moscow change in the years after 1771? Did the anti-contagion measures of the Russian state have an effect?

One particular feature of the Moscow epidemic calls out for a clearer explanation. It exacted a disproportionate death toll on the population of young adults, and especially young adult males. Why was that so? In what ways were young males at greater risk? Did a higher proportion of them remain in the city? Did their occupations (or habits) bring them in closer contact with rats and fleas? The contrasts with the experience of 1665 London, where females suffered disproportionately, are interesting.

The solutions to some other unresolved issues will probably remain speculative. It is tempting to say that the 1771 epidemic contributed to Russian fears of foreigners (especially the Turks), and that that xenophobia strengthened the Russian state's devotion to the practices of anti-contagion. Did the 1771 experience deepen Muscovite resentment of foreign, Westernized, cosmopolitan St. Petersburg, from whence came orders that imperiled Moscow's prosperity and peace?

REFERENCE AND SUGGESTED ADDITIONAL READING

This chapter has been based almost wholly on the source listed here, and English-speaking readers interested in more about the 1771 Moscow epidemic should consult it.

Alexander, John T. *Bubonic Plague in Early Modern Russia: Public Health and Urban Disaster.* New York: Oxford University Press, 2003. (Orig. pub. Baltimore: Johns Hopkins University Press, 1980.)

16

Yellow Fever in Hispaniola, 1793–1804

WHEN AND WHERE

Although yellow fever epidemics recurred in the islands of the Caribbean between the seventeenth and nineteenth centuries, serious outbreaks on the island of Hispaniola in the period between 1793 and 1804 had particularly important political consequences. Since the late seventeenth century, control of Hispaniola had been divided between Spain (Santo Domingo, on the eastern part of the island) and France (Saint Domingue, on the western). The French Revolution that began in 1789 precipitated a series of events in which yellow fever epidemics played a crucial role. By 1793 Great Britain and Spain were at war with the revolutionary French republic, and in September of that year Britain landed an army of occupation in Saint Domingue.

Those British forces arrived in the midst of political turmoil on the island. The French Revolution's promises of liberty had stirred the white planters (who hoped to be free of colonial restrictions), the mulattoes (who hoped for political rights), and the African-descended slaves (much the largest group, who hoped for freedom). Well-organized slave revolts had begun. Some of the slave leaders welcomed the British (and Spanish) as allies in their rebellion, but the French commissioner on the island proclaimed that all slaves were free, winning many of them back to French allegiance; then in February 1794 the French government entirely abolished slavery in its lands. The British attempt to control Saint Domingue now faced concerted opposition from a slave rebellion that became a war of liberation.

By June 1794, Britain landed about 4,000 troops on Saint Domingue, and in that summer a yellow fever epidemic began. Two newly arrived British regiments suffered over 40% mortality in three months, and by the end of the summer the epidemic had begun to spread from the town of Port au Prince (its original focus) to other places on the island. The disease abated somewhat at the end of 1794 and the beginning of 1795, but by the spring of 1795 it returned in strength and its effects on the British force in the summer of 1795 were horrific. One regiment newly arrived from Ireland in April had lost 41% of its members by July 1; it then suffered 23.6 deaths per 100 still-surviving members in July, 35.5 per 100 in August, and 42.4 in September. Another regiment experienced 60% mortality in October alone.

British losses continued through 1796 and 1797, although their numbers relating to mortality and causes of death are less clear. What was clear was that the British effort at the conquest of Saint Domingue had been frustrated by a combination of yellow fever mortality and the resistance of the ex-slaves led by Toussaint L'Ouverture. Army recruitments in Britain lagged, as men hesitated to join a force that would be sent to likely death in the West Indies. By 1797 the British government, needing recruits to face a potential French invasion of its homeland, decided to abandon its attempt to control Saint Domingue. In July 1798, the last British troops left. Of the total of 20,200 British troops sent there between 1793 and 1798, 12,700 had died, most from disease. Since Spain had ceded its part of Hispaniola to France when it made peace in 1795, the whole island was in theory loyal to France, but in effect it was independent and under the control of the black ex-slaves who had led the rebellion against their masters and the British invaders.

Yellow fever also savaged the next European effort to regain control of Saint Domingue, that of France in 1802 and 1803. Between 1798 and 1802, the island's practical independence stemmed from British control of the oceans, which prevented the nominal French overlords of Saint Domingue from reaching it. In March 1802, Britain and France made peace, and the French government attempted to reassert its control over Saint Domingue. Napoleon Bonaparte, who dominated France as First Consul, sent an army under the command of his brother-in-law Charles Leclerc. Leclerc's forces enjoyed initial success, but the French reimposition of slavery stirred resistance, resistance that allowed yellow fever to seriously weaken the French army. By November 1802, the original French force of 20,000 had been reduced to 2,000, and Leclerc himself died of yellow fever. Another French army was sent out in 1803, but yellow fever and popular resistance tore it apart as well. At the end of November 1803, the French evacuated, surrendering to a blockading British fleet. (Britain and France had again gone to war in May.) Although the numbers are uncertain, about 25,000 of the 35,000 French soldiers involved died in 1802 and 1803.

When the French left, the victorious revolutionaries led by Jean-Jacques Dessalines proclaimed Haiti an independent republic, the second one in the Western hemisphere, and the only state ever founded by a successful slave rebellion.

SIGNIFICANCE

These epidemics played a crucial role in the history of the Caribbean. Saint Domingue was the most important French colonial possession, the source of great wealth. Its ultimate surrender by France (and the failure of the earlier British attempt to take it over) marked the first extension of Robert Palmer's "age of the democratic revolution" to Middle and South America (Palmer 1964, 338, 514). The inability of the British and French to keep fever-ridden armies in the field, combined with the determined resistance of the resident black population, led to the defeat of the colonial powers and the independence of Haiti. To some unknown extent these events inspired revolutionary ideas elsewhere in the colonial Americas. When the French abandoned Haiti, they immediately sold their Louisiana territory in North America to the United States; it may be that yellow fever's depredations directly led to the Louisiana Purchase.

The yellow fever epidemics in the Caribbean in the 1790s and 1800s were part of a larger period of yellow fever attacks in the western Atlantic.

BACKGROUND

Yellow fever has been documented in the West Indies as early as the 1640s. Its causative virus likely evolved in east or central Africa; from there human traffic carried it first to west Africa, then across the Atlantic with the slave trade to the Caribbean. Yellow fever is carried from one person to another by a species of mosquito, *Aedes aegypti.* (The virus may also be found in populations of other primates as well as humans.) *Aedes aegypti* has a narrow range; it is found most often in urban or other dense settlements and prefers standing water (such as that in water casks and cisterns) for its breeding. Its habitat, so often human-centered, therefore differs considerably from the more wide-ranging swamp-dwelling mosquito species that transmit malaria. The severity of yellow fever varies considerably, but regardless of the severity of an individual case, one exposure confers immunity from further attacks.

That severity has depended on several factors, the most important being the presence of a densely settled population of people without previous exposure. Between the late seventeenth century and about 1770, periodic epidemics of the disease struck islands in the West Indies, most often on the heels of waves of settlement by Europeans and the African slave populations they imported. Europe offered little or no exposure to yellow fever, so almost all Europeans were vulnerable; while many African people may have been exposed to yellow fever, many others probably had not been. A fresh concentration of European settlers and planters, bringing more slaves, could create conditions favorable for an epidemic. Thus, yellow fever was especially serious in Barbados around 1700 and in Martinique in the 1730s, for example. And any time a large European military force (a dense population of unexposed people) appeared in the Caribbean, a major outbreak of yellow fever often accompanied it. When a British army made up of some Britons and some North American British colonists besieged Cartagena in 1741, an astonishing 70% of the force perished, mostly from disease; in taking Havana in 1762, the British lost 40% of their troops.

Few outbreaks of West Indian yellow fever occurred between about 1770 and 1793, and none of them were serious. Apparently, a high proportion of the resident population of the Caribbean islands (whether of European or African descent) had by then been infected by earlier cases; perhaps the virus was less lethal (for unknown reasons) in those years so that its cases did not attract attention. It became a not very serious, endemic disease, at least for the resident peoples.

The dramatic political situations created by the French Revolution changed all that, as can be seen earlier in the "When and Where" section. Large numbers of nonimmune people suddenly arrived from Europe: soldiers, sailors, officials, their wives, and servants. Most of them were housed in crowded military barracks in or on the edges of towns, located with no regard for the health of the troops (but see the "Responses" section). Those troops were generally poorly nourished, poorly clad against the wet climate, and too often consumed too much alcohol. Their barracks therefore promoted the spread of many diseases, including malaria, typhus, and dysentery, as well as yellow fever. Particular weather circumstances in the 1790s may have contributed as well. Years of high rainfall (even by West Indian standards) promoted mosquito populations; succeeding dry spells meant increasing human reliance on such standing water sources such as cisterns: ideal environments for *Aedes aegypti* mosquitoes.

And in 1793 a particularly lethal supply of those mosquitoes arrived, conveyed by a British ship that had become a nearly ideal floating environment for them. The *Hankey* had set out from England in 1792 carrying 120 passengers who intended to establish a settlement colony on the west coast of Africa; the intention was to cooperate with Africans, not enslave them. After about six months in the vicinity of the island of Bolama, the settlement failed and the *Hankey* departed, accompanied by a shipload of mosquitoes, who had found the tightly packed European crew, with their water barrels and jugs, an ideal environment. The vessel made its way into the Caribbean, stopping at Barbados, St. Vincent, and Grenada in the spring of 1793; these ports meant further exchanges of European crew members and ship environments, and therefore both serious disease propagation and enlistment of more vulnerable European sailors. The *Hankey,* still riddled with *Aedes aegypti,* arrived on the coast of Haiti, in the midst of revolutionary turmoil, in June 1793. Its next stop was to be Philadelphia, for which it set off carrying white planters now fleeing the Haitian revolution.

HOW IT WAS UNDERSTOOD AT THE TIME

Eighteenth-century thinkers still tended to group fevers within one large category that did not assume separate disease entities. But, by the time of the 1790s epidemics, the symptoms of yellow fever had been widely recognized, and those symptoms gave the ailment a clearly separate standing. Especially notable in victims were vomiting, often black or bloody, jaundice (hence the "yellow"), and high fever that led to delirium.

But while agreement might be possible about the identity of the disease, controversy persisted about its origins. Did it arise (or only exist) in particular places? Or could it be carried, contagiously, from one place to another? Eighteenth-century opinion, including opinion of Europeans in the West Indies where yellow fever was rife, often awkwardly maintained both; fear of contagion was general, but so too was the conviction that yellow fever was only imported from some dangerous other place. Communities did not want to admit, even to themselves, that yellow fever was native to them.

Some observations about the disease were also widely accepted: its highly localized, often urban character; the vulnerability of strangers (in the Caribbean) to it; its prevalence among seamen in the tropics; and the apparent greater vulnerability of the dissolute and the intemperate.

RESPONSES

British and French physicians in the West Indies responded to yellow fever somewhat differently in the 1790s. The French approach, more modest, attempted to ease the dramatic symptoms of the disease with warm baths and herbal concoctions. The British—notably the Saint Domingue hospital inspectors Hector McLean and Robert Jackson—urged more heroic measures in the hope of righting what they felt to be humoral imbalance in the victims' systems. British responses occasionally included bleeding or blistering to remove blood; more often bile was removed with purgatives such as calomel or other mercury (or arsenic) compounds. Laudanum (the imprecisely defined mixture of alcohol and opium) was frequently employed to ease the pain of many ailments, including yellow fever. Alcohol was also specifically prescribed to revive faltering pulses. (The contrasting French and British approaches to yellow fever in the West Indies may also be seen in the contemporary United States; see volume 2, chapter 17.)

The use of alcohol—in one form or another—as a specific remedy contradicted another common belief of the time: that drunkenness and the dissipation that stemmed from it were themselves aggravating factors or even causes of yellow fever. Certainly, the dosing of yellow fever patients with alcohol contributed to the generally wretched nursing care that characterized the British military infirmaries in Saint Domingue and elsewhere in the Caribbean.

Although some contemporary opinion recognized that higher elevations might be healthier, military conventions (or necessity) often prevented moving barracks out of sea-level cities. By 1797, however, a British commander, John Simcoe, began dispersing his forces out of Port au Prince, and that move may have lowered mortality, if too late to save the occupation mission.

UNRESOLVED HISTORICAL ISSUES

The precise mortality that can be ascribed to yellow fever in Hispaniola in the period 1793–1804 remains unknown, largely because the identification of the ailment remained imprecise. Many fevers swept through the West Indies in the eighteenth century; these particular major epidemics might have been dominated by yellow fever (which certainly could have dramatic symptoms), but malaria and typhus (and others) probably played a role as well. The possibility of variations in the virulence of yellow fever remains another variable in the medical detection of these diseases: Were the decades of the 1770s and 1780s in the West Indies free of yellow fever because most of the resident population had already been exposed to a case of it, or because it became in those years a mild infection of which people took no notice? Did the epidemics after 1793 simply result from an influx of nonimmunes (the European armies), or did their arrival coincide with an emerging and more virulent virus? Knowledge of the mortality rates suffered by the African descendants on Hispaniola is very imprecise. Did they suffer more from yellow fever after 1793 than they had in the 1770s and 1780s?

Some of the answers to such questions have had to rely on contemporary testimony, and that testimony itself is sometimes suspect. For example, a French author claimed in 1794 that yellow fever did not exist in Saint Domingue until that year; it had to have been imported from somewhere else. In 1796, the British government, fearing the adverse effects of the truth on the recruitment of soldiers, understated the frightful death toll of its troops in Saint Domingue. And subsequent historians, realizing the faulty nature of that evidence, have sometimes erred in the direction of exaggeration.

Western approaches to yellow fever remained in turmoil for the remainder of the nineteenth century, and the experience of Hispaniola did not contribute to a long-term resolution of disputes. Some argued that the British imposition of heroic medicine in Saint Domingue had reduced the mortality rate, and—together with the contemporary Philadelphia experience—that justified bleeding and purging. Whether yellow fever was contagious or local remained in contention. If the disease was particular to certain places, the unpopular quarantines (harmful for commerce) could not be justified.

The Caribbean yellow fever epidemics of the late eighteenth and early nineteenth centuries played an important role in some larger events, although whether they alone were sufficient cause for those events must remain an unanswerable "what if?" of history. Britain and France, the great Western maritime powers, were successively forced to withdraw from Hispaniola and cede control of it to a rebellious population of ex-slaves. In so doing, France surrendered its most important colony, one that in the 1770s had provided about 60% of France's Caribbean traffic. More than that, Napoleon reportedly said: "I am today more sorry than I like to confess for the expedition to St. Domingue. . . . Our national glory will never come from our marine," and he determined to sell Louisiana to the United States (Kukla 2003, 254). The enterprise and determination of the leaders of the Saint Domingue slave revolt might have defeated the British and the French in any case, and the expanding United States might have forced the cession of Louisiana. But would those events have happened without the yellow fever epidemics?

REFERENCES

Kukla, Jon. *A Wilderness So Immense: The Louisiana Purchase and the Destiny of America.* New York: Knopf, 2003.

Palmer, R. R. *The Age of the Democratic Revolution: A Political History of Europe and America, 1760–1800.* Vol. 2, *The Struggle.* Princeton, NJ: Princeton University Press, 1964.

SUGGESTED ADDITIONAL READING

Dubois, Laurent. *Avengers of the New World: The Story of the Haitian Revolution.* Cambridge, MA: Belknap Press of Harvard University Press, 2004.

Geggus, David. *Slavery, War, and Revolution: The British Occupation of Saint Domingue, 1793–1789.* Oxford: Clarendon, 1982.

Geggus, David. "Yellow Fever in the 1790s: The British Army in Occupied Saint Domingue." *Medical History* 23 (1979): 38–58.

James, C. L. R. *The Black Jacobins: Toussaint L'Ouverture and the San Domingo Revolution.* 2nd ed. New York: Vintage, 1963.

Kiple, Kenneth F. *The Caribbean Slave: A Biological History.* Cambridge: Cambridge University Press, 1984.

McNeill, J. R. *Mosquito Empires: Ecology and War in the Greater Caribbean, 1620–1914.* Cambridge: Cambridge University Press, 2010.

Smith, Billy G. *Ship of Death: A Voyage that Changed the Atlantic World.* New Haven, CT: Yale University Press, 2013.

17

Yellow Fever in Philadelphia, 1793

WHEN AND WHERE

In July 1793, an epidemic of yellow fever began in Philadelphia, the capital of the new United States. Yellow fever evidently reached Philadelphia on ships (especially the *Hankey*; see volume 2, chapter 16) that carried people fleeing from a revolution in the French Caribbean colony of Saint Domingue (Haiti). The epidemic reached its height in September and October 1793, dying out by November. Modern scholars estimate Philadelphia's population in 1793 as about 51,000; in the months of the epidemic perhaps as many as 5,000 of them died. At least 20,000 people fled the city during the epidemic, so the proportion of deaths among those who remained was quite high.

The actual mortality from yellow fever remains uncertain. In many of the deaths thought due to other causes, yellow fever may have contributed to the victim's vulnerability, either directly or by its effects on the networks of care for the sick.

Some groups of the population suffered higher mortality rates than others. Since yellow fever is often a relatively mild infection for the young, adults were at greater risk. Since previous exposure can confer immunity, those who had come to Philadelphia from southern homes (in the United States, the Caribbean, or western Africa) where yellow fever was more common enjoyed some relative advantage. The poor suffered disproportionately, if only because poverty limited their ability to flee and their diets may have meant general weakness. And males were at greater risk than females, for reasons that remain uncertain.

SIGNIFICANCE

The fact that this epidemic struck the capital city of a new and revolutionary republic gave it unusual significance to contemporaries, who read into it a variety of symbolic meanings (see the "How It Was Understood at the Time" and "Unresolved Historical Issues" sections). Medical and political interpretations of both the cause of the epidemic and possible remedies for it consistently overlapped, so the Philadelphia yellow fever remains a good case study for the interactions of medicine and politics.

Explanations of and responses to the epidemic illustrate many of the themes of eighteenth-century Western thought, especially its faith in science and its convictions about the importance of environments. Those responses also illustrate some of the contentions about disease that characterized the time, when old conceptions had been discredited and a single new model had not replaced them.

The epidemic demonstrates the growing importance of the trade links between the north Atlantic coasts of North America and Europe and the tropics in the eighteenth century, trade links that also extended into the American interior. That trade brought the Western world in ever-closer contact with the pathogens of tropical diseases such as yellow fever, as well as more generally altering environments in tropical and temperate zones alike.

BACKGROUND

As Europeans and their North American cousins reached into the Caribbean and along the western coast of Africa in the sixteenth, seventeenth, and eighteenth centuries, they encountered the *Aedes aegypti* mosquitoes that carried the causative virus of yellow fever from its usual hosts (monkeys as well as people) from one person to another. Yellow fever was a common disease of the tropics, originating in Africa. In the seventeenth and eighteenth centuries, the Caribbean was the chief focus of yellow fever for Europeans, and the ports engaged in the trades (especially slaves and sugar) involving that sea repeatedly suffered yellow fever outbreaks. If yellow fever began among people aboard a ship from a Caribbean port, the disease could be transmitted (by mosquitoes) from one person to another during the voyage, and thus reach a northern port. Yellow fever had broken out in Philadelphia as early as 1690 (only a few years after the city's original settlement); a yellow fever epidemic in 1699 took a higher toll (proportionally) than that of 1793. There had been periodic epidemics until 1762, and then there were 30 epidemic-free years, so that the population in 1793 had a high proportion of people without previous exposure. Yellow fever persisted in Philadelphia after 1793; the years between 1797 and 1799, for example, again saw serious mortality rates, while the disease also spread to other cities along the Atlantic seaboard.

HOW IT WAS UNDERSTOOD AT THE TIME

By the eighteenth century, the gruesome symptoms of yellow fever were well known in the Western world. Disturbing colors presented themselves: yellow eyes and skin, purple blotches under the skin where internal hemorrhages occurred, and black stools and vomit. High fever accompanied this colorful display, and death frequently followed. But the conception of a disease as a separate, discrete entity was less clear; might—for example—there exist degrees of "yellow fever," that might shade off into something else entirely?

Physicians also widely differed in their understandings of the fever's origins and causes, as well as therapies to be applied. Some believed that yellow fever arose from a troubled local atmosphere, a miasma; such a theory coincided well with more general eighteenth-century convictions about the importance of environments. Others believed that it passed contagiously from one person to another, and that its point of origin might therefore be some distance away from the site of the epidemic. Between these local miasma and contagion-over-a-distance theories ran a continuum of ideas that tried to incorporate elements of both.

In the 1793 Philadelphia epidemic these theories of origin very quickly became enmeshed in political controversy. The followers of Thomas Jefferson (coming to be called Democratic Republicans) distrusted city life in the new United States and so naturally concluded that the foul air (miasma) of the capital accounted for the disease. Their opponents, led by Alexander Hamilton (and called Federalists), feared the radical influence of the French Revolution on the new country and so blamed the disease on its importation from the French West Indies, especially Saint Domingue (Haiti) from whence contagious refugees had recently arrived.

Disagreement also marked thinking about the immediate cause of the body's symptoms. Did they result from an imbalance of the traditional humors? The yellow color of the skin and eyes certainly called attention to yellow bile, one of the ancient humours, and the black stools and vomit suggested an abundance of another, black bile. But modern thinking had been moving away from those ancient beliefs, and some physicians saw diseases arising from a disorder of solid tissues (such as blood vessels) rather than of the fluids (or humours) that coursed through them. Did yellow fever cause an overstimulation of the blood vessels?

These different theories of cause related to different possible therapies, as the next section ("Responses") discusses. But many other beliefs about yellow fever circulated through Philadelphia in 1793. Some called on other, new scientific ideas. Philadelphia was, of course, the home of Benjamin Franklin, who in addition to being a preeminent political figure of the early republic had also been one of the pioneers of electrical science. Might yellow fever be the product of atmospheric electricity? Still others insisted that God was punishing the city or the new nation for its sins.

And other contemporaries saw a racial component in yellow fever, noticing that African Americans seemed to have lower rates of infection. (It is likely that African Americans did experience lower rates of infection, but the explanation of that lay not in race but in past place of residence; those—whether white or black—who had spent their youth in southern latitudes were more likely to have gained immunity from a childhood exposure.)

RESPONSES

The most dramatic and immediate response to the yellow fever epidemic was flight. As many as 20,000 people—about 40% of the population—may have left the city while yellow fever raged. Those left behind included a higher proportion of the city's poor (whose living quarters adjoined the docks where the lethal ships lay, and who lacked the means to flee) and most of the city's African Americans (who performed a large share of the caregiving services that survived). And while flight may have been largely instinctive or unthinking, it in fact represented the surest chance of survival.

Other responses varied, and as is generally true in epidemics, depended on understandings of the origins or cause of the disease. Those who believed that yellow fever was imported from abroad—and more particularly from the French West Indies—called for a quarantine on traffic from those infected places. Within the eastern United States, quarantines were proclaimed against Philadelphia travelers and Philadelphia goods. Such internal quarantines might also appeal to those who feared the filth of the city and the possibility that its miasma might be spread elsewhere, an illustration of the ways in which theories of miasma and contagion from abroad might in practice overlap.

Strong believers in the role of miasma demanded a cleansing of the city. Some sanitation efforts commenced, but they were hampered both by a lack of resources (the hard-pressed city government had more immediate worries, including depletion of any possible sanitation workforce), and by the difficulty of knowing just what part of the environment (earth, air, water) needed attention. Particular complaints arose about a pile of coffee that rotted on a pier where it had been unloaded, but (apparently) no attempt was made to remove it. And one of the more bizarre theories called for firing guns into the air in the belief that such actions would help purify the atmosphere.

Some later opinion argued that during the epidemic the government of the city largely collapsed, and it is certainly true that the institutions of the federal government closed down and its members scattered. But some elements of the city government, with the assistance of an ad hoc citizens' board, successfully commandeered property for an isolation hospital, as well as an orphanage made necessary by the deaths of so many parents.

For many, the appropriate responses to the epidemic were prayer and appeals for divine mercy and forgiveness. But physicians claimed an important role as well, and their therapies depended on their views of cause. Benjamin Rush (1745–1813) occupied a particularly important place in Philadelphia's responses to yellow fever. Rush, prominent in the American Revolution and signer of the Declaration of Independence, was a leading Republican. The 1793 yellow fever epidemic strengthened his conviction (consistent with Republican principles) that the disease originated in a miasma, not from an imported contagion. It also confirmed his belief that yellow fever could best be treated by bleeding the veins and purging the bowels. In some cases, he proposed the removal of a high proportion (perhaps as much as 80%!) of the blood in the body. He also prescribed purgatives (especially calomel, a mercury compound) to empty the bowels. Rush's therapy, while based on a *solidist* interpretation of disease that saw overstimulated solid tissues at the root of fevers, in fact simply exaggerated that proposed by traditional humoral medicine.

Not everyone agreed with Rush's heroic measures. Some physicians favored a gentler therapeutic regimen that employed doses of cinchona bark and wine. And Rush's therapy was associated with Republican politics; therefore, the gentler alternative was Federalist medicine. Many physicians, however, fell between those two poles, employing bleeding, purging, and gentler stimulants and relaxants in different proportions. All the arguments, whether solidist or humoral, contained significant overlaps.

UNRESOLVED HISTORICAL ISSUES

Almost immediately after the 1793 Philadelphia yellow fever epidemic abated, a retrospective account of it appeared that framed later understandings of it. Mathew Carey, a Philadelphia printer, published his *A Short Account of the Malignant Fever lately Prevalent in Philadelphia* in early 1794. Carey saw the epidemic as a retribution for a people who had become luxuriously corrupt in the wake of the successful war for independence. As the epidemic proceeded, the heroic efforts of citizens such as the mayor, Matthew Clarkson, redeemed the city; civic virtue was reborn in the pressure of the tragedy. Carey also slighted the contributions (and sufferings) of the city's African Americans. For nearly two centuries, Carey's narrative dominated historical understanding of the epidemic. More recent historical accounts have attempted to present other perspectives, including those offered by another contemporary account, *A Narrative of the Proceedings of the Black People, during the Late Awful Calamity in Philadelphia*, by Absalom Jones and Richard Allen.

The political significance of the epidemic remains a subject of historical debate. John Adams, then the vice president, believed that the epidemic fatally weakened a Republican move for power and a potential revolution inspired by radical France. That extreme view of the epidemic's political impact has been debated by historians, who have softened the outline of political effects and raised other possibilities, including the weakening of Philadelphia's political and cultural primacy in the country.

Philadelphia's political leaders learned the importance of nursing care from the epidemic and attempted to provide it more carefully in the later epidemics of the 1790s. They also associated the prevention of yellow fever with sanitation and attempted to improve sanitary conditions. Rush's prestige in American medicine grew, and the measures he advocated in 1793 gave their name—Heroic—to a whole period of U.S. medical practice, when (in the early decades of the nineteenth century) physicians routinely prescribed violent bleedings and purgings.

Yellow fever remained a serious menace in U.S. cities through the nineteenth century, but it came to focus more on cities in the southern states—perhaps as trade from the Caribbean shifted more to such places as New Orleans. An understanding of the connections between the causative organism and a species of mosquito, *Aedes aegypti*, emerged in the last decades of the nineteenth century.

REFERENCE

Proceedings of the Black People, during the Late Awful Calamity in Philadelphia. Philadelphia: Independence National Historical Park. Reprint of 1794 pamphlet.

SUGGESTED ADDITIONAL READING

Estes, J. Worth, and Billy G. Smith, eds. *A Melancholy Scene of Devastation: The Public Response to the 1793 Philadelphia Yellow Fever Epidemic.* Canton, MA: Science History Publications, 1997.

Powell, J. H. *Bring Out Your Dead: The Great Plague of Yellow Fever in Philadelphia in 1793.* Philadelphia: University of Pennsylvania Press, 1949.

Smith, Billy G. *Ship of Death: A Voyage that Changed the Atlantic World.* New Haven, CT: Yale University Press, 2013.

18

Epidemics in the Napoleonic Wars, 1797–1815

WHEN AND WHERE

Repeated epidemics occurred in Europe during the prolonged periods of war that grew out of the epic French Revolution of 1789–1799 and the succeeding rise to power of Napoleon Bonaparte in 1799–1815. Those epidemics further illustrated the intimate relation between early modern warfare and epidemic disease. (See volume 1, chapter 10, and volume 2, chapter 8.)

By the late eighteenth century, European armies were less mercenary, more under the control of established governments, and hence under better discipline. They were perhaps less likely to pose safety or health hazards to civilians in the course of a campaign, although sieges continued to pose great danger to the besieged. And armies remained often poorly washed and nourished, and—with no clear understanding of the relation between dirt and disease—likely infested with lice. Typhus, as in the seventeenth century, was a constant danger. Plague had largely receded from at least western Europe, but dysentery and diarrhea remained. And the increased firepower of weaponry magnified the risk of septic infection.

Diseases especially followed regions of active military campaigns. In the 1790s, they concentrated in northern France, the adjoining Low Countries, and northern Italy. Napoleon's activities in the years after 1799 involved central German states, Moravia and Austria, Saxony, Prussia, Portugal, and northern Spain, and (most dramatically) his invasion from Lithuania into Russia.

As in the seventeenth century, the difficulties of separating epidemics from both the more general ravages of war and from continuing endemic mortalities frustrate any simple narrative of "an epidemic." Specific illustrative examples will follow:

1. Between 1806 and 1808, French military hospitals treated 421,000 patients. In 1807, the most serious of those years of warfare, only one-fourth of those suffered wounds, while illness accounted for the remainder. In the years between 1793 and 1815, British armies incurred 240,000 deaths, of whom only 27,000

fell in battle. Diseases led to two-thirds of the deaths in Wellington's armies between January 1811 and May 1814 (Muir 1998, 9).

2. More specifically, in Wellington's 1812 campaigns in Spain, 905 of his soldiers died of wounds, 35 suffered from gangrene, 4 from tetanus, while typhus felled 999 and dysentery a staggering 2,340 (Muir 1998, 299, n. 36).
3. Napoleon set off with perhaps 600,000 troops in his 1812 invasion of Russia. Although any estimate must be very imprecise, of that vast horde about 300,000 died from disease and related exposures and hardships (Muir 1998, 276, n. 18).
4. In the so-called Battle of the Nations fought at Leipzig in October 1813, perhaps 36,000 sick and wounded soldiers poured into the city, spreading contagion as they came; as they died, more followed, while the surrounding countryside had been devastated by pillaging that left surviving inhabitants impoverished, defenseless, and at the mercy of pathogens as winter set in. And the battered retreating French army carried "hundreds of wagons filled with unhappy wounded men who had no medical care since Leipzig . . . packed in with them were sick men suffering from dysentery, typhus fever, etc., almost all of them succumbing to inanition, weakness, and filth, as well as disease . . . with the result that they infected all the towns and villages along their route," thus conveying diseases and misery from Saxony back into northern France (Muir 1998, 264–265; quoted in Talty 2009, 264).

SIGNIFICANCE

While the wars of 1792–1815 offered vivid examples of significant loss of life from the confluence of violence and disease (as had the Thirty Years' War), the more prosperous and strongly governed states could now avert or cushion serious demographic collapse of the seventeenth-century sort. It also remains unclear to what extent disease was decisive in the outcome of any specific battle or campaign, but certainly any military history that neglects its effects is incomplete or misleading.

BACKGROUND

Warfare in the French Revolutionary and Napoleonic age remained hazardous to a population's health, and several new elements contributed to those dangers. Armies by the eighteenth century were generally better disciplined than their seventeenth-century predecessors, while the weapons with which they fought had not become significantly more destructive. What had changed were the scale of fighting, the size of armies, and their dramatically heightened zeal for victory. The French revolutionary governments had proclaimed a *levée en masse* that potentially could conscript the entire population for war, fought by citizens in defense of their ideals (or to extend their benefits to others). By 1812 Napoleon could assemble an army of about 600,000 troops, vastly larger than any force seen in previous

Western history. If it became disease-ridden, it therefore posed a proportionally greater risk of infection to whatever noncombatant population it encountered.

While some cities had benefited from central planning and improved building materials, they still suffered from haphazard methods of disposing human wastes. Their greater size simply magnified the dangers of waterborne disease, while urban density promoted person-to-person contagion. Rural populations were relatively defenseless in the presence of an army, which could move among the countryside with little hindrance from the walls and fortifications that might shelter cities.

HOW IT WAS UNDERSTOOD AT THE TIME

Central to the contemporary understanding of these epidemics was the persistent belief that "fevers" existed along a continuum and were thus not discrete entities. "Typhus" had many different names, sometimes called "famine fever," "hunger fever," "jail fever," "relapsing fever," the last term applied to an ailment that subsequently became recognized as distinct from typhus. The cause (or causes) of these fevers remained unknown, although in the Napoleonic world the dominant belief favored the role of "miasma," a corruption of the air, as opposed to "contagion" that spread from one victim to another. Once the fever had taken hold in a community, contagion was evidently involved, but it remained unclear just what agent passed the fever from one to another.

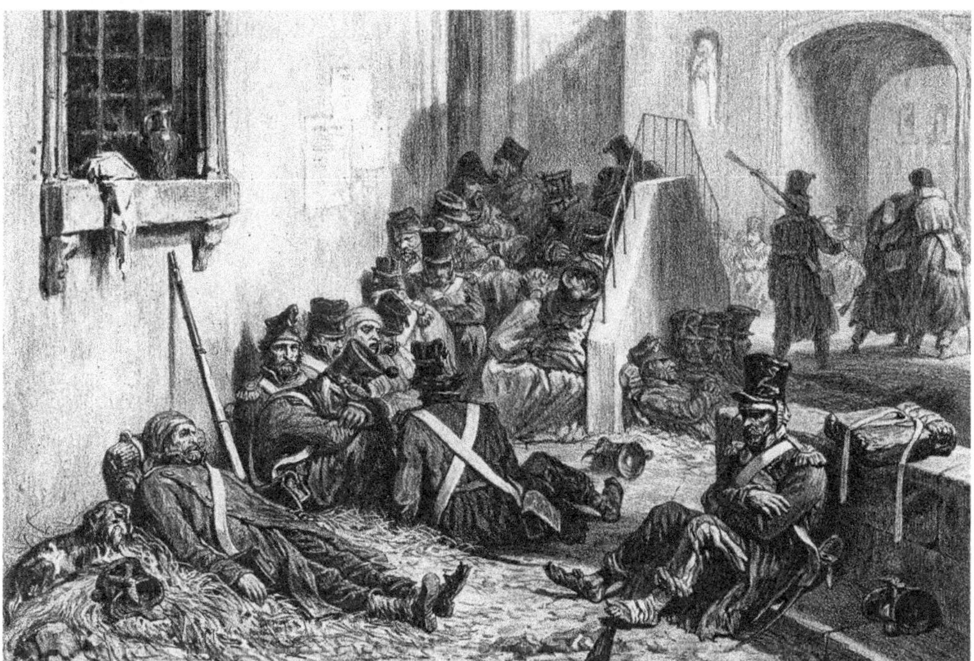

French soldiers suffering from typhus, lying in the streets of Mainz, Germany, during the Napoleonic Wars. (Wellcome Library)

RESPONSES

In military hospitals in the wake of a battle, wounds attracted immediate attention, being treated hastily, brutally, without any anesthetic relief apart from alcohol or laudanum, and with little or no attention to sanitation. Those of the wounded who survived that experience would remain in the crowded facility until recovery, joining a pool of those already infected by typhus or dysentery. Thus, the hospital itself could become a site of epidemic diffusion, both within its walls and in the surrounding regions.

In treating the diseases themselves, doctors (in or out of hospitals) continued to demonstrate that while the theoretical bases of humoral medicine had long been undercut, in practice therapies continued to rely on adjustments of the bodily fluids through bleeding and purging. The rashes that marked typhus called for bleeding; dysentery and diarrhea simply meant more purging. Some physicians might have recourse to herbal remedies for the relief of pain.

UNRESOLVED HISTORICAL ISSUES

As long as the cause of typhus remained uncertain, the disease would continue to haunt unsanitary situations where human lice could proliferate in dense human populations. Such conditions made typhus (and relapsing fever) major causes of death in the great Irish famine years of 1846–1850 and the local violence that accompanied the European revolutions of 1848–1849, for example. Although the transmission of typhus was successfully traced to an insect vector—the human louse—by Charles Nicolle in 1909–1910, the chaos of World War I meant that attempts to eradicate that insect vector would—and did—falter, and typhus thus remained (especially in eastern Europe) a major killer during and after the war.

REFERENCES

Muir, Rory. *Tactics and the Experience of Battle in the Age of Napoleon.* New Haven, CT: Yale University Press, 1998.

Talty, Stephan. *The Illustrious Dead: The Terrifying Story of How Typhus Killed Napoleon's Greatest Army.* New York: Three Rivers Press, 2009.

SUGGESTED ADDITIONAL READING

Horne, Alistair. *How Far from Austerlitz? Napoleon, 1805–1815.* New York: St. Martin's Press, 1996.

O Grada, Cormac. *Ireland before and after the Famine.* 2nd ed. Manchester: Manchester University Press, 1993.

Raoult, Didier, Olivier Dutour, Linda Houhamdi, Rimantas Jankauskas, Pierre-Edouard Fournier, Yann Ardagna, Michel Drancourt, et al. "Evidence for Louse-Transmitted Diseases in Soldiers of Napoleon's Grand Army in Vilnius." *Journal of Infectious Diseases* 1, no. 193 (January 2006): 112–120.

Zinsser, Hans. *Rats, Lice and History.* New York: Bantam Books, 1960. (Orig. ed. Boston: Little, Brown, 1935.)

19

Consumption in the Nineteenth Century

WHEN AND WHERE

In the nineteenth-century Western world, a disease most often called *consumption* was consistently the greatest single killer. Its peak mortality, reached at different times in different places, frequently exceeded 300 deaths per 100,000 people per year. (Only in its worst years, and only in a few places, did cholera mortality approach or exceed that figure in the West.) That disease went by several different names during the century: consumption, phthisis, and tuberculosis. Consumption was perhaps most frequently used earlier in the century, and tuberculosis gradually supplanted it as the century went on.

It is important to understand, however, that those terms do not necessarily refer to the same disease. "Consumption" and "phthisis" meant a wasting disease of the lungs and chest. *Tuberculosis* came to mean a disease involving a specific causative organism, *Mycobacterium tuberculosis*, especially when that organism affected the lungs. It is probable that many—perhaps most—of the cases of consumption did involve infection by that microorganism. But some may have been what later generations would call silicosis or even lung cancer, while some other diseases not associated with consumption at all (such as scrofula) did involve infection by *Mycobacterium tuberculosis*.

Consumption, whatever it was called, had been a major disease for several centuries before the nineteenth. Some factors to be discussed later (see the "Significance" and "Background" sections) suggest that it reached a peak in Europe in the nineteenth century, although reliable figures for its incidence really only begin in the years after about 1850. Those figures show that its decline began in Belgium (for example) in the 1860s, and in England in about 1870. The timing of that decline varied widely from country to country, and even from region to region within a country. The reasons for those variations are discussed later in this chapter; generally, declines in tuberculosis incidence occurred earliest in the most developed economies. But note again that those declines illustrate a change in tuberculosis incidence, not necessarily equivalent to consumption.

SIGNIFICANCE

Much of the significance of consumption at its height was cultural, although it was a preeminent killer. In the early nineteenth century, consumption was a major component of romanticism; death from consumption figured frequently in both the lives of the artists of the Romantic period, and in the artistic representations of suffering and death that those artists produced. Consumption was the disease that struck down the young, the gifted, and the beautiful. Percy Shelley wrote to the consumptive John Keats: "This consumption is a disease particularly fond of people who write such good verses as you have done" (Rollins 1965, 57). In fact, as René and Jean Dubos (1987) pointed out, the pale, wan, frail look of the consumptive became in the early and middle nineteenth century an ideal of beauty that the florid, the heavy, and the entirely healthy envied.

But as the nineteenth century wore on, other conceptions of the consumptive complicated the picture, as its associations with poverty, deprivation, and (perhaps) moral failure became more frequent. In the early part of the century, consumption was almost fashionable; by the latter part, tuberculosis was almost shameful. The evolution of the ways in which society constructed this disease, or gave it its meaning, forms another part of the epidemic's significance. Consumption and tuberculosis are cases that illustrate, with great clarity, the ways in which diseases are in part biological and pathological, and in part phenomena created by particular societies in particular places and times.

BACKGROUND

In modern understanding, the disease tuberculosis depends on the infection of the body by the microorganism *Mycobacterium tuberculosis.* This organism is airborne and easily transmitted from one person to another through the respiratory system. Infection, however, while necessary for tuberculosis, is not a sufficient explanation for the development of the clinical symptoms of the disease. Many people may be infected by the organism and remain healthy all their lives, betraying no signs of tuberculosis. Within their bodies, the infection is in effect walled off. In fact, some historians have speculated that almost everyone in nineteenth-century Europe was infected in that sense. In some infected individuals, however, the microorganisms are not contained, but spread into the body's organs. When the organs affected are the lungs, pulmonary tuberculosis results; that is the best-known form of the disease, and the one that certainly often lay behind consumption, but other organs may be affected as well. Why do some of the infected become tubercular? Why, that is, are their bodies unable to resist the spread of the microorganism? To answer that question, modern thinkers have considered a wide range of possibilities without being able to narrow that range. Those possibilities were also considered in the nineteenth century before the idea of the role of a *germ* entered the picture. (They are reviewed in the next section "How It Was Understood at the Time.")

We now believe that tuberculosis has been a human disease since the earliest stages of humanity's past and that its symptoms attracted the attention of writers of ancient Mediterranean, Chinese, and Indian civilizations. Probably always present, its importance in the Western world grew from the fourteenth or fifteenth century into the nineteenth. In the nineteenth century, social and economic conditions were favorable for both the spread of infection by the tuberculosis microorganism and the development of clinical cases of tuberculosis among those infected, thus, the rise of consumption as a nineteenth-century epidemic. Some of the nineteenth-century conditions that favored rapid infection by an airborne organism included the dramatic growth of congested cities in Europe; hastily constructed housing in those cities, which meant confined and sometimes windowless living quarters; smoky or fetid urban atmospheres that discouraged exposure to fresh air; crowded workplaces that brought large numbers of employees together under one roof, sometimes poorly ventilated; and the spread of state systems of compulsory education, which brought children together in crowded classrooms.

Some aspects of nineteenth-century urban life may have reduced human capacities to resist the breakout of the bacillus into the lungs. Diets for many lacked variety and quantity. Urban life, especially for newcomers, may have meant unusual levels of stress. More generally, poverty brought with it many of the possible conditions that made consumption more likely, and while historians have vigorously debated the standards of living of the nineteenth-century urban working classes, there is little doubt that many of those classes were very poor. One of the reasons that the disease's incidence began lessening late in the century may be that living conditions improved for at least some people.

HOW IT WAS UNDERSTOOD AT THE TIME

In the eighteenth and early nineteenth centuries, people understood consumption as a weakening, wasting, more or less gradually acting disease that affected the lungs, the chest, and the ability to breathe. Signs included a worsening pallor, frequent coughing, and the spitting-up of blood. And by the eighteenth century, autopsies had provided some understanding of the disease's pathology. Lesions, or tubercles, formed on lung tissue, and could be seen as the immediate cause of the progressive failure of the respiratory system.

But what caused such lesions to form? Why did they form in some people and not others? Eighteenth- and early nineteenth-century thinkers considered three broad possibilities, without reaching any sort of consensus about them: heredity, contagion, and irritation of the lung tissue. Consumption certainly ran through certain families, but did simple hereditary weakness explain that, or did the infected members of the family pass the disease on to others under the same roof? Examples of both possibilities abounded; while believers in one or the other could be found in all corners of the Western world, the theory of contagious consumption was more widely held in southern Europe, especially Italy.

The theories of heredity and contagion were both very old, while the "irritation of the tissue" theory was originally a product of the interest in mechanical philosophy that developed in the middle and late seventeenth century. That philosophy held that mechanical actions—pushes and pulls of one body or substance against another body or substance—accounted for all the changes in the natural world; one thing moved because another thing pushed it. If lesions were found on lung tissue, something—perhaps dirt particles or foul air—must have irritated that tissue. As the "irritation" explanation developed in the eighteenth century, other, less mechanical, possible irritants were considered as well, notably the effects of stress or exhaustion on the lung tissue.

Consumption was clearly a disease of weakness, and part of its explanation might focus on classes or groups of people who were naturally weak. In the eighteenth and early nineteenth century the weakness of one population—women—stood out as a marker for consumption. While certainly men suffered from it as well, women were thought to be especially vulnerable. Later in the nineteenth century, race and social class joined gender as explanations of why some were more prone to consumption. In the United States, African Americans were thought susceptible; in Europe, it was the lower or poorer classes. (As indeed they were, at least statistically. But were African Americans, or the European poor, naturally consumptive, or did environmental circumstances make them so?)

But for a time at least consumption was associated with gentility, not with poverty. According to a popular 1830 American medical writer: "Consumption spreads its ravages in the haunts of gaiety, fashion, and folly—but in the more humble walks of life where the busy hum of laborious industry is heard, it is seldom known" (Gunn 1986, 161).

RESPONSES

Consumption was a long-lasting, chronic disease. Physicians and others who treated it could advise a wide range of gradual palliatives without the pressure of demand for an immediate cure. Causal theories dictated most of those measures. If, for example, irritation of the lungs arose from dirty air, the sufferer should move to better air; so, by the late eighteenth century, sea air was often recommended, found either by residing on the seacoast or by taking an ocean voyage. By the mid-nineteenth century, the pure air of mountains became another favorite locale for the consumptive. These "find better air" solutions obviously applied chiefly to people with ample means.

If stress or exhaustion were the cause, then the solution—rest and relaxation—again applied mostly to those who could afford it. In the course of the nineteenth century, the sanatorium—a place of rest and relaxation (and perhaps healthful exercise as well) located in pure mountain or bracing sea air—emerged as a major response to consumption. The earliest such institution began at the end of the eighteenth century, but the sanatoria only spread rapidly after the 1850s, when Herman Brehmer opened a widely copied institution in Silesia. In subsequent decades, many other sanatoria were founded in both Europe and North America, all of them claiming the benefits of mountain or sea air for the consumptive patient. Their leaders did not agree, however, on the merits of rest or exercise. Brehmer originally believed that the weakness of the consumptive patient should be countered by a vigorous program of exercise; others (such as the American sanatorium leader Edward L. Trudeau) insisted on rest, a view with which Brehmer himself eventually agreed.

The practices of the sanatoria reflected another gradual change toward the end of the nineteenth century, as consumption, with its romantic overtones, gave way to "tuberculosis," which was associated more and more with poverty and even moral failure. In addition to providing rest, relaxation, or exercise, sanatoria (especially those in Britain and the United States) undertook to improve the habits of their inmates. Poverty was seen as the cause of tuberculosis, either directly (though the weakening of the body) or by bringing the victims into a hazardous environment of poor and confined air; training people in good work habits might in turn prevent tuberculosis by enabling them to better their standard of living. Some sanatoria therefore became corrective reformatories for the lazy.

The romantic image of consumption persisted, however, while that other (and more censorious) picture emerged. Henri Murger's *Scènes de la vie de Bohemè*, a story of the Bohemian life of Parisian artists, appeared in 1849, when its consumptive heroine illustrated the romantic view of the disease. But the story still resonated in 1896, when Giacomo Puccini's *La Bohemè*, a popular opera based on the story, was first performed.

To provide more immediate relief of the symptoms of consumption, physicians, other healers, and the general public had recourse to a very wide collection of remedies, in addition to the provision of a healthier environment. Because so many conceptions of the cause of the disease coexisted, and because consumption seemed to manifest such a variety of symptoms, a corresponding variety of therapies existed as well. Many were dietetic, urging (especially) the consumption of meat and dairy products. Cod liver oil enjoyed great popularity; so too did opium, or the tincture of opium and alcohol called laudanum, widely used for pain relief.

UNRESOLVED HISTORICAL ISSUES

During the nineteenth century, the immediate cause of consumption remained a subject of debate. In 1882 the German physician and microbiologist Robert Koch announced the discovery of a microorganism, the tubercle bacillus, that he claimed was responsible for the disease tuberculosis. This discovery came at a time when the germ theory, holding that specific microorganisms caused specific diseases, was rapidly making converts, thanks to the work of Koch and the French chemist Louis Pasteur. In fact, Koch's announcement of the tubercle bacillus was perhaps the greatest triumph of the new approach, since it apparently ended the mystery surrounding the century's most consistent killer. But Koch's discovery did not end the discussion of cause, for belief in general environmental or hereditary explanations of disease remained widely shared, and not just about tuberculosis. Koch's discovery of the cholera microbe was similarly resisted. Surely a violent ailment such as cholera, or a disease that ravaged the body such as tuberculosis, could not be solely the product of a microscopic germ. Other factors—the "soil" on which the "seed" fell—must play a role. Opponents of germ theory might concede that Koch's bacillus was a *necessary* cause of the disease, but not a *sufficient* one. And, as the "Background" section suggests, they were correct. When a test for the presence of the germ was developed (the tuberculin test, which grew out of an unsuccessful attempt by Koch to produce a vaccine for tuberculosis), many of those who tested positive (that is, infected by the bacillus) never developed disease symptoms.

Questions therefore remained about the most effective way to attack the disease. If the microorganism (eventually called *Mycobacterium tuberculosis*) were seen as primary, then bacteriological testing of individuals and the isolation of the positives to prevent the disease's spread were the proper responses. Ultimate success depended on eradicating the germ. But if the "soil" played an important role, then a broader attack on the social and economic factors that weakened the population was needed: environment, diets, housing, working conditions; physicians who treated those with symptoms, not bacteriologists who tested blood, would dominate.

In addition to the questions remaining unresolved at the end of the nineteenth century, consumption also poses one of the major unsettled questions in the history of human disease: Why did its incidence decline across most of the Western world between about 1870 and 1920? Did conscious human action against disease have any significant effect? It is generally agreed that explicit medical action, whether of prevention or cure, had little impact on the incidence or mortality of tuberculosis before the 1920s. The possible exception, which may have had an effect in some places, was the isolation of sufferers in sanatoria (and in Britain, in workhouses for the sick poor). That isolation may have reduced the airborne transmission of the germs from the sick to the healthy. But the number of consumptives so isolated was always a clear minority of the total body of the sick; most sanatoria catered to the well-to-do, and most of the sick were poor.

Improvements in living conditions provide a more likely explanation for the fall in tuberculosis mortality in the late nineteenth and early twentieth centuries. The British medical historian Thomas McKeown, in a series of books and articles, has argued very strongly that improvements in diets lay behind declining death rates in the period, including the decline in tuberculosis. Better nutrition, made possible by a combination of perhaps higher income levels, the opening of new agricultural lands, and a variety of changes in transportation and food preservation, may have enabled more people to remain healthy even when infected by tuberculosis germs. Not all scholars agree with McKeown, and they have doubted how widespread improvements in diet were, and added other possible explanations. By the late nineteenth century, some of the horrors of living in early industrial cities had been reduced; housing was more spacious and better ventilated, workplaces were perhaps more healthful than they had been, and any improvement in the quality of a city's air made it more likely that its residents would willingly open their windows. All those factors may have removed people from close and confined contact with others, and so reduced the chance of infection. The rapidly falling birth rates that characterized the developed industrial societies of western Europe and North America in the period may have played a role as well. Smaller families meant more resources for nutrition and less congested housing; fewer pregnancies meant greater powers of resistance for women.

The decline in tuberculosis that began in the late nineteenth century continued in the years after 1920 and became very steep after about 1950. In those years, deliberate medical intervention began to have an effect. The first moderately successful tuberculosis vaccine, BCG (*Bacille Calmette-Guérin*), began to be used in some countries (but not much in the United States and Britain) in the 1920s; after about 1950, antibiotics (especially streptomycin) emerged as dramatic cures for the disease, which subsequently seemed a thing of the past in the developed countries of the world.

But by the late twentieth century, tuberculosis was again one of the great killer diseases in the world, a development discussed in chapter 44 in this volume.

REFERENCES

Dubos, René, and Jean Dubos. *The White Plague: Tuberculosis, Man, and Society.* New Brunswick, NJ: Rutgers University Press, 1987. Reprint of a 1952 edition.

Gunn, John. *Gunn's Domestic Medicine.* Knoxville: University of Tennessee Press, 1986. Reprint of an 1830 edition.

Rollins, Hyder Edward, ed. *The Keats Circle: Letters and Papers and More Letters and Poems of the Keats Circle.* Cambridge, MA: Harvard University Press, 1965.

SUGGESTED ADDITIONAL READING

Barnes, David S. *The Making of a Social Disease: Tuberculosis in Nineteenth-Century France.* Berkeley: University of California Press, 1995.

Bates, Barbara. *Bargaining for Life: A Social History of Tuberculosis, 1876–1938.* Philadelphia: University of Pennsylvania Press, 1992.

Bynum, Helen. *Spitting Blood: The History of Tuberculosis.* Oxford: Oxford University Press, 2012.

de Almeida, Hermione. *Romantic Medicine and John Keats.* New York: Oxford University Press, 1991.

Feldberg, Georgina D. *Disease and Class: Tuberculosis and the Shaping of Modern North American Society.* New Brunswick, NJ: Rutgers University Press, 1996.

Hardy, Anne. *The Epidemic Streets: Infectious Disease and the Rise of Preventive Medicine, 1856–1900.* Oxford: Clarendon, 1993.

McKeown, Thomas. *The Modern Rise of Population.* New York: Academic Press, 1976.

Rothman, Sheila M. *Living in the Shadow of Death: Tuberculosis and the Social Experience of Illness in American History.* New York: Basic, 1994.

Smith, F. B. *The Retreat of Tuberculosis, 1850–1950.* London: Croom Helm, 1988.

Worboys, Michael. *Spreading Germs: Disease Theories and Medical Practice in Britain, 1865–1900.* Cambridge: Cambridge University Press, 2000.

Among the many contemporary accounts of "romantic" tubercular deaths are the following:

Dumas, Alexandre, *fils. The Lady of the Camellias.* Translated by Edmund Gosse. New York: P. F. Collier and Son, 1902. *A novel (originally published in 1848), in which pp. 318–323 describe the death of the title character.*

Huneker, James. *Chopin: The Man and His Music.* New York: Charles Scribner's Sons, 1927. *A biography that reprints (pp. 78–84) the letters of Fr. Alexander Jelowicki, recalling Chopin's final illness and death in 1849.*

20

First Cholera Pandemic, 1817–1824

WHEN AND WHERE

In 1817 cholera (or, as some Europeans called it, *Asiatic cholera*) began spreading beyond the areas of India where it had long been endemic, especially Bengal and the Ganges River delta. A serious outbreak in Calcutta (in Bengal) began in September 1817; within a year, the disease had spread to other places on the Indian subcontinent. Bombay experienced an epidemic in the summer of 1818. By March 1820, Siam (Thailand) was affected, beginning in Penang and then, in May 1820, in Bangkok. Manila, in the Philippines, suffered from cholera in 1820 as well. In the spring of 1821 cholera reached Java; in the same year, it appeared both in western Asia, first at Oman, and in eastern Asia, affecting Anhai in China. From those outposts, cholera advanced in 1822: in the east into Japan, via the port of Nagasaki, moving through much of western Honshu between Hiroshima and Osaka; in the west, into the Persian Gulf, up the Mesopotamian river valleys to Baghdad, from there into Syria. Persia was affected, and from there cholera moved into the Transcaucasus. By September 1823, cholera had reached Astrakhan, at the mouth of the Volga in the Russian Empire. Islands in the Indian Ocean—Zanzibar and Mauritius—were affected as well.

Although cholera epidemics persisted in some of these areas into 1824 (e.g., in Java), the pandemic seems to have halted by that year. Perhaps cold weather in the winter of 1823–1824 (in places such as central Japan and the Volga basin) prevented its advance into those areas. While the total death toll from the pandemic is not known, its depredations in some places were very severe. The Siamese capital, Bangkok, may have suffered 30,000 deaths (in a city population of about 150,000) in 1820. In the city of Semarang, in northern Java, 1,225 people died in 11 days in April 1821, and for the entire island of Java mortality for the year 1821 was estimated at 125,000 above normal. An early twentieth-century writer called this epidemic "probably the most terrible of all Indian cholera epidemics" (Rogers 1928, 8).

The vast majority of those affected by the first cholera pandemic were Asians. Cholera did disrupt the important military campaigns that extended British

First Cholera Pandemic, 1817–1824

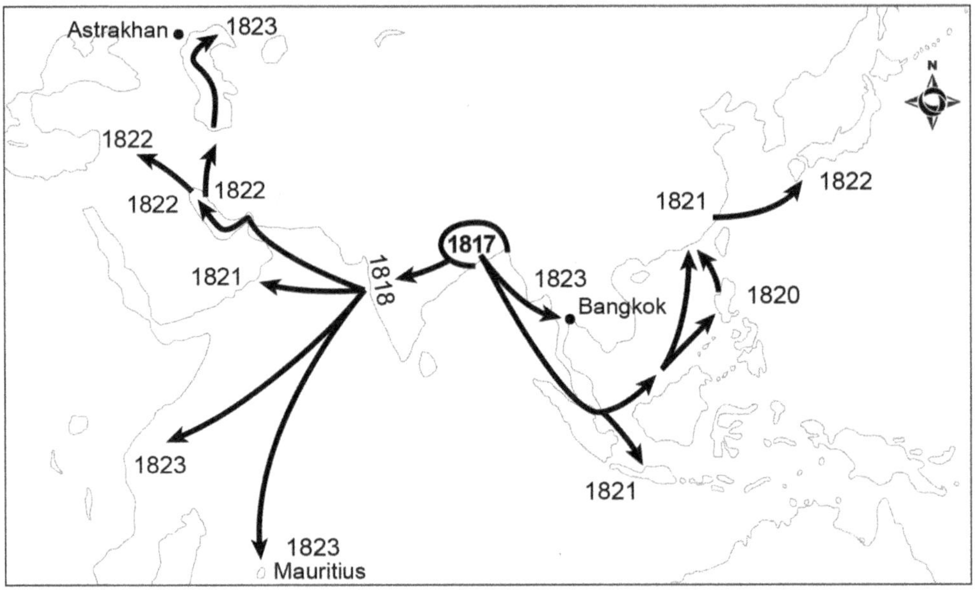

control in the Indian subcontinent; in one week in 1818, 764 soldiers (of a force of 11,500) died. About 200 deaths were reported in Russian Astrakhan.

SIGNIFICANCE

In the years 1817–1824, cholera moved, for the first time, out of the relatively confined areas of south Asia where it had long been endemic. Thus began a series of cholera pandemics that in many ways dominated the world's disease history in the nineteenth century. Its movement in those years illustrated, or was facilitated by, two important factors of nineteenth-century life, the spread of Western military and colonial power, and the rapid improvement in the speed (and frequency) of world traffic. By the first two decades of the century, much of the Indian subcontinent had fallen under British control, and that meant that India began to be more tightly drawn into an international political and economic network. British military and naval personnel more frequently moved to and from India and other places in west and southeast Asia, as part of the thickening web of control that tied India (to become, later in the century, the "Jewel in the Crown" of the British Empire) to Great Britain and to other British possessions. For example, cholera apparently moved with British military traffic from India to Oman and hence to western Asia in 1821. At the same time, the movement of Indian goods to other Asian locales (such as opium to China) increased, carried by increasingly dominant British shipping. The pattern of the classic cholera pandemic—following human traffic—was set with the 1817–1824 outbreak, sped on its way (if not actually caused) by the extension of Western economic and military power in Asia.

The mortality from the 1817–1824 pandemic will never be known, although it was certainly high. But it gained contemporary significance in part because Europeans in the 1820s made exaggerated estimates of that mortality, and those estimates inspired fears of a new Black Death in the West. Those fears in turn affected Western responses to the second cholera pandemic, which began in 1827 and, this time, spread to Europe and the Americas, becoming a true worldwide pandemic.

BACKGROUND

As now understood, cholera is caused by bacteria (*Vibrio cholerae*) that are most often transmitted through water supplies, although different foods may also be infected as well. They enter humans through the mouth. If the bacteria reach the intestines (most will be killed by stomach acids) very severe vomiting and diarrhea follow, with drastic dehydration and (frequently) an agonizing and rapid death. That disease is the one that had long been endemic in India, especially Bengal, before 1817. The word "cholera," however, had an older and more general meaning and was used to describe any severe diarrheal illness; sometimes such illnesses were called *cholera morbus* or (especially in infants) *summer cholera.* Apart from India, any reference to cholera before the nineteenth century certainly refers to a nonspecific description of severe diarrhea or dysentery.

HOW IT WAS UNDERSTOOD AT THE TIME

For Indians, the spread of cholera to parts of the subcontinent other than Bengal called for an explanation. Hindu, or *Ayurvedic,* medical traditions generally interpreted disease as a product of disorder in the three humours (wind, bile, and phlegm) of the body. That disorder sometimes had an environmental cause, for instance from the climate, and sometimes angry gods created disease, either by their direct intervention, or indirectly through the environment. Only divine intervention seemed adequate to explain the severe events in the years after 1817. Had gods been angered by, for example, the killing of sacred cattle to feed British troops? Had the lower castes been defying the gods by polluting water supplies? The extension of British power in Indian lands might itself have angered the gods, or perhaps deities were rebuking Hindus for their failure to resist the British more effectively than they did. Beginning in 1798, British rule in India had expanded very rapidly, overthrowing the sultanate of Mysore in the south, extending northwest from Bengal into the Ganges River Valley, and gaining control of the Maratha territories in central India. By 1818 Britain had ceased to be simply one of several Indian territorial powers and had become "master of India" (Metcalf and Metcalf 2002, 67). Hindu explanations of the spread of cholera frequently associated the disease with foreign rule.

Western understandings of Asiatic cholera remained largely nonspecific, as they would continue to be through much of the subsequent pandemics. Cholera lay on a continuum of diarrheal illnesses, the causes of which were vigorously disputed. And in 1818, the British were quick to blame the cholera that sickened their troops on the "dirty" Indian camp followers who accompanied their army. The British therefore regarded the disease as the product of a foreign enemy, just as the Indians did.

RESPONSES

As cholera spread outside Bengal, the number and variety of local Hindu responses increased. Different mediums (especially young women) offered themselves as mediators with the angry gods, and special ad hoc shrines appeared where the stricken gathered. Outside India, the Siamese monarchy, seeing the epidemic as punishment inflicted on the population by gods angry at human evil, ordered ceremonies to ward off that evil and attempted to promote meritorious conduct in the people.

The contagious character of cholera was a contentious topic from the start. British Indian opinion tended to deny that the disease was contagious, arguing rather that climate, environment, perhaps a fatal miasma led to cholera. The Russian state decided, as the disease lapped against its frontiers, that it was contagious and proposed a system of quarantine and isolation of victims, but the policy was not clearly implemented, perhaps because doubts about cholera's contagious nature persisted.

Immediate therapeutic responses had little effect, if only because cholera's symptoms developed so rapidly and death often intervened before any remedy could take hold. Perhaps for that reason, hospitals played little or no role in responses to the first cholera pandemic. Western and Ayurvedic therapies had much in common, for both were founded on humoral principles that attempted to relieve sickness by restoring humoral balance. Both therefore especially relied on modifications of diet, various purgatives and enemas, and (by some Western physicians) on the drawing of blood (*venesection*). In at least one case, the application of purgatives by foreign physicians contributed to a civil disturbance: in Manila in 1820, the populace, convinced that cholera came as a result of a plot to poison the city's water, rioted, and grievances about alcohol-based purgatives worsened the situation. Later cholera pandemics, especially that of 1827–1835, would feature frequent and serious such examples of civil disorder.

ISSUES RAISED FOR SUBSEQUENT CHOLERA PANDEMICS

The first cholera pandemic is also the least well documented, largely because it did not reach Europe or the Americas. But it raised important issues that would be dramatically illustrated in the succeeding cholera waves. The movement of soldiers and sailors remained an important vector of the disease. So too would international seaborne trade, especially as steamships were introduced from the 1830s on. Still another important movement of people probably also played a role in the first pandemic, although it was not then clearly realized: the traffic of religious pilgrimages, both toward Mecca from all over the Muslim world and within India as Hindus moved to religious sites. In 1831 a French author, Alexandre Moreau de Jonnès, associated pilgrimages with the spread of cholera in India, and the habits and customs of both Hindu and Muslim pilgrimages then came under attack by Western writers; Hindu pilgrimages especially were seen as primitive superstitions that menaced public health.

In the first cholera pandemic, Western and Asian medical responses had much in common. British medical practitioners in India still respected some Indian medical traditions, and a belief persisted that Asiatic cholera was a disease of a particular locality and so local knowledge of it should be honored. Should, for example, British local officials in India satisfy local beliefs by paying for Hindu anticholera ceremonies, with an eye to keeping the peace between themselves and their Indian subjects? In later cholera pandemics, such questions would become more difficult, as the gulf between Asian and Western practices grew and as Western opinion moved in the direction of contempt for Asian medicine and indeed almost everything Asian.

Another issue prefigured by the first cholera pandemic was the relation between disease and poverty. Contemporary Western observers made the connection in India, and when the later cholera pandemics reached the West, that relationship became a central point of discussion. Did the poor bring cholera on themselves by their irresponsible behavior, or did the very condition of poverty make cholera inevitable for them, regardless of what they did?

Finally, Western writers, horrified by the mortality of the pandemic in Asia, probably exaggerated it. Moreau de Jonnès (1831) put the death toll at about 18 million, and other writers increased their estimates to as many as 50 million. No evidence supports such beliefs, but their currency at the time when the second cholera pandemic was reaching Europe and North America helps explain the near-hysteria that it generated as it approached.

REFERENCES

Metcalf, Barbara D., and Thomas R. Metcalf. *A Concise History of India.* Cambridge: Cambridge University Press, 2002.

Moreau de Jonnès, Alexandre. *Rapport au conseil supérior de santé sur le choléra-morbus pestilentiel.* Paris: Cosson, 1831.

Rogers, Leonard. *The Incidence and Spread of Cholera in India: Forecasting and Control of Epidemics.* Indian Medical Research Memoirs, vol. 9. Calcutta: Indian Research Fund Association, 1928.

SUGGESTED ADDITIONAL READING

Arnold, David. *Colonizing the Body: State Medicine and Epidemic Disease in Nineteenth-Century India.* Berkeley: University of California Press, 1993.

Benedict, Carol. *Bubonic Plague in Nineteenth-Century China.* Stanford, CA: Stanford University Press, 1996.

De Bevoise, Ken. *Agents of Apocalypse: Epidemic Disease in the Colonial Philippines.* Princeton, NJ: Princeton University Press, 1995.

Hamlin, Christopher. *Cholera: The Biography.* Oxford: Oxford University Press, 2009.
Jannetta, Ann Bowman. *Epidemics and Mortality in Early Modern Japan.* Princeton, NJ: Princeton University Press, 1987.
McGrew, Roderick E. *Russia and the Cholera, 1823–1832.* Madison: University of Wisconsin Press, 1965.
Pollitzer, Robert. *Cholera.* Geneva: World Health Organization, 1959.
Owen, Norman G., ed. *Death and Disease in Southeast Asia: Explorations in Social, Medical and Demographic History.* Singapore: Oxford University Press, 1987.

21

Second Cholera Pandemic, 1827–1835

WHEN AND WHERE

The second cholera pandemic, like the first, had its origins in India, and especially in cholera's endemic home, Bengal. After the first pandemic had receded throughout Asia by 1824, the disease again began spreading from Bengal in 1827. By 1829 it had moved into Afghanistan and Persia (following one of the paths of the first pandemic), and in August of that year it surfaced in Orenburg, on the Ural River in the Russian Empire. But cholera did not stop, this time, on the frontiers of Russia. In July 1830 cholera cases broke out in Astrakhan, and the disease then rapidly followed human traffic up the Volga River and its tributaries: Tsaritzin and Saratov in August, Kazan and Moscow in September, and all the way to Archangel (on the White Sea) by November. In early 1831, epidemics of cholera first reached the western edges of the Russian Empire (Brest-Litovsk in January, Grodno in March, Warsaw in April); by June it arrived in St. Petersburg.

From western Russia, cholera moved into Europe. Berlin, to the west of Warsaw, was infected by August 1831, as was Vienna, Hamburg in October, and from there cholera moved across the North Sea to Sunderland, in northeastern England, in the same month. In 1832 more of western Europe fell under the epidemic, including the rest of the British Isles (London in February, Dublin in March) and France (Paris in March). By June 1832 oceanic traffic carried cholera across the Atlantic, as first Montreal and then New York had cholera cases that month, with Philadelphia following in July. In 1833 the epidemic spread to parts of Latin America, as well as the previously unaffected Iberian Peninsula.

In the first cholera pandemic, another tongue of infection had reached from India into western Asia, and that happened again with the second pandemic. By 1831 cholera had spread from Persia to Mesopotamia and the Arabian Peninsula. From the holy cities of the Hijaz (especially Mecca), Muslim pilgrims carried the disease in that year to Palestine, Syria, and Egypt. Further pilgrim traffic in the later years of the pandemic (until 1835) carried new epidemics from those places further into eastern Africa: Sudan, Ethiopia, Somalia, and Zanzibar.

The second cholera pandemic did not leave Southeast Asia untouched either, for Java suffered a serious epidemic in 1834–1835. East Asia, however, was apparently unaffected. No disease corresponding to cholera was reported in Japan in those years. And while serious epidemics occurred in China, the evidence suggests that cholera was not included in them.

As with the first cholera pandemic, no realistic estimate of total mortality is possible. But some places suffered very severely. Cairo may have lost 36,000 people (perhaps 15% of its population) to cholera in a few months; Paris reported 18,000 cholera deaths in 1832, and in April of that year the city lost over 700 people per week. The Hijaz cities of Mecca and Medina may have suffered between 12,000 and 30,000 deaths in the spring of 1831. New Orleans, not a very large city (about 75,000 people in 1840), had 5,000 deaths in this pandemic.

SIGNIFICANCE

The second cholera pandemic was the first one to reach Europe and North America. While reports of the first pandemic had reached (and frightened) the West, the reality of cholera's presence deeply affected Western ideas and emotions. Its immediate impact on Western culture probably exceeded that of any epidemic since the fourteenth-century plague, although its total mortality was far slighter and in fact was surpassed in Europe by the third cholera pandemic. In Asia its effects were less dramatic than those of the first pandemic.

Its impact and significance had less to do with its mortality and more to do with the particular social and political situation of the West in the early 1830s when it arrived, a situation that (as discussed later) led to dramatically different interpretations being given to the disease. Its appearance contributed to, and in some cases may have shaped, social tensions; it led to serious attacks on authorities, both political and medical; its presence led to a clearer view of poverty and poor living conditions. The particularly sudden and gruesome nature of its symptoms shattered many Romantic notions about death as a "beautiful" experience, and the evident helplessness of Western medicine in the face of the pandemic checked (but did not end) Western pride in the civilization's scientific accomplishments. At the same time, however, the second cholera pandemic provided some Western thinkers with further grounds for regarding the East as barbaric.

BACKGROUND

See volume 2, chapter 20 "First Cholera Pandemic, 1817–1824."

HOW IT WAS UNDERSTOOD AT THE TIME

Cholera made a great impression in part because of its dramatic symptoms. They overtook victims with frightening speed. A healthy young adult could begin a day with no sense of illness, yet be devastated or perhaps even dead by evening. Witnesses saw a massive dehydration of the body, profuse vomiting and excretion, the skin turning a deathly pale blue, the features of the face quickly pinched and gaunt. People were struck down in the street and collapsed in their own excrement. Roughly half of those who were stricken died.

The violence of the disease hung over all the contemporary understandings of it. But even more important in those understandings was the social and political context of the early 1830s. Many European societies in those years experienced social, economic, and political tensions. The great French Revolution of the previous generation still haunted European elites, many of whom feared another revolution. National aspirations had started to stir in the multinational empires and states preserved, or restored, by the Congress of Vienna; the Greeks had already risen against the Turks, and the American possessions of Spain and Portugal had won their independence through revolt. Economic and social change, particularly pronounced in Great Britain (the most advanced industrial society), likewise threatened to overthrow established order. In that general context occurred specific events. A liberal insurgency in Paris in July 1830 overthrew Charles X and replaced him with Louis Philippe, whose rule quickly disappointed many of those who had taken part in the uprising; French opinion was strongly divided between those wishing to restore order and those pressing for more liberty. In August, the Belgians, under the rule of the kingdom of the Netherlands, revolted and in October proclaimed national independence. Also on the heels of the French news was a nationalist revolution in Russian Poland, countered by a Russian army. In autumn 1830, the rulers of the German states of Brunswick, Saxony, and Hesse-Cassel abdicated and fled. In February 1831, liberal uprisings occurred in the Italian states of Parma and Modena, as well as within the Papal States, while a revolutionary society planned a revolt in Piedmont that it hoped (in vain) would spread throughout the Italian peninsula. Small wonder, then, that the British historian G. M. Young said (of an eminent earlier historian): "Niebuhr, who had seen one world revolution, sickened and died from fear of another" (Young 1936, 1).

No armed revolution occurred in Great Britain, but 1830–1832 were years of high political tension, ostensibly about the Reform Bill, legislation that would change the basis on which members of the House of Commons were chosen. Major riots shook several British cities in the course of that political struggle.

Little agreement existed within the Western medical community about either the underlying cause of cholera or about the nature of its disturbance of the human frame. Whether cholera was spread by contagion, or rooted in some environmental cause, or some awkward combination of those two possibilities, remained an important and contested theme. On a more immediate level, was cholera related to an inflamed gastric tract (as Broussais, perhaps the leading French medical authority, believed)? A failure of the circulatory system? A nervous disorder? Did it represent in some ways a humoral imbalance, in the old (but not yet entirely discredited) Galenic view? All those views had proponents. None commanded general assent. And that uncertainty increased the likelihood of political and social interpretations of the disease coming forward.

Those interpretations, for a start, surrounded the broad question of the contagiousness of cholera. The movement of the epidemic, seemingly along the paths of human traffic on land and sea, certainly argued its contagiousness, and as the second pandemic approached Europe from southwest Asia, most Western medical opinion assumed that it was contagious. With that in mind, the Russian government attempted to impose quarantines to stop cholera's progress. Cholera came anyway. The quarantines may have been inadequate, but for many the quarantine (and the notion of contagion that lay behind it) was politically unacceptable anyway. Liberal thinkers of the late eighteenth and early nineteenth centuries associated quarantines with a whole realm of aggressive and intrusive state measures that sometimes bore the name of medical police. Quarantines interfered with free human movement and especially with trade. Health passes, issued by governments to travelers, were similarly intrusive and restricting. Perhaps most menacing were the measures that a doctrine of contagion would impose on a city once a contagious disease infected it. Individuals would be isolated, perhaps in a special hospital, or in their boarded-up homes; their clothing and possessions might be burned. Any thoroughly applied policy based on contagion would surely meet heavy resistance, from the business community fearful of the disruption of trade and from individuals fearful of the disruption of their lives.

Quarantines, then, seemed both to fail and to stir resistance, as happened in Russia and then, as the epidemic moved west, in the Austrian Empire and in Prussia. Did governments wish to give populations that might already be politically tense still another grievance? Perhaps the key to cholera lay in the environment: in the atmosphere, in the waters, in the materials of everyday living. Environmentalist views of disease were very old; the Hippocratic writings of the ancient Greeks had conceived of diseases as associated with airs and places. British experts with experience in India inclined toward such an explanation of cholera. Quarantine, from this point of view, was useless. Environments must be cleansed.

But what made environments dangerous? Here, again, political views entered the picture. Were dirty environments hazardous? A lot of eighteenth-century thinking about disease had believed so, although the approach was often nonspecific, commending a general clean-up of airs, waters, and places. And whence came the dirt? In the second cholera pandemic, many of the people of the propertied classes found the source of dirt to be the poor or the marginal members of society. Perhaps their habits produced the dirt; perhaps their habits reflected their morals, or perhaps their irreligion. Why, in effect, were the poor the way they were? Were they inherently vicious or at least foolish? In the Europe of 1830, the poor were already widely feared as potential revolutionaries; cholera made them dangerous in another way as well.

Not all environmentalists reached the conclusion that ultimate responsibility for the epidemic rested on the poor. Some thinkers—fewer—saw poverty as a product of the society of the time. Especially in France, where a school of numerical medicine had been developing, cholera stimulated a collection of epidemiological statistics that clearly related disease incidence in Paris to poverty; the poorer the quarter of the city, the higher the incidence of cholera. The issue could be put starkly: Was poverty itself the problem, or were the poor and their habits the problem?

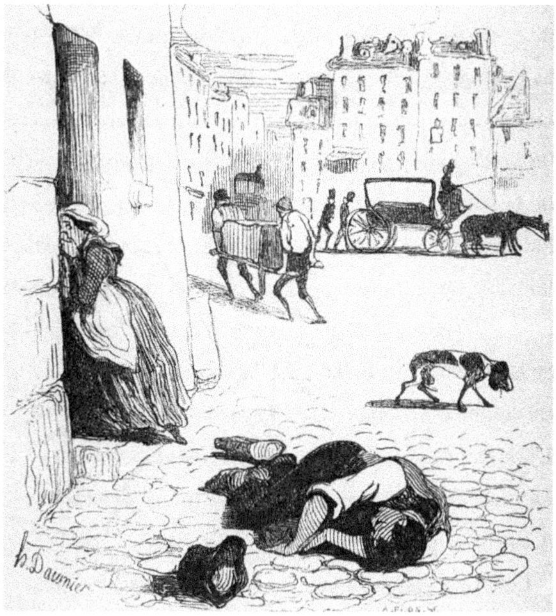

Illustration by Honoré Daumier titled *Cholera in Paris*, captures the horror of the 1832 epidemic. A man suddenly collapses in the street while a woman, entering her doorway, covers her mouth. In the background, caskets are taken away for burial. (National Library of Medicine)

Overlapping the elite's suspicions of the poor were fears of the "other." In the United States, cholera was associated with recent immigrants (especially Irish) and with African Americans. Ultimately cholera was Asian, and especially for British opinion, cholera and the Indian responses to it came (in the second pandemic) both to illustrate the unhealthiness of Asia and to prove that Indian responses, especially Hindu pilgrimages, stemmed from barbaric superstition. This view coincided with a gradual shift underway in British attitudes toward India, a shift symbolized by the policies of Lord William Bentinck, the British governor-general in India between 1828 and 1835. In that time, the British raj shifted away from respect for Indian traditions and toward contempt for Indian backwardness, joined with a conviction that India should be made as British as possible. Christian missions—forbidden by the British until 1813—were now to be actively encouraged; such "beastly" Indian religious customs as *thuggee* and *suttee* should be stamped out. Cholera, and approaches to it, both reflected this shift and contributed to it. In the second cholera pandemic connections began to be made between the spread of cholera and the massing of Indians (many of them poor) at places of Hindu pilgrimage. Those connections would be made more strongly in subsequent cholera pandemics, particularly the fourth.

Out of these different environmentalist and contagionist strands, in all of which political threads were woven, there came a widely accepted conflation often called *contingent contagionism.* Behind cholera lay some general, as-yet-unidentified, environmental cause. But it struck particular individuals, and was passed from

Second Cholera Pandemic, 1827–1835

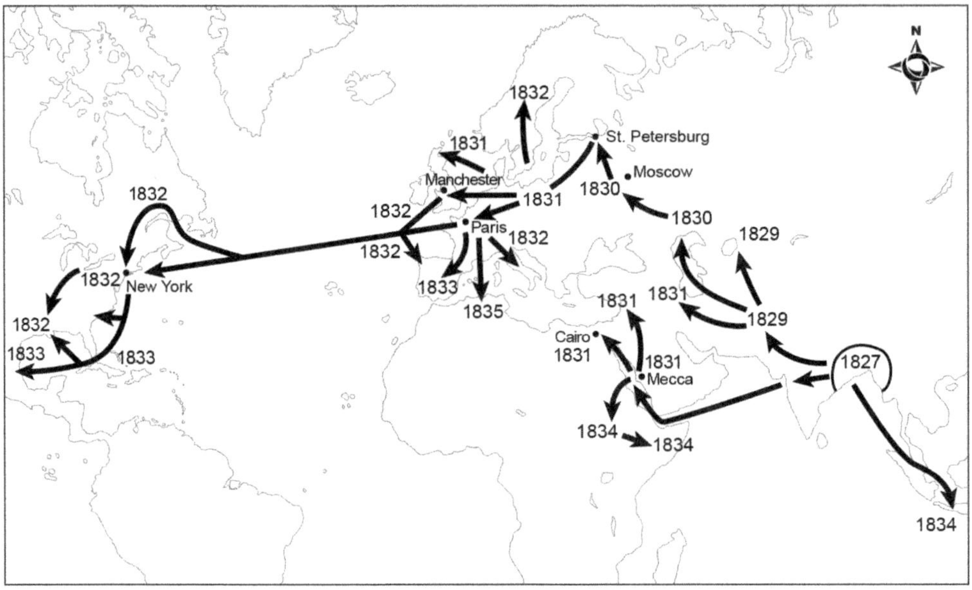

those individuals to others, for contingent reasons. Those contingencies could include a wide range of religious, moral, behavioral, and other possibilities. But because cholera was on some level contagious, and there did not exist an absolute correlation between those who fell ill and those who spurned middle-class religion and morality, the elites accepted—or urged—some measure of isolation of the sick.

Many people still believed that only God could be responsible for such a comprehensive scourging of sinful humanity. Divine services begging God's mercy were very common. In Great Britain, a fanatically religious member of Parliament moved to adopt a national day of prayer and fasting, and the government (perhaps embarrassed) agreed, declaring such a day on March 21, 1832. In the United States, many calls for similar action arose, but President Andrew Jackson, citing the principle of the separation of church and state, refused to support them. On a more general level, many people (especially those in the "proper" middle classes) saw cholera as a direct punishment inflicted on sinners.

Some poor populations understood cholera differently. In Paris, where perhaps the class warfare over the disease was sharpest, some believed that cholera was actually a plot organized by the elite to reduce the numbers (and hence threat) of the poor. The disease's drastic symptoms lent credence to rumors that people were being poisoned. The population doctrines of the English writer T. R. Malthus were seen as predicting a calamitous increase in numbers, to which the cruel response of the rich was a deliberate winnowing of the poor. Tension and at times violence therefore marked some reactions to public policies that demanded isolation of cholera victims.

OFFICIAL RESPONSES

Although some variation existed across the Western world, official responses and policies in different countries had many points in common. Quarantines and sanitary cordons, the establishment of ad hoc health boards to deal with the emergency, a variety of attempts to clean up an area, the isolation of victims, were all widely employed. Some purgative medical treatments were favorites. Some places officially appealed to divine mercy. While not an official policy, a very common response was flight. And very public—although certainly not official—was the popular resistance to many of the above measures, resistance that associated this cholera pandemic with social conflict.

Many Western governments had preexisting quarantine mechanisms, for the most part originally inspired by earlier plague epidemics. In Russia, when cholera appeared in Orenburg in 1829, such machinery was recommended. But questions immediately arose about its appropriateness. Were goods as well as people quarantined? For what period? The government's Central Medical Council, strongly contagionist in its views, urged a stricter quarantine, but the government itself, worried about both the prosperity of trade and the possibility of popular resistance, was not so sure. Cholera was contagious, but did it accompany goods or just people? And if it was passed through the air, quarantines were useless. Major riots occurred in the Black Sea port of Sevastopol in May 1830, stimulated by the extension of quarantine against a plague outbreak. Fear of recurring riots, combined with a clumsy bureaucracy, meant that the epidemic spread more rapidly than quarantines could handle. A strict quarantine, for example, was imposed around Moscow in September 1830, but the disease was already in the city.

Other cities in other countries had parallel experiences. New York declared a quarantine when cholera was reported in Montreal, but cholera arrived anyway. In Cairo, when cholera began spreading among Mecca pilgrims, a quarantine was proclaimed, but returning pilgrims simply overran it and the disease reached the city. Such experiences gave ammunition to Western writers who denounced quarantines as illiberal limits on human freedom, arguments that had particular weight in such liberal states as Britain, France, and the United States. One place apparently did impose a successful quarantine: Tunis, where the ruling bey, Hussain, decreed a 20-day quarantine on ships arriving at the port. Western merchants in the city opposed his move, but Tunis remained free of cholera during the second pandemic.

A common response to cholera was the appointment of central, and often local, boards of health. In some places these already existed, but many others quickly formed them on an ad hoc basis, giving them powers to direct sanitation efforts and organize the isolation of cholera victims. Sanitation attempts were unfocused; only with later cholera pandemics did authorities come to direct their attention to water supplies and sewage disposal. In the United States (where such boards remained local) and in Britain, the waning of the cholera pandemic often meant the end of the boards; only in later cholera pandemics did such boards become permanent.

The most obvious official actions were the isolation of cholera victims and the arrangements for disposal of the dead, illustrating the contingent contagionist conviction. Hospitals, some already existing, some hastily arranged for the occasion, were to isolate the victims from the healthy. And fear of cholera corpses led to the insistence on rapid interment, in special gravesites set apart from others, with bodies quickly and unceremoniously covered with quicklime.

Physicians throughout the Western world were generally helpless in the face of cholera, but they still tried many different therapies. Because the disease dramatically affected excretion, some of the more bizarre remedies involved either stopping excretion by blocking the rectum with beeswax or promoting excretion by using tobacco smoke as an enema. Fashionable new scientific techniques—electrical shocks—were deployed. But perhaps the most common single treatment was the administration of calomel, a mercury compound, as a purgative. (In retrospect, using a purgative to treat a disease whose effects included violent dehydration of the body seems a serious mistake.)

The facts that doctors differed in their approaches, that whatever they tried had little or no positive effect, and that many of their remedies brought more pain rather than less, all meant that many people sought relief (or hoped-for protection) from the wide range of irregular healers that could be found all over the Western world in the 1830s. Government regulation of healing professions varied widely from one country to another, but for the most part was still in its infancy. And even in France, where government recognition and licensing of doctors had perhaps proceeded the furthest, the state made no attempt in 1832 to limit access to irregular healers. In the United States, the 1830s were years of a bewildering variety of healing sects, and the cholera pandemic encouraged their further multiplication; the desperate were willing to try anything.

POPULAR RESPONSES

Moscow, the first large European city to be affected by cholera, awaited the disease with considerable dread, for it had also been the last major European city to suffer a plague epidemic, in 1771. That experience had entered into the popular imaginations and collective memory of Muscovites. As cholera approached in the autumn of 1830, an estimated 50,000 people (of a population of about 300,000) fled the city; those who remained quickly bought out the apothecaries' supplies of reputed preventive goods, such as camphor. When the disease actually began claiming victims in Moscow, the city developed a fairly effective public health bureaucracy, although it was hampered by the interference of the central government. Some quarantine was attempted, and in principle the city determined that all cases of cholera should be reported. But the authorities also wisely (in Roderick McGrew's view) did not insist on the universal application of that reporting rule, and in doing so probably prevented major social tensions. Many Muscovites (as many in other cities) dreaded reporting cholera in their families, for they feared the isolation of the sick, the destruction of belongings, and the degrading disposal of bodies that followed official intervention. Moscow was spared the major riots that occurred elsewhere, although the final death toll from cholera, between September 1830 and January 1831, was put at about 4,600.

St. Petersburg, the Russian capital, had a different experience. Cholera reached that city in June 1831, while the Russian army was struggling to subdue the Polish rebellion. Perhaps because the Poles (and others in Europe) blamed the advance of cholera into the Polish lands on the Russian soldiers, St. Petersburg authorities were alive to the possibility of "Polish poison" in their city. Whether for that reason or others, those authorities gave the police the task of suppressing cholera. The epidemic was "treated like a crime wave . . . [T]he sick and the well, the inebriates and the infirm, were collared, dumped unceremoniously into the dreaded cholera carts, and hauled off willy-nilly to the lazzarettes [special isolation hospitals]" (McGrew 1965, 109). The populace reacted furiously, blaming the police, physicians, and foreigners for the cholera deaths, and cried poison. After a series of special religious services asking God to deliver them from the epidemic, crowds stormed a hospital and liberated the patients (as well as the deceased), and battered a German physician to death. Troops eventually dispersed the crowds (and the angry czar, Nicholas I, lectured a crowd on its misbehavior), but the government was frightened: so much so that it quietly softened its approach to cholera control in St. Petersburg.

In Paris, two strands of popular violence flowed together during March and April 1832, while cholera raged in the city. One strand related only tangentially to the epidemic: the attacks of scavengers (*chiffonniers*) who had been angered by the city's new garbage and trash removal policies. Those policies, motivated by a desire to clean the city's environment more efficiently, provided for the more rapid and thorough removal of trash. But they also left fewer opportunities for the scavengers, who regarded their traditional livelihood as imperiled. The scavengers rioted in early April, throwing the new garbage carts into the Seine. The other strand, more directly related to cholera, stemmed from the widespread and popular beliefs that cholera was a hoax, the product of an elite that was determined to reduce the revolutionary threat of the lower orders by poisoning them. Also, in early April, angry crowds moved through Paris streets, seeking those responsible, especially doctors and hospitals. Perhaps five or six people were actually killed by these crowds, but (according to Catherine Kudlick) the horror of these events deeply impressed the upper and middle classes, who saw the "hideous underworld of revolutionary disorder" of the worst phase of the great French Revolution looming before them again (Kudlick 1996, 180). Cholera was thus associated in the minds of the poor with a government plot, while to the elites it was synonymous with disorder and dangerous revolution.

Something of the same fears expressed themselves in Great Britain, but there (as in Paris) particular local issues also shaped events. The rapid expansion of medical education in the early nineteenth century, and the increased emphasis placed on direct experience with human anatomy in that education, had led to a critical shortage of corpses for such demonstrative dissection. Hence arose the celebrated trade of grave robbing. Anatomy schools purchased bodies illegally unearthed by these "resurrectionists." These actions deeply offended popular ideas about proper burial of the dead and respect for their remains, and doctors were generally blamed. And in 1828 two Edinburgh criminals, William Burke and

William Hare, were found to have been selling fresh corpses of people whom they had murdered to an anatomy school. Doctors seemed, if not murderers themselves, in league with murderers. Doctors would now be greeted with cries of "Burkers."

These resentments of doctors were magnified by other political circumstances in the early 1830s. Widespread belief in, and disgust with, political corruption existed, forming part of the pressure for reform that mobilized mass support for the Reform Bill. Cholera, according to many supporters of reform, was at least a distraction from reform efforts, on another level a humbug to give politically connected healers more jobs, and (most disturbing) an opportunity for doctors to gain more corpses for dissection. To these different interpretations, British official policy, urging localities to create isolation hospitals and provide for the rapid disposal of cholera's victims, seemed a menace to traditional and deeply held beliefs.

In September 1832 (after some months of rising tensions in the city), a Manchester man discovered that his grandson, four years old, had died in an isolation hospital. When the coffin was opened a brick was found in place of the child's head. Had the head been given to the anatomists? An angry crowd carried the coffin through the city, shouting execrations against doctors and cholera hospitals; the crowd stormed a hospital, broke its windows, tore down a wall, broke up cholera vans, and liberated the patients. When the police intervened, a police station was attacked. But R. J. Morris, who retells this story, also notes that British authorities—with the Russian experiences in mind—did not insist on a strict application of quarantine and isolation rules; if possible, they hoped to avoid such disturbances as the Manchester riot.

UNRESOLVED HISTORICAL ISSUES

In the series of cholera pandemics that affected the world in the nineteenth and early twentieth centuries, the second pandemic made the greatest single psychological impact on the West. But many issues that it raised would only be resolved with later pandemics. Many theories existed about its cause (or causes); the causes would become clearer by the time of the fourth pandemic (1863–1875), but some doubts remained into the fifth (1881–1896).

The social tensions associated with the second pandemic have drawn considerable historical attention; for a variety of reasons those tensions were less severe in subsequent cholera pandemics. But the attention paid to the second pandemic should not obscure the fact that in the West, the third cholera pandemic was more demographically significant than the second, and (more generally) that the cholera story in the world was only beginning.

Historical writing about cholera has also speculated about the connection between the second pandemic and the development of Western (and especially British) sanitation practices and ideas. Modern historical opinion now downplays the relation of the second pandemic, for all its impact on the popular mind, and the ideas subsequently advocated by the British sanitary reformers such as Edwin Chadwick and Thomas Southwood Smith. Truer connections between the gospel of integrated sewage and clean water systems may be seen in the third cholera pandemic (1839–1856).

REFERENCES

Kudlick, Catherine J. *Cholera in Post-Revolutionary Paris: A Cultural History.* Berkeley: University of California Press, 1996.

McGrew, Roderick. *Russia and the Cholera, 1823–1832.* Madison: University of Wisconsin Press, 1965.

Young, G. M. *Victorian England: Portrait of an Age.* Oxford: Oxford University Press, 1936.

SUGGESTED ADDITIONAL READING

Arnold, David. *Colonizing the Body: State Medicine and Epidemic Disease in Nineteenth Century India.* Berkeley: University of California Press, 1993.

Briggs, Asa. "Cholera and Society in the Nineteenth Century." *Past and Present* 19 (1961): 76–96.

Coleman, William. *Death Is a Social Disease: Public Health and Political Economy in Early Industrial France.* Madison: University of Wisconsin Press, 1982.

Delaporte, François. *Disease and Civilization: The Cholera in Paris, 1832.* Cambridge, MA: MIT Press, 1986.

Durey, Michael. *The Return of the Plague: British Society and the Cholera, 1831–32.* Dublin: Gill and Macmillan, 1979.

Evans, Richard J. "Epidemics and Revolutions: Cholera in Nineteenth-Century Europe." *Past and Present* 120 (1988): 123–146.

Gallagher, Nancy E. *Medicine and Power in Tunisia, 1780–1900.* Cambridge: Cambridge University Press, 1983.

Hamlin, Christopher. *Cholera: The Biography.* Oxford: Oxford University Press, 2009.

Kuhnke, LaVerne. *Lives at Risk: Public Health in Nineteenth-Century Egypt.* Berkeley: University of California Press, 1990.

Morris, R. J. *Cholera 1832: The Social Response to an Epidemic.* New York: Holmes and Meier, 1976.

Owen, Norman G., ed. *Death and Disease in Southeast Asia: Explorations in Social, Medical and Demographic History.* Singapore: Oxford University Press, 1987.

Pollitzer, Robert. *Cholera.* Geneva: World Health Organization, 1959.

Rosenberg, Charles E. *The Cholera Years: The United States in 1832, 1849, and 1866.* Chicago: University of Chicago Press, 1962.

22

Third Cholera Pandemic, 1839–1856

WHEN AND WHERE

The third of the great nineteenth-century cholera pandemics began spreading from Bengal (India) in 1839. Its spread was even more nearly worldwide than the second pandemic had been; for the first time the disease reached deeply into Latin America, as well as returning to Europe and North America.

Cholera was endemic in India, and there has been some disagreement among historians about when the second cholera pandemic ended and the third began. All the cholera pandemics radiated outward from Bengal; it may be helpful to regard their movements as a series of concentric waves, which sometimes overlapped in different parts of the world. The effects of one pandemic might still have been felt in some distant places at the time when another pandemic wave was beginning to spread out. At least one older historical account that still commands respect (Pollitzer 1959) defined the second cholera pandemic as lasting until about 1850, and the third beginning in 1852. This chapter follows other arguments that see a break in Indian cholera between 1836 and 1839; the center of the pond was relatively calm in those years, although waves generated earlier still moved elsewhere. A new surge began in Bengal in 1839.

The third pandemic first reached out to southeast and eastern Asia, when Malaysia, Singapore, and southeastern China became infected with cholera in 1840. It is likely that British troops and Anglo-Indian trade carried the disease to those places with the outbreak of the so-called Opium War between Britain and China in 1840. From the south China coast cholera then moved inland and began a march westward that eventually infected Burma (reached from China, not adjacent Bengal as one might assume), western China, and from there (by 1844–1845) to central Asia, Afghanistan, and Persia.

Another chain of infection spread westward across India from Bengal to Bombay, and from there jumped by sea to Mesopotamia (Iraq) and Aden (Yemen) by 1846. This chain had a long and active career. From Mesopotamia and Arabia cholera advanced to Persia and the shores of the Caspian Sea; from there it followed one of the paths of the second pandemic, to Astrakhan and Orenburg in the

Russian Empire, to Moscow (in September 1847), and from there to northern and western Europe in 1848.

One important node for its further diffusion was Mecca, in Arabia, the world center of pilgrimage for Muslims. In the summer of 1848, Egypt was infected as a result of pilgrim traffic; in 1849 cholera advanced across North Africa, reaching Tunisia by November and becoming serious there in early 1850.

By the end of 1848, cholera had also moved across the Atlantic from Europe to the United States. A ship from Le Havre (France) carried the disease to New York in December, while in the same month, vessels from the German ports of Hamburg and Bremen brought it to New Orleans. Cholera then followed the still-dominant water lines of communication into the American interior, quickly moving up the Mississippi River and its tributaries from New Orleans to St. Louis, Louisville, and Cincinnati in December, Nashville in January 1849, Quincy (Illinois) in March, and from there to Chicago in April. Further water traffic carried cholera from Chicago through the Great Lakes to Detroit in August. From St. Louis cholera began traveling west on the trails with the gold seekers (and others) to California. San Francisco had cholera by the end of 1850. Cholera moved more slowly out from New York, thanks to winter cold, but it reached Philadelphia and Baltimore in May 1849 and Boston in June.

The pandemic spread from the United States to the Caribbean. Cuba, the only Caribbean place brushed by the second pandemic, started suffering from the third in March 1850; from there cholera moved to Jamaica in October. And cholera kept reappearing in the United States, spreading renewed infections to other Caribbean places (including the Bahamas, Barbados, and Puerto Rico) between 1852 and 1855. Still another finger had reached out from the United States as well, for traffic from New Orleans to Panama carried cholera in 1849; from there it passed to Colombia and perhaps Ecuador in 1850.

Continuing infections from India led to another wave of cholera reaching Persia, Mesopotamia, and eventually Europe in 1853. In 1854 this branch of the third pandemic moved from southern France back eastward to Greece and Turkey, carried by the troops moving to the Baltic Sea for the Crimean War. And a particularly important tongue of this late stage of the third pandemic saw cholera carried in 1855 from Portuguese ports to Brazil, where perhaps the greatest mortalities of the pandemic (apart from India) occurred. After 1855 cholera abated across much of the world, with one significant exception. Japan, whose isolation had successfully kept the second cholera pandemic away from its shores, had what Ann Bowman Jannetta calls its worst cholera epidemic in 1858 (Jannetta 1987). The disease first reached Japan through Nagasaki, the traditional port of entry for foreigners; Japanese sources claimed that cholera was brought on an American warship, and more generally the Japanese associated this outbreak with the new openness to trade more or less forced on them by Western (initially American) pressure. Asiatic cholera had thus, by the end of the third pandemic, spanned the globe to reach Asian territory from the West.

No estimate has been made of total world mortality in the third cholera pandemic, but very serious death tolls occurred in many different places. For some locales, the third pandemic was the worst of the century. That was certainly true of Brazil and the Caribbean, many places in the United States, and most places in Europe. The high levels of mortality in Europe between 1848 and 1854, however, were accompanied by far less social and political turmoil than had accompanied the second cholera pandemic, and that circumstance has posed a problem for historians (see the sections "Responses" and "Unresolved Historical Issues" that follow).

Some notion of the pandemic's severity may be gained by considering important examples of the mortality it inflicted on different continents. In western Asia and North Africa, 15,000 died of cholera in the pilgrimage city of Mecca in November 1846, 6,000 in Cairo in 1848, and 7,600 in Tunis in 1849–1850. The last, likely an underestimate, occurred in a city whose total population was about 150,000. The mortality rate for Tunis, therefore, might have been about 50 deaths per 1,000 population, or 5%. For Tunisia as a whole the mortality may have been closer to 10%, a very serious rate for any epidemic.

In England and France, death totals exceeded those of the second pandemic. England, where cholera was more widespread than in 1831–1832, about 61,000 people died of it in 1848–1849, and a further 26,000 in 1853–1854, 10,000 of those in London. In Paris 20,000 died of cholera in 1849, a larger total (but a slightly lower mortality rate, about 2%) than in 1832. Norway suffered the most serious cholera epidemic in its history in 1853, as about 1,600 people (of a total population of 49,000) in Oslo died of cholera between July and November.

In the United States, 5,000 people in New York City died between May and August 1849, and by the time the epidemic had ended that total had risen to about 15,000. New York's mortality rate was therefore about 3%, comparable to Oslo's and slightly higher than Paris's. But some of the smaller American cities of the Mississippi and Ohio river valleys, where the epidemic came earlier and lingered longer through the year, were hurt much more severely. St. Louis and Cincinnati may have lost 10% of their populations.

Some of the most appalling mortalities, however, occurred in the lands of the Caribbean and in Brazil. In some of those places, slavery was still legal, and the cholera death toll among the slave populations was especially high. In Puerto Rico, the official death toll (probably too low) from cholera in 1855 was about 25,900, about 5% of the population. But a very high proportion of the dead were male slaves, 14% of whom died. In Cuba between 26,000 and 34,000 slaves perished, between 8% and 10% of their population.

Even Caribbean places where slavery had been abolished suffered very severely, and the fact that those places had high proportions of ex-slaves suggested that people of African descent were especially vulnerable (see the "Unresolved Historical Issues" section). Thus, Kingston (Jamaica) had between 4,000 and 6,000 deaths in late 1850, between 10% and 15% of its population; Barbados lost between 20,000 and 25,000 in 1854, also about 15% of the population of the island. Horrific mortality was reached in some smaller communities: in Soufrière, a village on St. Lucia, 400 people of a total of 900 perished.

In 1855 and 1856, cholera reached Brazil for the first time in its history, and serious epidemics spread from three different landing points along the coast: Belém in May 1855, from whence the disease moved up the Amazon River; Bahia in July; and the capital, Rio de Janeiro, also in July. From the latter two cities the adjoining northeastern (Bahia) and southern (Rio de Janeiro) hinterlands were infected. In all over 200,000 Brazilians, two-thirds of them African descendants, died. Some particular places suffered more than others. The small city of Porto Alegre lost 10% of its population; in the village of Assemblea, "334 persons out of 700 died within two weeks" (Cooper 1986, 476). In Brazil, as in the Caribbean, the disease especially affected the poor segments of the population, slave and free.

SIGNIFICANCE

The third cholera pandemic was the first one to spread widely into Middle and South America, in addition to North America, Europe, northern Africa, and Asia. The mortality that resulted there made it one of Latin America's major disease disasters. While it generated much less comment and social turmoil in Europe than the second pandemic had done, its mortality there was heavier as well. For most places in Europe, the third cholera pandemic resulted in the highest number of deaths of any of the six cholera pandemics.

The spread of the pandemic also provided some vivid illustrations of the tightening political and economic connections of the world in the age of European imperial domination.

Did the pandemic mark a significant shift in thinking about the cause (and prevention) of cholera? Not clearly so. But the evolution of thought in the direction of understanding cholera as a discrete specific disease continued, and important doubts had begun to develop about the association of cholera and personal moral failure (see the "How It Was Understood at the Time" section later in the chapter.)

BACKGROUND

By the mid-nineteenth century, environmental changes were underway in some parts of the world that eased the path of the third cholera pandemic. In part those changes grew out of changing economic relationships between different areas; in part they reflected the determination of Europeans to master the globe.

Egypt provides a good illustration of the importance of environmental change, and of the relation between that environmental change and economic pressure. LaVerne Kuhnke (1990) argues that by the late 1840s Egypt was undertaking a new system of irrigation, one that directed more water from town water supplies to agricultural lands. The khedive of Egypt, Muhammed Ali (in power from 1805 to 1849), was determined to bring his country closer to the economic level of Europe. This led him to promote cotton as a cash crop that would bring Egypt money, and hence to the construction of new irrigation systems to water the cotton. The resultant low levels of water supplied to towns increased the risk of cholera infection, as town dwellers were forced to reuse their limited supplies in which some human excretions (carrying cholera bacteria) were more likely to be found.

European imperial ambitions also contributed to facilitating cholera's spread in the third pandemic. Two major movements of troops, one at the beginning of the pandemic, the other at its end, both carried cholera to new places. British forces moved from India through the East Indies to attack Canton (China) in 1840, and cholera followed. Sizable numbers of French (and British) troops sailed from southern France into the Black Sea in 1854 during the Crimean War against Russia; the last phases of the third pandemic were thus carried to Greece and Turkey.

Even more than the second pandemic, the third cholera pandemic coincided with a major period of political unrest and revolution in Europe.

HOW IT WAS UNDERSTOOD AT THE TIME

Cholera continued to inspire fear almost everywhere, thanks to the violence of its symptoms, its unpredictability, and the strong likelihood that it meant death. For example, Egyptians who made light of bubonic plague found cholera frightening. And perhaps because people found it so terrifying, many different peoples continued to blame its presence on the behavior, or simple presence, of an "other." In the West (and especially in the United States) cholera continued to be associated with the moral failures of other groups, such as immigrants, or with the sinful (or perhaps just stupid) behavior of those thought to be vicious. In both the United States and the Caribbean, cholera was associated with race, with Africans carrying the blame. And in Tunisia, some felt that Europeans were at fault for the appearance of a disease that their country had previously avoided.

But, in general, the understanding of cholera during the third pandemic was dominated by two unsettled questions. First, was cholera spread contagiously from one individual to another, or was it the product of a more general environmental pollution? Second, did the responsibility for cholera lie with individuals and their behavior, or did the society as a whole create conditions that spread the disease? Underlying these questions was a widespread realization that the poor suffered disproportionately, but why was that so? Did their individual habits—their viciousness, or their carelessness—create conditions that allowed a contagion to spread, or create a miasmatic environment? Or were the poor trapped by a social system that made contagion inevitable (in crowded quarters) or where economic forces created noxious environments? In many places where the third pandemic struck, governments and medical personnel alike wrestled with those questions, revealing uncertainty and sometimes conflict over the appropriate responses to the disease.

In Great Britain, the medical profession remained largely contagionist in its interpretation of cholera, although government policies were not so certain. In both France and the United States, anti-contagionist arguments were more widely accepted by physicians, politicians, and the general public, although American belief in the role of individual moral failure remained more insistent. In both countries, however, important doubts began to be raised about whether individuals and their moral failings could be held accountable. Did God punish individuals for their disobedience of His laws? And if so, what laws: those demanding

THIRD CHOLERA PANDEMIC, 1839–1856

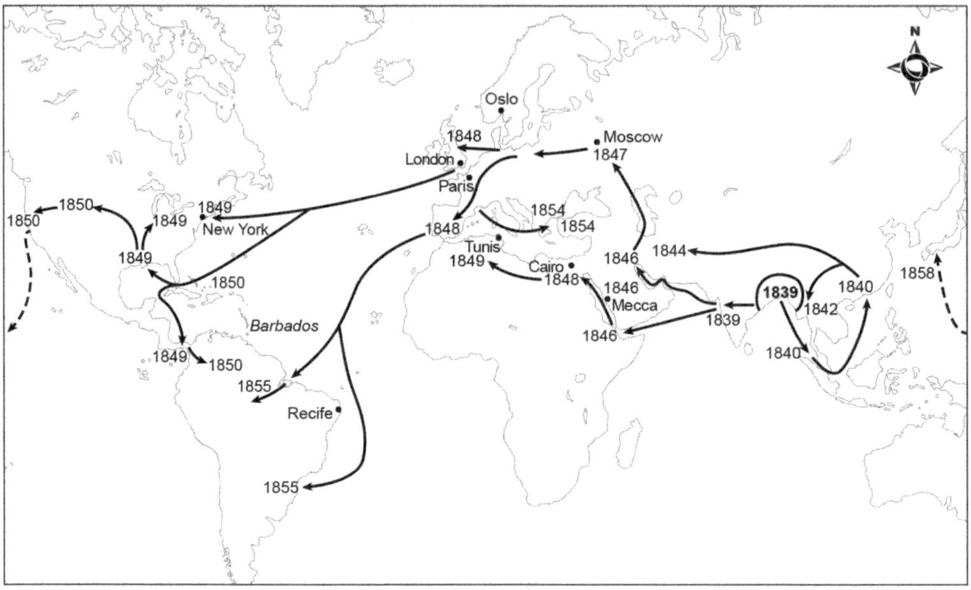

observance of a particular creed's Sabbath or more universal laws of nature? Were the poor responsible for their own misery and squalor (conditions that presumably generated cholera), or did society as a whole have a responsibility to clean up such squalor?

Outside Europe and North America some of the same themes were repeated. In Brazil, the medical community remained sharply divided about cholera's contagiousness, while in Tunisia some arguments blamed the miasma and general lack of sanitation for the epidemic.

Almost everywhere, too, divine powers were seen as playing a role. Westerners might regard the people of Bali (Indonesia) who regarded cholera as the product of a "demonic, protective deity" (Owen 1987, 117–141) as superstitious, but President Zachary Taylor of the United States had no qualms about proclaiming a day of "national prayer, fasting, and humiliation" (Rosenberg 1962, 121) when the third pandemic arrived.

RESPONSES

The responses of public authorities followed their convictions about what spread cholera. Anti-contagionist measures focused on sanitation and were often led by standing or ad hoc boards of health created to enforce sanitation measures. In Great Britain, a central board of health had been created in 1848, just before the third cholera pandemic arrived. But because it still had to rely on the willingness of local government bodies to adopt its policies, those policies remained suggestions. The board's zealous belief in the merits of sanitation—meaning the provision of clean water, the removal of human wastes and other nuisances—was opposed by many British physicians, who believed that cutting contagion by isolating the victims made more sense. Local governments often followed the lead of local physicians. By the later stages of the epidemic (1853–1854), however, more British local governments had adopted the General Board of Health's advice. (British medical opinion was in part being swayed by the views of British doctors in India, who were resolutely anti-contagionist; because of their presumed greater experience with cholera, their views had weight.) The official British enthusiasm for sanitation (even though it may have been stronger in theory than in practice) was mirrored in other places in Europe and beyond, especially in places such as Tunisia and Egypt where the rulers aspired to prove themselves to be modern with sanitary codes and commissions.

Quarantines, the first line of defense against a contagion, had become very controversial. Many European states had abandoned them after their apparent failure to halt the second cholera pandemic. Russia was one such state, and the presence (in 1830) or absence (in 1848) of quarantines against cholera seemed to make no difference. A conference called in Paris 1851 to discuss cholera quarantines failed. In America, New York City had no quarantine mechanism in place in 1848–1849. And even in places where quarantines were proclaimed—such as Egypt and Brazil—they proved almost impossible to enforce. Pilgrim traffic through and into Egypt was too great to be controlled in that way; trade between Brazil and (especially) Britain was too important for such interference.

Special isolation hospitals for cholera victims were sometimes undertaken, as another response to cholera's possible contagion. The rapidity of the disease's assault made their application difficult, for the victim might be dead before he reached the hospital. Memories of the 1832 fears of such hospitals during the Second Cholera Pandemic also lingered, and property owners resisted the provision of such a hospital on an ad hoc basis. Whose property would be used? Not mine. New York's first cholera hospital in 1849 was above a tavern.

Official responses also included appeals to the Deity. In Tunis the ruling bey arranged an invocation, in which Koranic verses (and other compositions) were read daily by *sharifs* (descendants of the Prophet). Nancy Gallagher (1983, 55–56) notes that "Just after the invocation was made at the Great Mosque, the disease abated and soon disappeared. The apparent effectiveness of this measure was such that Mustafa Khaznadar [a minister of Ahmed Bey, the ruler] announced that the men who participated in the invocation no longer needed proof of their holy descent."

As in the second cholera pandemic, fear generated many popular responses. Rumors spread; bodies were hastily disposed of before their contagion could take hold; people fled cities and towns if they could. But unlike the experience of 1832, civil unrest did not follow in the wake of cholera in the third pandemic. Some communities, notably in Brazil, fell into near chaos; government functions stopped, patients were abandoned, the dead rotted in their homes in Cachoeira, a district of Brazil's Bahia province. But the sort of near-revolutionary violence against officials and doctors that occurred in the second cholera pandemic was absent. (See the "Unresolved Historical Issues" section.)

Medical therapies for cholera resembled those of the second pandemic, which is to say that they remained ineffective or actually harmful. Western physicians remained wedded to drastic purgatives such as calomel; as a response to a disease that was accompanied by drastic loss of body fluids such a remedy was disastrous. The long tradition of bleeding had weakened by the mid-nineteenth century, however. Alternative and folk medicine relied on herbs and oils, gentle treatments that at least did no harm.

UNRESOLVED HISTORICAL ISSUES

The cause of cholera remained unknown at the conclusion of the third pandemic, and conflict continued over whether a contagious agent or a more general environmental poison spread the disease. Generally, the impact of the third pandemic strengthened the arguments of the sanitationists, not the contagionists. The answers to the prevention of cholera could be found, it was believed, in the broad approach of civil engineering, one that would provide clean water, remove human wastes, garbage, trash, and the dead animals that fouled city streets, and perhaps regulate the noxious emissions of industry.

It is therefore ironic that an experiment performed in the late stages of the third cholera pandemic suggested how the cholera contagion worked, although it also illustrated the importance of water as a cholera source. In 1854 John Snow, a London physician, compared two adjoining London districts that seemed economically and socially similar in most important respects (e.g., levels of income and housing density). They differed in two ways: one had a far higher rate of cholera than the other, and they were served by different sources of water. Snow argued that one difference explained the other, and that therefore cholera was somehow carried in the water supply that served one of the communities. Snow's observation would begin to carry weight in the next (fourth) cholera pandemic, in the 1860s.

Other arguments persisted as well, especially those concerning the role of individual responsibility for avoiding cholera. Those arguments have in a sense never been resolved, but the germ theory of cholera would shift their grounds in important ways.

The experiences of the third pandemic also clearly raised questions about the relationship between cholera and race. The differential mortality observed in Middle and South America, where people of African descent suffered higher rates than those of European descent, led some nineteenth-century Europeans (and white Americans) to conclude that cholera provided another illustration of white supremacy; either God, or the forces of Darwinian natural selection, had given white bodies more ability to withstand diseases. But even in the nineteenth century, this argument was countered by one that considered the conditions under which the African descendants (especially slaves) lived.

Kenneth Kiple, a modern historian, has concluded that those of African descent were at many environmental disadvantages in the Americas (Kiple 1985). They lived in crowded and dirty conditions where infected water supplies were more likely; they often lived along the waterfronts where cholera cases would be transported by sea; and their poor nutrition may have had the particular effect of weakening the stomach acids that (in most cases) kill cholera germs.

Unlike the second cholera pandemic, the third was not accompanied by dramatic social unrest. That fact has raised some historical questions, of the "why didn't the dog bark?" type. The third pandemic inflicted, if anything, higher mortality than the second; it occurred in years (1848–1849) marked by widespread political unrest and even revolution across Europe, but the cholera epidemics do not seem to have figured in those revolts. Why? Perhaps the higher mortality was less concentrated in poor quarters; if so, the middle class could not as easily stigmatize the poor, and the poor could less easily regard cholera as a middle-class plot. Perhaps the medical profession was held in higher esteem by the late 1840s, although that was clearly not the case, for example, in the United States. Perhaps the greater emphasis on sanitation, and the reduction of efforts at quarantine and isolation, removed some grievances. Perhaps European grievances in 1848–1849 were more overtly and plainly political (a point made by Richard Evans 1988), and needed no fuel from an epidemic. Perhaps, as Catherine Kudlick argues for France, the bourgeoisie had become more secure by 1848 and felt less threatened by the lower orders (Kudlick 1996).

REFERENCES

Cooper, Donald B. "The New 'Black Death': Cholera in Brazil, 1855–1856." *Social Science History* 10 (1986): 467–488.

Evans, Richard J. "Epidemics and Revolutions: Cholera in Nineteenth-Century Europe." *Past and Present* 120 (1988): 123–146.

Gallagher, Nancy E. *Medicine and Power in Tunisia, 1780–1900.* Cambridge: Cambridge University Press, 1983.

Jannetta, Ann Bowman. *Epidemics and Mortality in Early Modern Japan.* Princeton, NJ: Princeton University Press, 1987.

Kiple, Kenneth F. "Cholera and Race in the Caribbean." *Journal of Latin American Studies* 17 (1985): 157–177.

Kudlick, Catherine J. *Cholera in Post-Revolutionary Paris: A Cultural History.* Berkeley: University of California Press, 1996.

Kuhnke, LaVerne. *Lives at Risk: Public Health in Nineteenth-Century Egypt.* Berkeley: University of California Press, 1990.

Owen, Norman G., ed. *Death and Disease in Southeast Asia: Explorations in Social, Medical and Demographic History.* Singapore: Oxford University Press, 1987.

Pollitzer, Robert. *Cholera.* Geneva: World Health Organization, 1959.

Rosenberg, Charles E. *The Cholera Years: The United States in 1832, 1849, and 1866.* Chicago: University of Chicago Press, 1962.

SUGGESTED ADDITIONAL READING

Coleman, William. *Death Is a Social Disease: Public Health and Political Economy in Early Industrial France.* Madison: University of Wisconsin Press, 1982.

Hamlin, Christopher. *Cholera: The Biography.* Oxford: Oxford University Press, 2009.

Hamlin, Christopher. *Public Health and Social Justice in the Age of Chadwick: Britain, 1800–1854.* Cambridge: Cambridge University Press, 1998.

Maglen, Krista. *The English System: Quarantine, Immigration and the Making of a Port Sanitary Zone.* Manchester: Manchester University Press, 2014.

Pyle, G. F. "The Diffusion of Cholera in the United States in the Nineteenth Century." *Geographical Analysis* 1 (1969): 59–75.

23

Typhoid Fever in Cities, 1850–1920

WHEN AND WHERE

Typhoid fever, a common and dangerous intestinal infection, became an important endemic problem in American and European cities of the nineteenth century, and in some times and places rose to dangerous epidemic levels. Those epidemic outbreaks were the product of particular local causes, and typhoid epidemics did not therefore sweep across wide areas or move from one city to another. Briefly, contamination of water supplies most often produced those epidemic situations, and in the nineteenth century the rapid growth of cities in the early age of industrialization concentrated people around water supplies that could quickly become infected, especially when breaches connected water supplies to sewage. (See "Background" section later in the chapter.)

In the middle of the century, urban death rates from typhoid fever could range between 50 and 100 deaths per 100,000 people per year. For example, London's average across the decade of the 1850s was 87 and that rose to 89 in the 1860s, with some years worse than others. In 1870 the typhoid mortality rate in Milwaukee (much smaller and much newer) was about 67.

But between one city and another, wide variations existed, which suggested that some cities were consistently more dangerous than others. Those variations tended to widen later in the nineteenth century and into the early twentieth, as cities responded to the problem with differing levels of success. Between 1888 and 1912, Kansas City (Kansas) averaged a typhoid mortality rate of about 67, while Kansas City (Missouri), across the river, recorded an average of about 23. Among large cities in the same years the rate in Philadelphia was nearly 43, while New York's had fallen to 19 and London's to less than 9.

Some even wider variations existed within single cities, illustrating that typhoid epidemics could bear much more heavily on some populations than on others. In London in the 1860s, typhoid carried off an average of 152 per 100,000 per year from the St. George in the East district, and only 31 from the Hampstead district. In Pittsburgh, perhaps the most typhoid-ridden city in North America, the typhoid mortality rate between 1899 and 1907 was about 130, but in 1907 that number was a frightening 315 in one ward of the city and only 22 in another.

Other figures show that mortality rates from typhoid began declining in the late nineteenth and early twentieth centuries, although at different times in different places. Generally British and European cities improved before their American counterparts, as the London number cited earlier suggests (and typhoid incidence in Berlin and Paris had fallen even lower than London's). For London the steep decline in typhoid mortality began in the 1870s and continued into the early twentieth century. In 1900, 4,300 Londoners succumbed to typhoid, and at that point typhoid mortality rates were only about one-sixth of those of the 1860s. By 1923 that toll had fallen to about 250.

In American cities, the crucial decades were after 1890 or even after 1900. Chicago changed its water system by reversing the flow of a river by 1900; New York dramatically improved between 1900 and 1930; Milwaukee's typhoid rates fell sharply after 1910, and Pittsburgh's in the decade of the 1910s. By 1930 typhoid had ceased to be a major disease problem in the cities of North America and Europe.

(For examples of particular epidemics and their connection to local conditions, see the "Background" section.)

SIGNIFICANCE

Typhoid fever was an epidemic disease that rose rapidly in popular consciousness with industrial urbanization, when critical masses of people found themselves at risk from it. It was brought under control relatively quickly as a result of changes in sanitation that were not necessarily, or entirely, undertaken with a clear understanding of why they worked. Its story is therefore an important example of the indirect or inadvertent relations between epidemic disease and social change.

Typhoid fever was a serious disease in nineteenth-century Western cities and attracted much attention at the time. Its demographic impact should not be exaggerated, however; the mortality rates quoted above for epidemics rarely or never approached the annual death toll from tuberculosis. Such exaggerations still appear in some modern works: for example, Erik Larson's claim that "in 1885 fouled water had ignited an outbreak of cholera and typhoid that killed ten percent of [Chicago's] population" (Larson 2003, 109). No nineteenth-century epidemic in the Western world remotely approached a death rate of 10,000 per 100,000.

The understanding of typhoid fever that emerged in the nineteenth century has led one historian to label it the "exemplary disease" (Stevenson 1982). Arguments about it foreshadowed more general discussions about the causes and courses of disease. For example, in the course of the concern with typhoid fever the idea of the *asymptomatic carrier* (a person infected by a germ who displays no symptoms) was advanced and then applied to other diseases. And typhoid fever figured in the most dramatic episode in the popular conceptions of the healthy carrier—the "epidemics" caused by Typhoid Mary.

BACKGROUND

According to modern views, typhoid fever is caused by the infection of the digestive tract by the bacterium called *Salmonella typhi.* This germ is present in water (or food) contaminated by the excretions of people already infected by it. It therefore spreads most often as a result of water supplies being mixed with human wastes. Although *Salmonella typhi* is one of a large class of *Salmonella* bacteria, unlike most of the others it only lives in humans, not other species. But it can live and grow in different foods, and so can pass from contaminated water to food, and hence to more people. Another possible transmission route involves the fly, which may carry the bacterium from excretions to food (although this possibility has not yet been proven). Water mixed with sewage, food in contact with such water, and a swarm of flies, are therefore all background factors in the spread of typhoid fever; the first, mixing water and sewage, is especially important.

Many examples of these factors at work exist in the generation of typhoid fever epidemics in the nineteenth and early twentieth centuries. Pittsburgh took its water from its rivers (as did many other cities in Europe and America); neighboring communities dumped untreated sewage into the same rivers. When Newark replaced water from the Passaic River with that from the Pequannock in 1893, a typhoid mortality rate that had approached 100 per 100,000 in 1890 and 1891 fell almost immediately to about 30. Meanwhile adjacent Jersey City continued to draw its water from the Passaic, and its typhoid mortality rate remained at about 80.

Chicago drew water from Lake Michigan, using an intake two-and-one-half miles offshore that had been constructed in 1867. The rapid growth of the city in subsequent years meant that the capacities of that intake became inadequate, and another intake was opened in 1890. But that new intake was placed only 1,500 feet from the shoreline of the lake into which Chicago also dumped its sewage. In 1891 Chicago suffered nearly 2,000 typhoid fever deaths, a mortality rate of 174.

Even later, when cities had significantly lowered typhoid rates, sudden epidemic surges could follow an unexpected contamination. In New York in the decade of the 1920s, an average of about 950 people fell ill (and about 125 died) from typhoid annually, representing a very low morbidity rate when compared with earlier times. But in 1924 and 1925, over 3,100 cases occurred when a water source became contaminated and oysters were polluted.

The rapid growth of cities, illustrated by the Chicago example, could strain water supplies and lead to less healthy sources. The same growth also meant vast increases in the volume of sewage, and the corresponding difficulty of disposing of it. And in the late nineteenth century, the density of flies was simply staggering. In part flies were attracted to the vast urban population of horses and the manure they deposited. In 1902 Great Britain had about 3.5 million horses; those horses may have produced *21 million tons* of manure annually, of which a fair proportion landed on city streets and drew flies.

Social conditions in cities also contributed to higher typhoid rates. Many cities in both America and Europe drew migrants from rural areas where typhoid fever was not considered a problem. Perhaps for that reason, when officials issued precautionary advice (see the "How It Was Understood at the Time" and "Responses" sections), the advice was not heeded; in the United States the additional problem of language complicated the advice given to recent immigrants. Some of these difficulties probably explain why, while typhoid rates declined dramatically in London in the 1870s when a better water and sewer system was in place, further reductions in the disease only occurred gradually. Anne Hardy (1993, 170–172) argues that neither the professional skill of plumbers nor the domestic habits of the urban population could be changed as rapidly as the relatively simple provision of clean water, and that a lot of opportunities for typhoid infection thus persisted.

HOW IT WAS UNDERSTOOD AT THE TIME

The identification of typhoid fever as a separate disease emerged only slowly in the course of the nineteenth century. Its symptoms were common to many ailments: fever, headaches, digestive upsets and abdominal pain, red rashes all characterized a continuum of fevers. For that reason, any estimates of mortality and morbidity rates before the middle or later nineteenth century must be only guesses. One of the diseases with which it was long confused was typhus—an American physician, William Gerhard, differentiated the two in 1837, but his arguments gained ground only after 1850. And even then other confusions remained. The term "enteric fever," meaning simply intestinal fever, included both typhoid fever and the later-identified paratyphoid fever, caused in fact by a different bacterium.

The association of the disease with water or food contamination was made before any understanding of the responsible bacterium. The English physician William Budd made such arguments in the 1840s, but his water contamination theory contended with others for several decades. Some believed that the disease came from an agent that appeared by spontaneous generation in the body; others argued that the presence of a general miasma, or bad atmosphere, caused the disease. (In those ways, the arguments about the cause of typhoid fever mirrored those of other diseases in the middle nineteenth century, a period of dispute about disease causes. (See, e.g., the chapters on cholera pandemics in this volume.)

Budd's arguments for water transmission did support the growing sanitation movement in Great Britain, one of whose goals was providing clean water. Sanitary reform had other motives in addition to the prevention of disease, including political pride and aesthetic sensibility. But whatever those motives, improvements in water cleanliness did result in declining mortality from typhoid, and the perception of that reduction lent support to Budd's theory.

Then in 1880 the German microbiologist Carl Eberth identified what he claimed was the causative microorganism, and four years later Georg Gaffky isolated it and studied its properties. As was true of other germ discoveries in those years, acceptance of the Eberth-Gaffky organism as the cause of typhoid fever only took place gradually, as general environmental notions gave way slowly. Eberth's germ did, however, explain the mechanism of transmission through water, closing the gaps in Budd's argument. By 1896 blood tests could show the presence of *Salmonella typhi* in a person, and so place the diagnosis of typhoid fever on a more precise basis.

Understanding another aspect of typhoid fever also began in the late nineteenth century: that the healthy or asymptomatic carrier might exist. Budd had advanced such an idea in 1873; early germ theorists, in the 1880s, showed that diphtheria could be spread by such carriers, and by the 1890s—if not sooner—such a cause could explain the beginnings of a local typhoid epidemic where no obvious case had previously existed.

RESPONSES

In the long run, the important response to the presence of typhoid fever was to provide clean water supplies clearly separated from human wastes. London had made great improvements in that respect by the 1870s. In part reacting to its 1890–1892 typhoid epidemics, Chicago, under increasing pressure from doctors and germ theorists, undertook the massive engineering project that reversed its river's flow, carrying the city's sewage not into the lake from which it drew its water but toward the interior of the country. Pittsburgh installed a water filtration system between 1908 and 1912. For years after 1900, such engineering improvements were therefore undertaken in part as direct responses to the threat of typhoid fever.

In a related category, there were improvements in domestic sanitation. In 1871 Edward, Prince of Wales (the future Edward VII), Queen Victoria's eldest son, fell ill of typhoid fever while staying at a lodge in Yorkshire. (And, in fact, his father, Prince Albert, had died of typhoid in 1861.) Prince Edward recovered, although two other guests at the lodge did not. William H. Corfield, a sanitary expert, concluded (a bit hesitantly) that the disease could be traced to a defective toilet. The popular furor over the prince's health made Corfield a celebrity, and he subsequently became an authority on the healthy home, whose books sold widely and inspired other works that urged attention to health in home construction and plumbing. With that also came slow changes in domestic personal habits of cleanliness such as washing hands and boiling water for safety.

The attitudes of political authorities also evolved. Although as late as 1891, the health officer of Newark vigorously denied that a typhoid epidemic was present in the city, calling reports about it a "press fabrication" (Galishoff 1988, 105), other city governments moved toward more action. By 1918, for example, Chicago had chlorinated its water, made typhoid a reportable disease (meaning that the city was to receive notice of all cases), placed warning placards on infected houses, restricted food handling processes, and quarantined identified healthy carriers.

Medical responses to typhoid fever also evolved. In the middle of the nineteenth century, physicians were still largely helpless in the face of the wide variety of fevers, and many urged letting nature take its course. (That course, in the case of typhoid fever, might last three or four weeks, with death intervening in about 10% of the cases.) Behind that approach lay centuries of Hippocratic tradition, and the belief that a fever was part of a natural and healing response to an illness. Other physicians attempted more active intervention with traditional bleeding and purging. As the century wore on, interest in reducing the fever itself grew, with the idea that fever was itself harmful, not healthful. Immersion in cold water was the most obvious method, and water cures had a long history that enjoyed a revival in the nineteenth-century movement called *hydropathy.* In the 1870s quinine, which had become the most important antimalarial treatment, was also applied to reduce typhoid fever. Attempts to produce synthetic substitutes for quinine in the

1880s briefly had exciting prospects but proved to be dangerous to circulatory systems. And the discovery of the responsible bacterium led to hopes of a preventive vaccine, and by the time of World War I (1914–1918) troops were receiving a fairly effective vaccine.

The application of antibiotics to typhoid fever, beginning in the late 1940s, drastically reduced the disease's seriousness and mortality.

UNRESOLVED HISTORICAL ISSUES

Typhoid ceased to be an epidemic problem in the Western world for a complex variety of reasons, and historians may still debate the relative roles of water purification, food inspections, domestic habits, and the control of healthy carriers in bringing the disease to a halt. Was any one measure decisive? Probably not, although water purification was certainly central.

Another uncertain historical matter relates to the importance of poverty as a marker for typhoid. Did the poor quarters of a city suffer disproportionately? In many cases, certainly yes, but did other variables, such gender, occupation, or age, play a role as well?

A truly effective cure for typhoid fever waited until the development of antibiotics in the 1940s. But now—as with many bacterial diseases—strains of *Salmonella typhi* are appearing that have higher resistance to antibiotic treatment. "*Salmonella* serotypes adapt happily into new ecological niches. They are resourceful and resilient; they do not respect human boundaries. As long as there is animal life on earth, the *Salmonella* family will have a future" (Hardy 2015, 230).

REFERENCES

Galishoff, Stuart. *Newark: The Nation's Unhealthiest City, 1832–1895.* New Brunswick, NJ: Rutgers University Press, 1988.

Hardy, Anne. *The Epidemic Streets: Infectious Disease and the Rise of Preventive Medicine, 1856–1900.* Oxford: Clarendon, 1993.

Hardy, Anne. *Salmonella Infections, Networks of Knowledge, and Public Health in Britain, 1880–1975.* Oxford: Oxford University Press, 2015.

Larson, Erik. *The Devil in the White City: Murder, Magic, and Madness at the Fair That Changed America.* New York: Crown, 2003.

Stevenson, Lloyd G. "Exemplary Disease: The Typhoid Pattern." *Journal of the History of Medicine and Allied Sciences* 37 (1982): 159–181.

SUGGESTED ADDITIONAL READING

Cliff, Andrew, Peter Haggett, and Matthew Smallman-Raynor. *Deciphering Global Epidemics: Analytical Approaches to the Disease Records of World Cities, 1888–1912.* Cambridge: Cambridge University Press, 1998.

Duffy, John. *A History of Public Health in New York City, 1866–1966.* New York: Russell Sage Foundation, 1974.

Koppes, Clayton R., and William P. Norris. "Ethnicity, Class, and Mortality in the Industrial City: A Case Study of Typhoid Fever in Pittsburgh, 1890–1910." *Journal of Urban History* 11 (1985): 259–279.

Leavitt, Judith Walzer. *The Healthiest City: Milwaukee and the Politics of Health Reform.* Princeton, NJ: Princeton University Press, 1982.

McTavish, Jan R. "Antipyretic Treatment and Typhoid Fever: 1860–1900." *Journal of the History of Medicine and Allied Sciences* 42 (1987): 486–506.

Platt, Harold L. *Shock Cities: The Environmental Transformation and Reform of Manchester and Chicago.* Chicago: University of Chicago Press, 2005.

Tarr, Joel A., James McCurley III, Francis C. McMichael, and Terry Yosie. "Water and Wastes: A Retrospective Assessment of Wastewater Technology in the United States, 1800–1932." *Technology and Culture* 25 (1984): 226–263.

24

Yellow Fever in New Orleans, 1853

WHEN AND WHERE

In the summer of 1853, New Orleans, which had repeatedly endured yellow fever outbreaks, suffered its worst yellow fever epidemic. Over about five months somewhere between 9,000 and 11,000 people in New Orleans died of yellow fever; as many as 40,000 cases of the disease developed in a population that (in the summer) may have been about 100,000. Yellow fever caused about half of the deaths recorded in the whole of 1853 in New Orleans.

Physicians first noticed cases of yellow fever in late May. Through June, the disease remained confined to the poorer quarters of the city near the Mississippi River and its docks, and the number of cases created no alarm. Then in July mortality and morbidity began increasing, and fears grew. By the end of July, many of those who could flee the city had done so, and the hospitals were full. Deaths began occurring in embarrassingly public places. By early August, the condition of cemeteries was becoming scandalous, as bodies hastily buried in shallow graves were exposed to the elements, decomposed, and emitted rank odors into the surrounding air. In the third week of August, the epidemic reached its peak, claiming over 250 victims per day. By about the same time, the city had mobilized its services (both those of government and voluntary philanthropy) more effectively. The crisis clearly eased by the first week of September, and the city's board of health declared the epidemic over on October 13. In December, 254 deaths were reported from cholera, and none from yellow fever.

SIGNIFICANCE

Many yellow fever epidemics in nineteenth-century cities were especially disruptive of the community's life, and the 1853 New Orleans episode was one of the most vivid examples of yellow fever's destructive power. The rapid onset of drastically gruesome symptoms and the potentially (if erratically) high levels of mortality made the disease deeply feared; part of its disruptive power stemmed from the general acceptance of flight as the only recourse. A yellow fever epidemic could therefore bring the economy of a city to a halt, as people fled from it and quarantines were hastily proclaimed against commerce from it. Cities in the southern United States were particularly vulnerable in the nineteenth century, for they had become the receiving points for imports of such goods as coffee and sugar that originated in lands where yellow fever was endemic.

The ravages of 1853 in New Orleans contributed strongly to a real (though gradual) shift in views of public responsibility for health in the United States. At the start of the 1853 epidemic, New Orleans had a board of health, but its activity and powers were minimal. That began to change during 1853. When yellow fever returned to the city in 1854, the state of Louisiana responded by creating a permanent state board of health and erecting a state quarantine system, both for the first time.

The horrors of 1853 also contributed to the widespread American opinion of New Orleans as a chaotic, pestilential city that was best avoided. That image proved difficult to shake.

BACKGROUND

New Orleans had the most consistent and troublesome history of yellow fever of any American city. Between 1825 and 1860, it suffered through 12 epidemics, of which 1853 was only the worst; for example, yellow fever accounted for over 30% of the city's deaths in 1841, about 15% in 1843, and about 25% in 1847, while 1854–1855 were bad yellow fever years as well. Although yellow fever never became endemic in New Orleans (its winters were just cold enough to halt the *Aedes aegypti* mosquitoes that carried the virus), some nineteenth-century thinkers feared that the city might sustain the disease indigenously. The location of the city contributed to its troubles, for it was (and is) exceptionally low-lying and surrounded by swampy ground; malaria *was* endemic there. Although the connection between yellow fever and mosquitoes had not been made in 1853, New Orleans citizens had long complained about the fetid air, smells, and unsanitary messes that characterized their environment.

The social structure and the economy of New Orleans contributed to its vulnerability. It received large numbers of immigrants from Europe (especially Ireland and Germany) in the mid-nineteenth century, people from northern latitudes who had no previous exposure to yellow fever. It conducted a large amount of trade with Caribbean and South American ports where yellow fever was endemic. (See volume 2, chapter 16.) The importance of that commerce to its economy meant that quarantines were a particularly sensitive political issue; instituting them would be fiercely resisted.

The people of New Orleans regularly fled the city—if they could afford to do so—to escape yellow fever epidemics. Some of them left in the summer anyway, hoping to escape heat. But the massive exodus of 1853 certainly skewed the death toll heavily in the direction of the poorer classes, and perhaps (to some slight extent) contributed to diffusing yellow fever elsewhere.

HOW IT WAS UNDERSTOOD AT THE TIME

The symptoms of yellow fever had been long known in 1853. A number of its names referred to those symptoms, including *yellow jack* (reflecting the bilious color of the skin and eyes) and *black vomit* (self-explanatory). While doctors generally recognized it from those symptoms, they were less sure of its cause, and indeed unsure of whether its cause differed from other fevers. Yellow fever was one of the central diseases at stake in nineteenth-century discussions of the relative importance of contagion and environment. In 1853 New Orleans (and elsewhere), most expert opinion held that yellow fever was a miasmatic disease, borne on (and perhaps originating in) a foul atmosphere. That atmosphere perhaps teemed with tiny organisms that caused the disease. Although no such specific yellow fever organisms had been identified, popular belief imagined that such tiny living particles attached themselves to bedding and clothing.

Near-unanimous agreement existed on another environmental point: that yellow fever did not survive the first frost in the autumn or winter. It was, therefore, strictly a hot-weather disease.

The conviction that yellow fever was an environmental product meant that flight was a logical response to its threat: escape the dangerous environment. But nineteenth-century opinion could not entirely break free of behavioral explanations of yellow fever; dissolute conduct was to be avoided if flight were not possible; the apparently higher toll in poorer quarters of cities might, after all, be related to the faulty habits of the poor as well as to the atmosphere in which everyone lived. Contemporaries also recognized the relative immunity enjoyed by people of African origin or descent, a fact that had been used to argue the existence of essential racial differences between whites and blacks.

In 1853, orthodox American medicine was still heavily influenced by the heroic interpretations and therapies of Benjamin Rush, while against that tradition a variety of alternative medical systems and therapies had arisen. Generally, the orthodox beliefs of the time saw all fevers as related, and all (including yellow fever) manifested themselves in over-tension (or over-relaxation) of the nerves and muscles of the body.

RESPONSES

The predominance of the environmental view of yellow fever governed many of the responses to it. Those responses aimed chiefly at prevention, or (if that failed) at containment, of the disease. The city government took such action only slowly, for the notion of individual responsibility for health was especially strong in mid-nineteenth-century America. The surest prevention of yellow fever seemed to be flight from the afflicted area, and that response was an individual matter. A reluctance to admit the presence of yellow fever also delayed government action. If other cities learned of yellow fever in New Orleans, they might proclaim quarantines that would hurt New Orleans business; both city officials and city journalists therefore hesitated to admit that yellow fever had arrived.

For some combination of those causes, the New Orleans city council took few steps against yellow fever until the epidemic was well established in late July. One earlier step—in late June—suggested that city officials knew that a crisis was at hand: the council abruptly cancelled the long-standing arrangements with private contractors for street cleaning. Corruption had long characterized the contract cleaning system, resulting in high levels of public dirt and smelly nuisances such as dead animals. With another yellow fever epidemic on the horizon, the city council decided to assume street cleaning as a government responsibility. But while New Orleans theoretically possessed a standing board of health, its powers and actions were minimal. And the city council actually adjourned for the summer at the end of July; just as the epidemic was obviously becoming serious many members of the council left the city.

While the council left, the board of health began asserting itself. It ordered streets to be flushed with water and vital statistics to be collected. By mid-August, the board had begun a number of other public health initiatives to clean the environment: the scandal of rotting corpses in the overloaded cemeteries was confronted by hiring more laborers; lime was spread around the city, bedding and clothing of the sick were burned, citizens were urged to don nose bags filled with spices to keep the miasma from their lungs. In a curious attempt to purge the atmosphere, cannon fire was ordered and tar was burned in the vicinity of cemeteries to overcome the supposedly deadly exhalations that surrounded them.

Care of the sick was less clearly a public responsibility, and much of it fell to voluntary and charitable organizations. New Orleans had one large hospital, staffed by the Sisters of Charity; in August the board of health did commission some temporary infirmaries as well. The Howard Association, a private philanthropic group that commenced a national appeal for relief funds, organized much of the medical and nursing services.

Although medicine in fact could offer no effective remedy for yellow fever, hopeful alternatives existed. Many orthodox physicians remained committed to a heroic treatment, calling for bleeding the veins and purging the bowels. Behind that approach ultimately lay the theory of the four humours, but in nineteenth-century America, bleeding and purging were intended to relieve fever-inducing tension in the muscles and nerves. Quinine, now increasingly recognized as an effective specific remedy for malaria, was also employed to fight yellow fever. The historic connection between New Orleans and France meant that some members of its medical community, educated not in American but in French traditions, were less enthusiastic about heroic bleedings and purgings, and more inclined to gentler therapies. And the broad variety of other medical sects, such as homeopathy (emphasizing minute doses) and Thomsonianism (emphasizing botanical medicine), offered other gentler therapies as well.

Prayer was another important response. Some members of the city's clergy remained very active throughout the epidemic. They appealed to the board of health for the proclamation of an official day of prayer, and the mayor designated September 2; on that day the city came to an almost total stop as the population flocked to the churches to beg God's mercy. That the epidemic was waning by that date might have been seen as evidence of divine favor; the subsequent rapid decline in mortality, as evidence of prayer's efficacy.

UNRESOLVED HISTORICAL ISSUES

Because the epidemiological path of yellow fever remained unknown until the very end of the nineteenth century, important questions lingered after the 1853 epidemic in New Orleans. Agreement about quarantines remained politically difficult, and their effects remained uncertain. Cities continued to use quarantines as weapons to cripple the commerce of their rivals. For instance, Galveston or Mobile (which vied with New Orleans for shipping on the Gulf of Mexico) could quarantine traffic from New Orleans; if yellow fever beset all three cities, each could offer shorter quarantine periods to importing merchants, hoping to seem more attractive. Those commercial pressures continued to mean that declaring a quarantine was a political act; partly for that reason, the effect of quarantines remained unclear, for too many people had too many reasons to evade them even if they were proclaimed. Another yellow fever outbreak in 1878, and the quarantines that accompanied it, particularly crippled New Orleans merchants. In the subsequent years, those merchants increasingly pushed for some federal quarantine policy that would override sectional interests. (The Marine Hospital Service, a "quasi-national" [Humphreys 1992, 128] agency, was given some quarantine powers in the 1890s, but political issues persisted, and the discovery of the role of mosquitoes lessened interest in quarantines after 1900.)

Behind the question of quarantine lay the unresolved debate between contagion and miasma theorists. By 1855 the state of Louisiana had created a permanent standing board of health and asserted its powers to quarantine. Since the major tasks of boards of health involved cleansing the environment, while quarantine clearly responded to fears of contagion, the state's actions reflected continued ambivalence about how yellow fever spread. Margaret Humphreys, however, argues convincingly that fear of yellow fever remained the most important force driving the extension of public health systems in the southern United States, and most public health measures of the nineteenth century proceeded from environmentalist assumptions.

The frequency of yellow fever epidemics in New Orleans, and in the American South generally, declined in the last quarter of the nineteenth century, and the role of the strengthening systems of public health in that decline might still be debated. The mosquito transmission theory was only applied after 1900, so the gradually weakening presence of yellow fever in the 25 years before that requires other and more complex explanations. The last American yellow fever epidemic was in 1905, and certainly the final banishment of the disease did follow the discovery of the role of *Aedes aegypti* mosquitoes in its transmission. Campaigns against mosquitoes, pioneered in Caribbean areas that fell under American political control (notably Cuba and Panama), involved a combination of pouring oil on such standing water locales as cisterns, draining wet places, and screening yellow fever patients from mosquitoes. Although New Orleans began acting (at first inconclusively) against mosquitoes in 1901, the 1905 epidemic convinced doubters, and the city undertook systematic mosquito eradication.

REFERENCES AND SUGGESTED ADDITIONAL READING

Carrigan, JoAnn. *The Saffron Scourge: A History of Yellow Fever in Louisiana, 1796–1905.* Lafayette: University of Louisiana at Lafayette Press, 1994.

Duffy, John. *Sword of Pestilence: The New Orleans Yellow Fever Epidemic of 1853.* Baton Rouge: Louisiana State University Press, 1966.

Humphreys, Margaret. *Yellow Fever and the South.* New Brunswick, NJ: Rutgers University Press, 1992.

25

Fourth Cholera Pandemic, 1863–1875

WHERE AND WHEN

The world's fourth cholera pandemic began, as the earlier ones had, in the Indian subcontinent. In 1863 cholera again spread from Bengal across India, reaching Bombay on the west coast in 1864. From that port it began its ocean travels around the world. Of particular importance was its passage through western Asia to the Mediterranean lands and beyond, a path of infection that earlier cholera pandemics had followed as well, but one that in the mid-1860s attracted special attention.

The port of Aden, in southern Arabia, was a stopping point for ocean traffic between India and the Red Sea, and hence between India and Europe, especially Great Britain. The volume of traffic between India and Aden made it certain that cholera would arrive there, as indeed it did in 1864. In early 1865, traffic from Aden began carrying cholera onward, to (for instance) Somalia, and from there the disease moved on into Ethiopia. But the important move from Aden in 1865 was up the Red Sea to the Hijaz, that section of western Arabia that includes the Muslim pilgrimage center of Mecca and its seaport, Jidda. To Mecca came Muslims from all over the world, including India, Malaysia, and the East Indies, who might be carrying cholera; from Mecca others went back home, to Egypt, Syria, Palestine, and North Africa, passing cholera along as they moved. Mecca suffered a major cholera epidemic in April 1865, apparently brought by a shipload of pilgrims whose journey had begun in Singapore. Of the 90,000 pilgrims in Mecca at the time, 15,000 died of cholera.

From the Hijaz cities, cholera moved to Egypt, where over 60,000 deaths occurred in June and July 1865, months during which Egyptian society nearly came to a halt. Egypt was in turn the conduit for cholera's passage over the Mediterranean to European ports. Naples had about 5,600 cholera deaths in 1865 and 1866. Such European ports themselves became the foci of new infections of other European points; by the end of 1865, cholera had spread to Great Britain, the Netherlands, the German states, and Russia. Europe in turn passed the disease to the Americas. In 1865 vessels from Marseilles carried cholera to Guadeloupe, in the West Indies; one source claims that 12,000 people on that island died in the

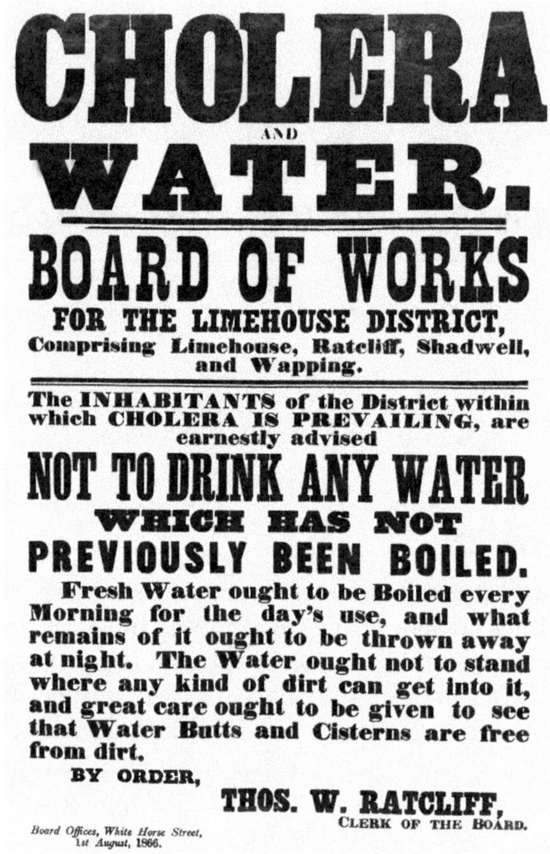

Broadsheet warns residents of London's Limehouse district against drinking water that has not been boiled or that has been contaminated by dirt, 1866. Opinions about the cause of cholera differed at this time—some said contaminated water alone was the problem, while others argued that surely additional factors must be involved. (Wellcome Library)

resulting epidemic. And in October 1865 a vessel from London brought cholera to New York; while that episode was contained without an epidemic, another steamer, carrying nearly 1,100 poor immigrants, arrived in April 1866 and cholera began to spread in the city. New York recorded 591 cholera deaths that year. From New York, cholera fanned into the interior of the United States in the summer of 1866; by the mid-1860s, the American network of railways was dense enough to provide rapid movement of both people and their infections through at least the eastern part of the country.

American places served as further centers for cholera's diffusion. The disease moved from Guadeloupe to Hispaniola in 1866 and from there to Cuba, where 4,400 deaths from cholera occurred in 1867 and 1868. And from New Orleans other 1866 ocean traffic carried cholera to Nicaragua.

Meanwhile cholera had jumped into the African continent from several directions. By 1869 the infection of Ethiopia (from Aden) had spread down the East African coast to Zanzibar, Mozambique, and Madagascar. Cholera reached North

Africa both directly from Egypt—true of Algeria and Morocco—and also from Europe; Tunisia managed to keep contacts with Egypt safe, but in April 1867 cholera appeared, probably brought from Sicily by smugglers. By June 1867, 150 people were dying daily in Tunis. Cholera also moved overland in Africa, accompanying caravans across the Sahara. Such traffic carried cholera to Senegal in 1868, and from there it moved elsewhere in West Africa.

The years of the fourth pandemic were especially severe ones in India itself where cholera was endemic. At times cholera coincided with years of famine, with terrible results for the Indian people. Famine occurred in years of drought, when Indians were more likely to drink from contaminated wells; famine drove villagers into cities, straining water supplies and the removal of excrement. Madras in 1866 provided an example of such suffering. And India, like Mecca, showed the apparent hazards of crowds gathered for religious pilgrimage. In April 1867 a Hindu pilgrimage site at Hardwar drew three million pilgrims to gather in a camp along the Ganges River that was roughly nine miles long and three miles deep. Cholera started affecting them on April 13; the pilgrims began dispersing with "inconceivable" rapidity (Malleson 1868, 10) and within two days the camp had almost emptied. Traveling by roads, the vast throng, now infected, spread cholera throughout northwestern India. About 250,000 had been stricken, half of them fatally.

SIGNIFICANCE

During the fourth cholera pandemic Western opinion explicitly associated the disease with the religious pilgrimages central to Hinduism and Islam. European governments, acting on that belief, began efforts to regulate and control such pilgrimages in the non-Western world, and so the fourth cholera pandemic stands at a crucial point in the developing connections between medicine, disease, and Western imperial power. (See the "Responses" section.)

The fourth cholera pandemic also led to greater general conviction that cholera moved with human traffic, that it had to be imported from someplace else. This conviction went together with a growing, and somewhat different, belief that water pollution and cholera were related. Only by the time of the fifth cholera pandemic would the specific agent in polluted water be identified, however.

BACKGROUND

By the 1860s, steam-powered transportation made possible a great expansion of human traffic in some important places that were involved in the fourth cholera pandemic. Two notable examples are within India and within Egypt. In India, the British rulers had encouraged heavy investment in railroads by British capital. In 1857 less than 300 miles of railroad existed in India; by 1870 the mileage exceeded 5,000, and by 1880 it neared 10,000. Both the numbers of Hindu pilgrims who could move, and the speed with which they could travel, increased dramatically. Such sites as Hardwar, Allahabad, and Puri could rapidly fill with pilgrims, and the pilgrims could just as rapidly diffuse throughout the country at the conclusion

Fourth Cholera Pandemic, 1863–1875

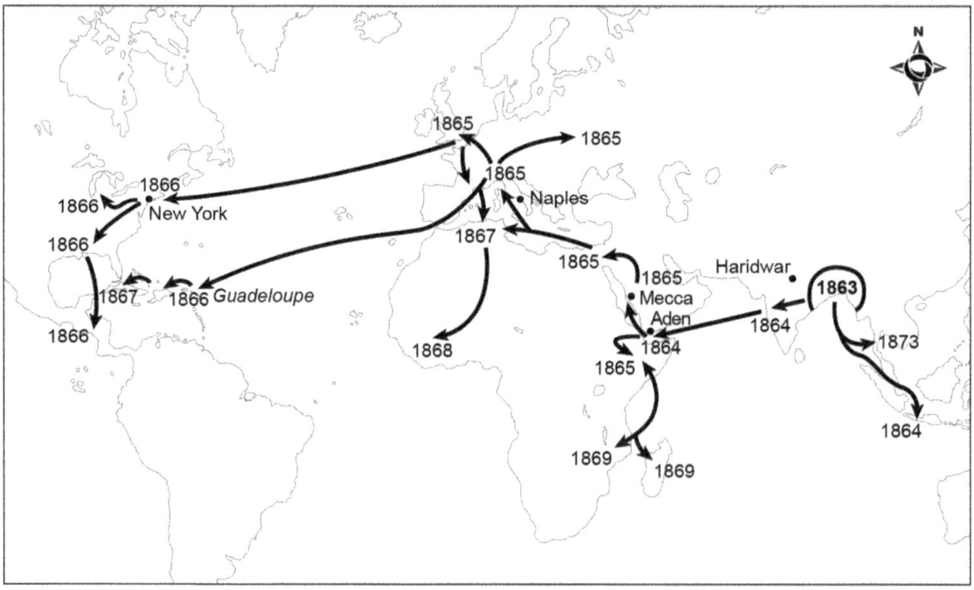

of their stay. Indian railroads could also quickly speed Muslims to seaports such as Bombay on their way to a Mecca pilgrimage, and steamships now made that journey quickly and reliably.

Pious Muslims bound for Mecca from the Mediterranean lands could also travel by steamship to Alexandria and could then move to Suez (on the Red Sea) by means of a railroad (built in 1858) that connected that city with Cairo and Alexandria. In 1869 the Suez Canal opened, and steamships could move directly from Mediterranean ports to Jidda, on the Red Sea adjoining Mecca.

These changes in transportation infrastructure, which so dramatically transformed world disease environments, were part of the dynamic Western industrial economy's expansion into the world. That expansion, perhaps more than ever by the 1860s, was also driving important social and political changes, and those changes too might affect the spread of epidemics. For example, Japan (under significant Western pressure, initially American) opened its country to world trade in the late 1850s, and cholera immediately arrived. By the 1860s, the government of Tunisia had in effect collapsed, and European power was able to dictate medical and public health measures (see the "Responses" section).

Rapid economic and technological changes might now occur in many places in the world, and the consequences of those changes for epidemics were often mixed or unclear. Western-dominated change might both give and take away. The construction of port facilities and the Suez Canal brought shantytowns where diseases such as cholera could spread rapidly to Egyptian cities. But by the late 1860s and 1870s improved (and safer) water supplies had begun to come to some large Indian cities.

HOW IT WAS UNDERSTOOD AT THE TIME

Many of the uncertainties about cholera that had existed in the earlier pandemics of the nineteenth century still remained during the fourth pandemic. In particular, the debate about whether the disease spread by contagion or through environmental pollution had not been settled. The *gospel of sanitation* (urging environmental purification) that had gained ground in the second and third pandemics now confronted the evidence of water transmission, which might be environmental but which also suggested a route of contagion. That evidence, put forward by John Snow in 1854, had gained some powerful allies, especially the Munich sanitation expert Max von Pettenkofer. Pettenkofer argued that polluted water was at least a necessary cause of cholera, even though he was unwilling to call it a *sufficient* cause.

The result, during the fourth pandemic, was a growing belief in what Peter Baldwin (1999) calls *neocontagionism*, particularly applied to cholera. Baldwin's neocontagionism included a more sharply focused attempt to prevent the movement of disease from one place to another. It emphasized inspecting victims and their symptoms to identify the presence of a disease; promptly notifying authorities when a disease was present; isolating the sick; medically surveilling travelers; and disinfecting individuals, their dwellings, and their goods. This approach recognized that total quarantines and sanitary cordons were increasingly impractical (or would be impossibly expensive) in an age of mass steam-powered transportation.

Some authorities (e.g., the Italians) remained contagionist in their approach, continuing to emphasize quarantines; others (such as the British) remained convinced of the importance of sanitation. But the differences, as illustrated in the "Responses" section, were those of degree. British leaders took part in quarantine efforts; Italians agreed that sanitation was important.

But if many accepted the role of water pollution in spreading cholera, they remained uncertain about the immediate primary cause of the disease. Did some poison precipitate out of the atmosphere and hence into the water? Or did a similar poison originate in an individual?

Other more general beliefs about cholera also existed, some on a more popular level. The fourth pandemic led to a Western conviction that the pilgrimages of other religions (especially Islam and Hinduism) were inherently dangerous, and perhaps symbolic of backward superstition.

But for some non-Westerners, the actions of Europeans and North Americans led to cholera. Japanese opinion associated cholera's appearance with the intrusion into their country of Western trade; some Indians believed that cholera came in the wake of disturbances in the social order such as the Sepoy Revolts of 1857, which were a response to the disruptive presence of the British.

RESPONSES

Official responses by governments included different mixes of efforts to improve sanitation and attempts to control contagion. In general, European cities and states tried to inspect victims to verify the presence of cholera, notify the world that cholera was present, isolate the victims, and inspect and quarantine travelers. At the same time, they also took sanitary steps, mandating street cleaning, and—combining their fear of contagion and their fear of dirt—ordering the disinfection or destruction of the property of the sick.

New York's response illustrated a firmer commitment to sanitation, and a greater hesitancy to control contagion. News of the fourth pandemic's arrival in Europe in 1865 spurred the state of New York to create a board of health for the city, and to confer on it sweeping powers to order sanitation measures. Its composition was designed to keep it free from the political influence of the city government, for city political corruption had, it was felt, nullified earlier attempts at sanitary reform. This board of health began a vigorous street cleaning program to dispose of noxious "nuisances" that might either cause cholera (if your view of the disease was environmentalist) or contribute to its spread (if you were a contagionist). Once cholera did enter the city in 1866, the board destroyed bedding and clothing, and lavishly spread disinfectants such as lime on property. Quarantine or isolation facilities, however, remained harder to find; private owners resisted attempts to commandeer their property for such purposes. But New Yorkers generally praised the efforts of the board of health, and credited it with the striking reduction in cholera mortality (officially given as 591) since the 1849 epidemic, when over 5,000 had died. Some American cities without such boards of health suffered much higher losses in proportion to their populations than did New York.

European powers set an important precedent in the International Sanitary Conference that met in Constantinople in February 1866. This conference, called in direct response to the fourth cholera pandemic, created an international sanitary commission to monitor Muslim pilgrimage to the Hijaz. The commission was to regulate quarantines and the embarkation conditions of the sea traffic of pilgrims. The governments of Ottoman Turkey (the titular ruler of the Hijaz), Egypt, and British India promised to cooperate with the commission. In the 1860s and 1870s, the framework of this international control remained very sketchy and incomplete, but by the 1880s it had become more elaborate.

Egypt and British India, two of the principal targets of such measures, found obeying the rules difficult. Egypt set up rigid military cordons to control traffic, but they proved inadequate to handle the volume of people that could move through the country by rail or (after 1869) through the Suez Canal. The Egyptian government also attempted to destroy the property of the sick, but doing so inspired popular resentment and resistance (as did, if they were effective, the military cordons). And the Egyptian government's resources were not great, as its modernizing projects had by the early 1870s brought it to the edge of bankruptcy. Desperate for money, it sometimes levied taxes (on the burial of animals, for instance) that undercut sanitation.

The British government of India likewise promised cooperation with the international commission and likewise did so only lukewarmly. British attitudes toward epidemics leaned more in the direction of sanitation anyway, and those attitudes were especially prevalent in Anglo-India. Too much of the prosperity of British India depended on the free movement of international trade, so any quarantine was suspect. International quarantines to control Muslim pilgrim traffic might offend millions of Indian Muslims, and a rigorous policing of internal Hindu pilgrimages would stir other resentments. In the years after the 1857 Sepoy Revolt, the British were especially leery of seeming to interfere with Indian religious beliefs. So while an 1868 Indian government report called the Puri "temple car" (a huge wagon carrying an image of the Hindu divinity Jagannath, the origin of the word *juggernaut*) "tawdry and contemptible" (Arnold 1993, 187), in fact the Indian government only reluctantly and incompletely regulated pilgrim traffic.

Where sanitation improvements were undertaken in Asia or Africa, they sometimes were intended to benefit European communities. Thus, the Indian government, pushed by the notions of Snow about water transmission of cholera, gradually introduced improved water and sewer systems in Calcutta and Bombay that probably contributed to lowering the horrific cholera toll in those cities in the 1870s. Even more striking reductions in mortality were achieved in British military installations in India, where much more thorough sanitary work occurred. The experience of Tunisia was similar. The bey's government had earlier ceded power over public health to a European-run commission, and in the fourth cholera pandemic that commission concerned itself largely with the health of the resident European community. And for some Europeans in North Africa, flight remained an option when cholera approached. (As indeed it was for the North African elites as well: the Egyptian Khedive Ismail fled to Constantinople in 1865.)

Medical responses to cholera were still largely powerless. The disease remained a sudden, violent irruption in a person's life, one that resulted in a rapid death for about half of those stricken. Western medicine, which had been positively harmful for cholera victims earlier, had at least moderated its purging and bleeding, but it offered no effective therapy.

UNRESOLVED HISTORICAL ISSUES

Some immediate issues about cholera remained unresolved in the 1870s. The precise causative agent was still unknown. Some argued that no such single causative agent could exist, and that a devastating ailment such as cholera could only be explained by the interaction of a number of environmental and personal factors. And because no such single agent had been found, and the number of possible contributing factors might be limitless, how should the efforts of sanitation (or of contagion control) be focused?

The experiences of the fourth pandemic strengthened the claims of both sanitation and contagion in different ways. Especially in the United States, where the apparent success of the anti-cholera efforts of the Metropolitan Board of Health of New York became a model for other cities to undertake similar campaigns against dirt, interest in sanitation and hygiene grew rapidly in the years after 1866. But at the same time, Europeans became convinced by the fourth pandemic that cholera was above all an alien Asian import, carried to them by human traffic.

Still unknown in 1875 was how far Western power over the policies and independence of Asian and African countries would extend in the name of public health. Apart from actual colonial possessions (India), such powers were increasingly affecting nominally independent Turkey, Tunisia, and Egypt. Would they be extended to (for example) China and Japan? Western powers feared not only epidemic disease but also subversive or revolutionary religious zealotry of the kind that was soon to shake the Sudan. Would the Western powers use the fear of disease, and their medical response to it, as a tool of empire to extend their powers? That question was still open in the 1870s, and it has revived as a disputed point in recent historical writing.

REFERENCES

Arnold, David. *Colonizing the Body: State Medicine and Epidemic Disease in Nineteenth-Century India.* Berkeley: University of California Press, 1993.

Baldwin, Peter. *Contagion and the State in Europe, 1830–1930.* Cambridge: Cambridge University Press, 1999.

Malleson, G. B. *Report on the Cholera Epidemic of 1867 in North India.* Calcutta: Office of the Superintendent of Government Printing, 1868.

SUGGESTED ADDITIONAL READING

Gallagher, Nancy E. *Medicine and Power in Tunisia, 1780–1900.* Cambridge: Cambridge University Press, 1983.

Hamlin, Christopher. *Cholera: The Biography.* Oxford: Oxford University Press, 2009.

Harrison, Mark. "A Question of Locality: The Identity of Cholera in British India, 1860–1890." In *Warm Climates and Western Medicine: The Emergence of Tropical Medicine, 1500–1900,* edited by David Arnold, 133–159. Amsterdam: Rodopi, 1996.

Jannetta, Ann Bowman. *Epidemics and Mortality in Early Modern Japan.* Princeton, NJ: Princeton University Press, 1987.

Kiple, Kenneth F. "Cholera and Race in the Caribbean." *Journal of Latin American Studies* 17 (1985): 157–177.

Kuhnke, LaVerne. *Lives at Risk: Public Health in Nineteenth-Century Egypt.* Berkeley: University of California Press, 1990.

Maglen, Krista. *The English System: Quarantine, Immigration and the Making of a Port Sanitary Zone.* Manchester: Manchester University Press, 2014.

Pollitzer, Robert. *Cholera.* Geneva: World Health Organization, 1959.

Pyle, G. F. "The Diffusion of Cholera in the United States in the Nineteenth Century." *Geographical Analysis* 1 (1969): 59–75.

Roff, William R. "Sanitation and Security: The Imperial Powers and the Nineteenth Century Hajj." *Arabian Studies* 6 (1982): 143–160.

Rosenberg, Charles E. *The Cholera Years: The United States in 1832, 1849, and 1866.* Chicago: University of Chicago Press, 1962.

26

Smallpox in Europe, 1870–1875

WHEN AND WHERE

Epidemic smallpox spread through Europe (and beyond) in the years between 1870 and 1875 in the worst Western outbreak of the disease in the nineteenth century. At the end of the six years, about 500,000 Europeans had succumbed to smallpox, and many thousands of others had been scarred by it.

The epidemic apparently began in France, which had to that date made no attempt to compel vaccination of its people. Although many of the French had been vaccinated, and many French physicians (and much French educated opinion) favored the practice, perhaps one-third of the French population had never been vaccinated at all, while many others had only been vaccinated in childhood and not revaccinated later. In the 1860s, therefore, a fairly high level of endemic smallpox persisted in the country, including in its largest city, Paris.

When the Franco-Prussian War began in July 1870, it created conditions favorable to the spread of an epidemic. Large numbers of French troops—many of them unvaccinated—assembled, and smallpox cases multiplied. The war quickly became a military disaster for the French forces, 373,000 of whom were imprisoned in Germany, perhaps 14,000 of them suffering from smallpox. In that way the disease gained an epidemic foothold among the civilian population of Germany. Meanwhile the victorious Prussian army pushed into France, besieging Paris. French people fleeing from the war added to the spread of smallpox infections.

The epidemic moved out from its French center in the next several years. For France 1870 was the worst year, one in which 10,500 smallpox deaths occurred in Paris alone. (There had been fewer than 600 in the whole country in 1866.) Estimates of the total number of French smallpox deaths in 1870–1871 range from 60,000 to 90,000. Smallpox also quickly moved into the German civilian population, beginning in September 1870. It continued to rage there through 1871 and 1872: over 5,000 deaths in Berlin in 1871, over 3,600 in Hamburg in the same year, and a peak of 65,000 in Prussia as a whole in 1872. The total number of German deaths—over 160,000—exceeded even the French.

One interesting contrast existed between the two countries. The Prussian monarchy, earlier in the nineteenth century, had begun the systematic vaccination of the members of its army. During this epidemic, German troops suffered about 8,500 cases of smallpox, and something over 400 deaths; in the same period about 125,000 French troops contracted smallpox, and of them about 28,000 died. Those dramatic figures became strong evidence in support of those who urged compulsory vaccination as an appropriate preventive response to smallpox (see the "How It Was Understood at the Time" and "Responses" sections).

By late 1870, the epidemic had begun to spread elsewhere in western Europe, as the number of smallpox cases in Great Britain, Belgium, and the Netherlands accelerated in 1870 and then peaked in 1871. In that year Great Britain had 23,100 smallpox deaths, Belgium 21,300, and the Netherlands 12,400. Over the course of the epidemic, 8,000 Londoners died of smallpox. It continued in western Europe in the next year as well, with a further 19,000 deaths in Great Britain, and it also began to reach central Europe. Between 1872 and 1874, the Austrian domains may have suffered 140,000 smallpox deaths, and in 1874 the epidemic wave peaked in Sweden, where over 4,000 died. The number of dead in Russia remains unknown but was likely large.

This European smallpox epidemic also reached across the Atlantic. Emigration from Europe to the Americas, an important feature of the period, generated heavy passenger traffic and some of that carried smallpox infection with it. In 1871 Philadelphia, an important emigrant destination, had about 2,000 smallpox deaths; in the next year Buenos Aires had over 8,400. Other cities in both North and South America were affected as well.

By the 1880s, smallpox had receded to less epidemic (but still serious) levels in southern and central Europe, and been dramatically reduced in some other states. Thus, while the German Empire suffered a total of 155 smallpox deaths in 1886, Genoa alone had 275, Rome 470, and Budapest over 1,500. Sweden reported none.

And while this European epidemic existed independent of Asian events, it is worth remembering that in roughly the same period of the century severe smallpox epidemics recurred in East and South Asia. India averaged nearly 170,000 smallpox deaths annually through the 1870s; Bombay alone recorded over 3,000 deaths in 1876, and its annual toll frequently rose to over 1,000.

SIGNIFICANCE

The epidemic of smallpox in Europe in the early 1870s was the most serious attack of the disease in the Western world in the nineteenth century, and it remains the most serious such epidemic in the West since Edward Jenner developed his vaccination in 1798. As such, it illustrates the incomplete extent of preventive vaccination that still existed at that date, and it also reminds us that the history of smallpox in the West did not end suddenly with Jenner, despite the praise lavished on him during his lifetime.

The epidemic of the 1870s served as an important spur to changes in national responses to the threat of smallpox. In particular, it led to greater efforts at compulsory vaccination, and those efforts in turn stimulated discussion of the coercive powers of the state. (See the "Responses" section.)

BACKGROUND

Edward Jenner had announced his smallpox vaccine in 1798, and it had rapidly gained both popular and official favor in many places in the Western world. Its use had some immediately dramatic effects. Sweden, where vaccination was made compulsory in 1816, saw its number of smallpox deaths fall from about 12,000 in 1800 to a mere eleven in 1822.

But epidemics persisted. Ireland was shaken by smallpox (and other diseases in the midst of a famine) in 1817. The late 1820s were bad smallpox years in many places, and in 1837, 2,100 Londoners died of the disease. A period of slightly declining virulence of smallpox then intervened, but by the late 1850s smallpox had again become dangerous. Russia may have had over 100,000 deaths in 1856; in Berlin in 1858 there were 4,500 cases of the disease, and in London another serious outbreak occurred between 1861 and 1863.

Official responses to smallpox varied from one country to the next. At one extreme stood France, where the technique of Jennerian vaccination remained controversial. Despite the fact that Napoleon I had admired Jenner, France's different nineteenth-century governments never attempted to compel vaccination for its population, and in fact only did so in 1902. France's rural population, especially, continued to regard smallpox as an inevitable childhood disease; French traditionalists and conservatives associated vaccination with the French Revolution that they disliked. It is not therefore surprising that the serious epidemic of the 1870s had its origins in France, for smallpox had remained present there almost continuously.

At the opposite pole to French policy were a number of states that made vaccination compulsory. Bavaria was apparently the first, in 1807; Denmark followed in 1810, Norway in 1811, Russia in 1812. The fact that smallpox persisted in some of these states may have been due to the ineffectiveness of their decrees; it was one thing for the Russian government to compel vaccination of its far-flung population, and quite another to actually accomplish it. All over Europe the skill of the vaccinators varied, as did the quality of the vaccine. And an important background point was the question of a vaccination's permanence. Did one vaccination confer a lifelong immunity, as Jenner himself had believed? Or did it wear off after an unknown time, leaving the individual once again vulnerable? The German state of Württemberg was the first to act on the latter belief, when it introduced revaccination in 1829.

The policies of some states occupied a range between the voluntary approach of France and the compulsory path of the Scandinavian countries. Great Britain's approach illustrated a middle ground. Jenner, of course, was an Englishman, and his innovation was widely hailed there. But its application remained entirely voluntary until 1840, and compulsion then only proceeded by fits and starts. In that year Parliament required the local officials called Poor Law Guardians (who had charge of public welfare relief) to pay medical practitioners to serve as vaccinators for the population receiving public relief. In 1853 a new measure required that all children in the care of the poor relief authorities be vaccinated within their first three months, but no practical government mechanism existed to enforce this rule. Slowly a government department improved the training of vaccinators and began paying local authorities on the basis of the vaccinations they performed. But no revaccination provision existed. Smallpox hospitals were created, but every epidemic surge overwhelmed them and thus defeated attempts to isolate the victims.

Meanwhile, the Kingdom of Prussia followed another halfway policy about compulsory vaccination. It imposed no blanket compulsion on its population as a whole, but did require it (including revaccination) of its soldiers (as well as prisoners and inmates of state workhouses) in 1834. It also pursued a series of positive reinforcements designed to convince people of the vaccination's worth, holding out rewards to employers who had their employees vaccinated, making parents liable for damages if their unvaccinated children became ill, and the like.

At the outbreak of the epidemic wave of 1870, therefore, European states had evolved an uneven pattern of preventive vaccination. The fact that the toll in epidemics from the 1830s on was heaviest among adults, and among the poor of all ages, suggested first that adults who had been vaccinated earlier had lost their immunity in the intervening years and second that the expense of vaccination (in those countries where it remained voluntary) denied access to it for many.

That inconsistent pattern of vaccination also could be found in other parts of the world where the technique had been introduced, in many places under more-or-less forceful Western pressure. Both Great Britain and Spain vigorously promoted vaccination in their far-flung imperial possessions and met only indifferent success. In India—the most populous imperial territory—smallpox had long been present, a long tradition of Ayurvedic medicine existed that countered Western medical beliefs, a Hindu goddess presided over smallpox, and the practice of inoculation had been strongly established. British attempts to promote vaccination also faced technical difficulties. The arm-to-arm transfer of cowpox vaccine from one person to another could be conveyed from Britain to India, obviously expensive and time-consuming; attempting the involvement of Indians directly in this transfer would face resistance grounded on caste beliefs, while taking cowpox matter directly from cattle would offend Hindus. And by the 1850s many Indians had become convinced that the British intended to convert them to Christianity. Despite these obstacles, British authorities persisted in campaigns of vaccination, for reasons that surely involved a humane desire to prevent disease (as well as an illustration of Western cultural superiority), but much of India remained unvaccinated.

The rapid urbanization of much of Europe in the nineteenth century certainly contributed to maintaining smallpox epidemics, for the disease could move swiftly through congested urban quarters. The greater speed and reliability that railroads made possible may have also played a role; what became a major smallpox epidemic in Montreal in 1885 apparently reached the city by rail from Chicago in the United States.

HOW IT WAS UNDERSTOOD AT THE TIME

As had been true earlier, nearly universal agreement existed that smallpox was a contagious disease that spread from one victim to others. Less agreement existed about the actual mechanism of contagion, a point that would in fact remain a mystery throughout the century.

Although the benefits of Jenner's vaccination as a preventive measure were widely accepted, much argument still raged about it. Many objections to it—some religious, some medical, and some practical—had been raised in its early years, and by 1870 those objections had been joined by political ones (see the "Responses" section). The necessity or desirability of revaccination remained uncertain.

As the sections "Background" and "Responses" discuss, authorities pursued conflicting approaches to smallpox epidemics, some emphasizing general prevention with widespread vaccination, others addressing the immediate epidemic threat by systems of isolating the sick. Did isolation hospitals help contain infection, or did their concentration of the sick simply make them centers for the disease?

Overhanging some of these uncertainties was a lingering conflict of opinion about whether environment played any role in smallpox's diffusion. That it was contagious no one doubted, but was contagion in some way contingent on the environment? Many, for instance, held the habits of the poor—and the environment those habits generated—responsible for the persistence of the disease.

RESPONSES

One set of responses was insistence on more compulsory (and free) vaccination, more with the thought of preventing future epidemics than stopping this one. The British government passed a Vaccination Act in 1871 that appointed officers to enforce the rules compelling vaccinations for children. Harsh penalties awaited parents who resisted. Vaccination stations in London were organized, beginning what a historian has called the "consummation of the state vaccination program" (Hardy 1993, 126), but no provision was made for revaccination.

Meanwhile in the German states the political structure had been altered by the creation of the federal German Empire in 1871 under Prussian leadership. A new imperial law in 1874 required vaccination of all children and offered free vaccination. The measure also provided that all children be revaccinated at the age of 12. The subsequent contrasts between smallpox incidence in Britain and Germany were striking. In England and Wales, the death rate from smallpox peaked at 1,012 deaths per million population, in 1871; in Germany, the highest rate was 2,624 deaths per million, in 1872. By 1877, when the rate in England and Wales was still an appreciable 173, it had fallen to under 5 in Germany. The continuing success of the German vaccination policy owed something to government efforts to convince the population that the procedure was safe; partly for that reason a serious anti-vaccination movement never developed in Germany as it did in Great Britain (see the "Unresolved Historical Issues" section).

Another response pattern addressed the epidemic more directly, aimed at stopping its spread. Authorities demanded notification of cases of smallpox; victims, when found, would be isolated in smallpox hospitals; their contacts would be traced and also isolated; their property would be disinfected. This approach, while seemingly a more direct assault on an epidemic, proved difficult to implement in practice. Compelling notification from physicians, for example, contradicted the ethics of medical communities that were, by the 1870s, becoming sensitive to professional codes of conduct. People in general still feared the stigma of smallpox and so might hide its presence if they could. Disinfection disrupted households. Neighborhoods resisted the creation of smallpox hospitals in their midst, fearing—perhaps with some reason—that they were centers of infection. It was only in 1882 that London smallpox hospitals were sited away from residential areas; only in 1889 did Great Britain make notification of smallpox's presence compulsory.

Nevertheless, some attempts were made in the 1870s to adopt this immediately reactive approach. The Leicester Experiment, so-called from the English city that pursued it, was the best-known example. The approach deemphasized the universal vaccination of the population and aimed at selective control in the hope of isolating smallpox from contact with new victims, thus allowing the epidemic to die out. (As Hopkins [2002, 305] notes, the Leicester Experiment anticipated the methods adopted by the World Health Organization campaigns of the 1960s and 1970s that led to smallpox's eradication, finally announced in 1977.)

The responses to the smallpox epidemics of the 1870s left many unanswered questions, and in fact stimulated new and more vigorous political objections to government policies.

UNRESOLVED HISTORICAL ISSUES

By the end of the epidemics of the 1870s, the most serious unresolved questions about smallpox revolved around the wisdom, safety, and political morality of vaccination. Even before Jenner had developed his vaccine based on cowpox, controversy surrounded the earlier method of inoculation. In the nineteenth century, the objections to inoculation had persisted about vaccination, and other objections had arisen as well.

Some religious believers feared that vaccination (or the earlier inoculation) represented interference with the will of God. To that was added a concern that vaccination, involving as it did an animal disease (cowpox), was in some way degrading, inhuman, and bestial. That concern was kept alive by continuing arguments about the best method of preparing the vaccine. Jenner had transferred cowpox matter from one person's arm to another and thus gained his supply, but doing so may have both lowered the vaccine's effectiveness and created problems with adequate supplies. In the 1840s a new technique (developed initially in Italy) began using lymph obtained directly from calves. That technique only spread very slowly through the rest of the century, despite the advantages it offered; it kept the animal nature of the process in the public mind.

A number of physicians, and many others, continued to raise questions about the safety of vaccination. Inoculation had involved the deliberate transfer of smallpox from one person to another, obviously dangerous. Did vaccination lead to other diseases as bad or worse than smallpox? Throughout much of the nineteenth century, many believed that vaccination led to secondary transmission of syphilis. Occasional disasters strengthened such fears; one such happened in Montreal in 1885, when the administration of a contaminated vaccine led to an outbreak (including fatalities) of erysipelas. Other medical opposition to vaccination stemmed from anti-contagionist beliefs. Diseases, these views maintained, could not be explained simply as contagions; the environment in which they spread should be considered too, and focusing on the mode of transmission from one to another could not be the whole answer.

All these arguments became political ones as well, especially in Great Britain, when governments moved in the direction of compelling vaccination of their people. Should governments have the power to dictate to parents what should be done for the health of their children? British pamphlets began appearing in the 1850s that opposed such state power, and during the smallpox epidemics of the 1870s, anti-vaccination associations formed in many parts of Great Britain. These associations argued both that vaccination was dangerous and that state compulsion was philosophically wrong and an affront to human liberties.

In some ways the Leicester Experiment at least overlapped with such concerns, and its popularity in Great Britain may illustrate their depth. The reduced threat of smallpox after the 1870s may have also led to disregard of vaccination. Certainly, vaccination was not universal in many places in the Western world even after the 1870s epidemics. In the 1890s over half of the children in some east London districts remained unvaccinated. In Montreal in 1885 vaccination was especially resisted by the French-Canadian population, in part because they saw it as an imposition of the ruling Anglo-Canadians; recent immigrants to the United States were similarly reluctant. In 1898 the pressure of the anti-vaccination groups led the British government to modify its insistence on compulsion; from that date British parents could win exemption for their children by invoking a conscience clause. In India, vaccination became "compulsory" in 1880, but subsequent argument persisted about whether that meant "prescriptive" or "permissive." In the early twentieth century, some American states adopted similar policies.

Some historical uncertainties also remain about the role of compulsory vaccination in the decline of smallpox in Europe. In the nineteenth century, levels of infant vaccination did not always coincide with levels of smallpox infection, nor did compulsion always correlate with lower smallpox levels. And some evidence suggests that threatening legal penalties for failure to vaccinate did not always result in higher levels of compliance with the law. The relative effects of legal compulsion (on the one hand) and of popular acceptance of a technique (on the other) are still the subjects of historical research, with interesting implications for contemporary public health policy.

A final uncertainty concerns the role of varieties of the causative organism of smallpox in the waxing and waning of the disease throughout history. In the 1860s, a much milder version of the disease was first clearly described. We now say that this version is caused by the virus *Variola minor*, while the much more dangerous smallpox virus is *Variola major*. At what different points in the past (if ever) did *Variola minor* become widespread, and in doing so confer immunity from attacks by its lethal *Variola major* relative?

REFERENCES

Hardy, Anne. *The Epidemic Streets: Infectious Disease and the Rise of Preventive Medicine, 1856–1900*. Oxford: Clarendon, 1993.

Hopkins, Donald R. *The Greatest Killer: Smallpox in History*. Chicago: University of Chicago Press, 2002. (Orig. pub. as *Princes and Peasants: Smallpox in History*. Chicago: University of Chicago Press, 1983.)

SUGGESTED ADDITIONAL READING

Ackerman, Evelyn B. *Health Care in the Parisian Countryside, 1800–1914*. New Brunswick, NJ: Rutgers University Press, 1990.

Arnold, David. *Colonizing the Body: State Medicine and Epidemic Disease in Nineteenth Century India*. Berkeley: University of California Press, 1993.

Bliss, Michael. *Plague: A Story of Smallpox in Montreal*. Toronto: HarperCollins, 1991.

Durbach, Nadia. *Bodily Matters: The Anti-Vaccination Movement in England, 1853–1907*. Durham, NC: Duke University Press, 2005.

Glynn, Ian, and Jenifer Glynn. *The Life and Death of Smallpox*. Cambridge: Cambridge University Press, 2004.

Hennock, E. P. "Vaccination Policy against Smallpox, 1835–1914: A Comparison of England with Prussia and Imperial Germany." *Social History of Medicine* 11 (1998): 49–71.

Huerkamp, Claudia. "The History of Smallpox Vaccination in Germany: A First Step in the Medicalization of the General Public." *Journal of Contemporary History* 20 (1985): 617–635.

Porter, Dorothy, and Roy Porter. "The Politics of Prevention: Anti-Vaccinationism and Public Health in Nineteenth-Century England." *Medical History* 32 (1988): 231–252.

Williams, Naomi. "The Implementation of Compulsory Health Legislation: Infant Smallpox Vaccination in England and Wales, 1840–1880." *Journal of Historical Geography* 20 (1994): 396–412.

27

Measles in Fiji, 1875

WHEN AND WHERE

In January 1875, a British warship HMS *Dido* arrived in the Fiji Islands, in the south-central Pacific Ocean. Among its passengers were a prominent Fijian chief and his retinue, members of which had caught measles in Australia and carried still-contagious cases of the disease with them to their home islands. The Fijian population had never before been exposed to measles, and when the disease started moving through the islands its effects were terrifying. By February 1875 measles had spread through most of the Fiji Island chain, and for the next several months the disease ravaged the population. By June 1875, the measles epidemic had largely burned itself out.

The population of the Fiji Islands in 1875 may have numbered about 135,000. In the six months of the measles epidemic perhaps 36,000 of them died, over one-quarter of the population.

SIGNIFICANCE

This episode stands as a classic and well-documented case of a virgin soil epidemic that occurs when a population that has been previously isolated from contact with a particular disease pathogen is suddenly exposed to it. Without immunities (whether inherited or acquired) such a population is especially vulnerable, and rates of both sickness and death may be very high. Since the nineteenth century, such epidemics have most often struck island populations or groups isolated in some other way from contact with the larger world; tragically such groups included North American Native Indian communities. The Fiji measles epidemic of 1875 is a particularly vivid example of the result. In an earlier period, and on a far larger scale, the epidemics that afflicted the Americas in the sixteenth and seventeenth centuries may also be regarded as virgin soil events.

This Fijian epidemic also clearly illustrates the diffusing power, for diseases, of Western trade and transportation in the nineteenth century, power that made the elimination of disease-free havens much more likely.

And, of course, the epidemic was a major event in the history of the Fiji Islands. The massive death toll came just after the previously independent islands had fallen under British sovereignty; although the epidemic was not responsible for that political change, it certainly weakened indigenous traditions and authority, making more likely the perpetuation of colonial rule.

BACKGROUND

In the course of the nineteenth century, Western commercial interests and cultural outreach broke down the previous isolation of the Fiji Islands, and in the process exposed its population to a series of new diseases. Although European mariners had first reached Fiji in the 1640s, consistent Western contact only began after the 1790s. European traders sought sandalwood and the sea animal called the *trepan* (a relation of the starfish); Christian missionaries arrived as well. On the heels of these contacts, starting in the 1790s, the islands suffered a series of epidemics, probably including tuberculosis, dysentery, and influenza, some of them very serious. After the 1850s, a new element, which changed both the population and the disease environment, entered the picture: Western interests acquired land for plantation agriculture, first growing cotton, and then sugar. The plantations needed labor, which was supplied by importing field hands from other Pacific Islands, and then increasingly from India. (Nearly half of the modern population of the Republic of Fiji is of south Asian descent.)

Some facts about measles and how it spreads may contribute to an understanding of the 1875 epidemic. Measles is a very contagious infection, carried by a virus, which spreads from person to person both through the air and through direct contact. One case of measles confers lifelong immunity from further infection. Measles, similar to smallpox, is therefore a disease that maintains itself in a population by finding people free of previous infection. Such a population is most obviously found among young children, and so measles has traditionally been a childhood infection. The sick are contagious for a period of 9 or 10 days after their symptoms (a rash and fever) develop. These circumstances may explain why measles, a common childhood disease through much of the world, was slow to reach islands such as the Fijis. The vast distances of the Pacific Ocean meant that most voyages to Fiji were prolonged, perhaps two or three months in duration. Most mariners—whether from Europe, North America, or Asia—had probably long since contracted measles. If a voyage began with a rare case of measles on board, the sufferer would likely cease to be contagious within 10 days, and only if there were another unexposed mariner could the disease persist. By the end of a 60-day voyage, the disease would long since have exhausted the possibilities. So while tuberculosis, influenza, venereal disease, and dysentery could all be carried on long voyages, and thus reach Fiji earlier, measles only made the trip when a ship carried a number of Fijians—all unexposed—with it. One Fijian could contract measles in Australia, and then the disease could be passed through the Fijian passengers who were still contagious when the ship reached the islands.

HMS *Dido*, as it happened, was returning Fijian leaders to their home after a meeting in Sydney where the British assumption of sovereignty over the Fijis had been arranged. Other tribal and island chiefs therefore greeted the Fijian delegation when it arrived home; a large meeting of leaders took place to explain the new arrangements; the delegations then scattered to their home islands and villages. They carried measles with them.

HOW IT WAS UNDERSTOOD AT THE TIME

Western and mainland Asian societies had long experience with measles, and some early Chinese and Arabic authors had differentiated it from smallpox, with which it could easily be confused. By the seventeenth century, some European physicians had also identified the differences between the two diseases. No clear understanding of its cause existed in the nineteenth century, although its contagiousness was easily recognized. Its resemblance to smallpox, for which preventive inoculation techniques had long existed, led to experiments on similar techniques for measles, but they had been unsuccessful. Physicians could only attempt to relieve the symptoms of fever and the itch of a rash.

For the Fijians, the disease came as an unexplainable catastrophe, for which malign or vengeful gods must be responsible.

RESPONSES

For a period of several months, this epidemic reduced Fijian society to near collapse. Such a severe epidemic may be made worse by the resulting failure of social services to care for the sick. A later British report noted that "there was no one left to gather food or carry water, to attend to the necessary wants of their fellows, or even, in many cases, to bury the dead" (McArthur 1968, 9). Desperate to relieve their fevers, Fijians lay in water to cool themselves.

The increasing importation of labor into the Fiji Islands meant that measles became established in the population. Steamships took over the trade in laborers, completing their voyages from India to Fiji much more quickly; thus, the chances of moving more active measles cases to the islands increased. Notable epidemics recurred in 1903 and 1910–1914, during which many Fijians fell ill, but their death rates were much lower. That fact illustrates that measles no longer fell on Fiji as virgin soil, but instead gradually became a relatively mild childhood disease. And after the 1875 disaster, ships arriving in the Fiji Islands were subject to a more careful quarantine.

UNRESOLVED HISTORICAL ISSUES

The more general problem of disease's role in the depopulation of isolated islands, especially in the Pacific, has become a persistent theme in historical writing about the area in the period when Westerners began moving into and through the Pacific. The 1875 measles epidemic in Fiji is an especially vivid example of a more general phenomenon; much modern historical literature has seen the Western incursion into the Pacific as a disaster for the islanders, and diseases have contradicted the idea that the arrival of the developed West represented progress for the Pacific peoples.

Why the captain of HMS *Dido* did not impose a self-quarantine on his ship when it approached Fiji remains an open question. The contagious character of measles was well known. Were Fijian lives of no significance?

REFERENCE

McArthur, Norma. *Island Populations of the Pacific.* Canberra: Australian National University Press, 1968.

SUGGESTED ADDITIONAL READING

Ahuja, Neel. *Bioinsecurities: Disease Interventions, Empire, and the Government of Species.* Durham, NC: Duke University Press, 2016.

Bushnell, O. A. *The Gifts of Civilization: Germs and Genocide in Hawai'i.* Honolulu: University of Hawaii Press, 1993.

Cliff, Andrew D., and Peter Haggett. *The Spread of Measles in Fiji and the Pacific: Spatial Components in the Transmission of Epidemic Waves through Island Communities.* Canberra: Australian National University Research School of Pacific Studies, 1985.

Crosby, A. W. "Hawaiian Depopulation as a Model for the Amerindian Experience." In *Epidemics and Ideas: Essays on the Historical Perception of Pestilence,* edited by Terence Ranger and Paul Slack, 175–201. Cambridge: Cambridge University Press, 1992.

Stannard, David E. *Before the Horror: The Population of Hawai'i on the Eve of Western Contact.* Honolulu: University of Hawaii Social Science Research Institute, 1989.

28

Fifth Cholera Pandemic, 1881–1896

WHEN AND WHERE

Another widespread cholera pandemic began in south Asia in 1881, and persisted (although in several somewhat distinct spurts) from that date until 1896. The pandemic's first incursion outside the Indian subcontinent reached Java, Borneo, and the Philippines late in the summer of 1882. The death tolls in Batavia and Surabaya (Java) and Manila (Philippines) were especially severe; perhaps 10% of Manila's population died between August and October 1882, three times the normal mortality rate. Cholera moved west as well, and fears of its spread into Arabia prompted the Egyptian government to impose strict quarantines.

In 1883 cholera became very serious in western Asia, again infecting the Muslim pilgrims who moved annually to the Hijaz region of Arabia. The area of Mecca suffered a major epidemic in that year, and from there cholera broke through the Egyptian attempts at quarantine; 58,000 Egyptians died of cholera in 1883. On the other side of Asia, quarantines were also imposed in the Shantou province of China.

The fifth cholera pandemic reached the West in 1884, as the disease moved across the Mediterranean to seaports in Italy and France. Naples officially recorded about 7,100 cholera deaths, beginning in August and peaking in September; in fact, the true toll may have been between 10,000 and 20,000, and the epidemic resulted in major civil unrest in the city (see the "How It Was Understood at the Time" and "Responses" sections). In France, the disease first reached Toulon, then jumped to nearby Marseille before spreading inland to Paris, where nearly 1,000 cholera deaths occurred. In 1885 cholera reached Spain, and as many as 60,000 Spaniards (especially in Valencia and Murcia) perished.

By 1886 the pandemic crossed the Atlantic, infecting Argentina. And on the other side of the world, 155,000 cases of cholera were reported in Japan. More cases occurred in the Americas in 1887, as Chile experienced an outbreak. The spread of cholera across oceans had by this time become an obvious issue (see the "Responses" section), and North America was not immune. It did, however, resist, for by the time of the fifth pandemic a more precise conception of the cause of cholera was gaining ground, a conception that justified careful quarantines and rigorous laboratory testing. When a ship from Marseille and Naples docked in New York with cholera cases, a rigorous quarantine was imposed, backed by bacteriological testing, and it kept the disease from coming ashore.

In the years between 1888 and 1891, the fifth pandemic retreated to its Asian homelands, where new outbreaks occurred in the East Indies and the Philippines in 1888 (the latter was thought to have arrived with sea traffic from Hong Kong) and the Arabian pilgrimage sites again suffered in 1889 and 1891.

But then in 1892 cholera reappeared in Europe, following the path of infection that it had taken as early as the second pandemic more than 60 years earlier: into Russia from the Caspian Sea, moving up the Volga River from Astrakhan with human traffic in the summer months. The result was a new period of serious social disruption in some Russian communities (see the "Responses" and "How It Was Understood at the Time" sections), as perhaps 215,000 Russians died of cholera in 1892. Not all of Russia was affected equally; Moscow, the scene of a major cholera epidemic in 1830, was largely spared in 1892.

The subsequent course of the pandemic in Europe in 1892 was important both for what happened and what did not happen. Cholera in Russia led to one major outbreak in western Europe, as the German city of Hamburg suffered an important epidemic in August and September; but while earlier cholera pandemics (notably the second) had spread widely across Europe and into North America, new understanding of the cause of the disease led to a partial success in averting more widespread cholera attacks in the West. Some cholera deaths did occur, however; Paris, for example, suffered about 1,000.

Cholera continued to linger in Russia in 1893 (with 39,000 further deaths), but its main activity that year was a renewed assault on western Asia and on the sites of Muslim pilgrimage. Mecca alone recorded about 13,400 cholera deaths, and one estimate suggests that over 30,000 pilgrims succumbed to cholera in the Hijaz as a whole in 1893. It was one of the worst cholera years for the Arabian Peninsula. The fifth cholera pandemic lingered through 1896 in some other places, notably Morocco and Egypt (where a further 16,000 died in 1896), but it then came to an end.

SIGNIFICANCE

The discovery of the *Vibrio cholera* microorganism believed to be responsible for the disease occurred during the fifth pandemic. From that point, cholera seemed to some to be the product of a germ, so the fifth cholera pandemic became a test of the germ theory, not just as it applied to cholera but to other diseases as well. Some vivid illustrations and contrasts of disease theories therefore occurred.

The fifth cholera pandemic also provided evidence for the continuing power of epidemics to stimulate civil disturbances in European society, and those disturbances in some cases had important political and social consequences. The recurrence of cholera epidemics in the Muslim pilgrimage sites of western Asia contributed to revived (and controversial) attempts to impose international quarantines.

BACKGROUND

The fifth cholera pandemic, even more than the fourth, occurred at a time when transportation changes had linked the continents of the world together more closely than ever. Steamship voyages now regularly consumed days instead of the weeks or months previously needed. A dense network of railroads existed in Europe and in much of North America; a similar network was spreading in India, which was of particular importance for the continuing diffusion of cholera.

Several other general circumstances affected the fifth cholera pandemic. A dramatic new period of large-scale emigration from southern and eastern Europe to the Americas was underway in those decades. And although agricultural and transportation technologies had reduced the threat of famine in many places of the world, that threat was still very real in others. Hunger could (and did) drive much migration, both within countries and across oceans. Poor, hungry people could be important disease carriers, and they could strain systems of sanitation as they crowded into cities when rural food failed.

The last decades of the nineteenth century were also years of accelerating Western imperial competition, especially (but not solely) in Africa. Western imperial powers showed themselves increasingly, if erratically, concerned about the spread of epidemics in the territories to which they laid claim (whether formally or informally). For example, by the 1880s, the western European powers began appointing consuls at Jidda, Arabia, to monitor threats both to imperial security and to imperial health that might come from the annual Muslim pilgrimages. A quarantine station was in operation off the coast of Yemen by 1881, and more attention began to be paid to the conditions of life (and death) aboard ships carrying emigrants or pilgrims.

HOW IT WAS UNDERSTOOD AT THE TIME

When cholera again became epidemic in Egypt in the summer of 1883, both French and German governments dispatched teams of scientific investigation to Alexandria. Robert Koch, the great German microbiologist who led the German team, soon identified a microorganism in the intestinal walls of cholera victims that he thought might be responsible for the disease; he was unable, however, to induce cholera symptoms in animals when he infected them with the microorganism. As the cholera epidemic waned in Egypt, Koch moved on to Calcutta, where cholera victims abounded. He found the same microorganism in 70 subjects. Although Koch was still unable to produce cholera symptoms in test animals using the germ, in a series of papers published in early 1884 he announced his conviction that his discovery, the bacterium called *Vibrio cholerae,* caused cholera.

Koch believed that this germ infected primarily water supplies (and some foods), and that it entered into those water supplies from the excretions of people infected by it. If Koch was right, the presence of such germs in the human body indicated that a person was infected by cholera; if the spread of cholera was to be prevented, water supplies and food sources should be kept free from contact with the excretions of the infected. If Koch was right, therefore, isolation and sanitation measures should be taken against specific targets.

Koch's discovery came in a period of growing enthusiasm for the germ theory of disease, which Koch and Louis Pasteur had powerfully revived in the mid-1870s. By 1883 a growing number of germs thought responsible for major diseases had been identified, perhaps most sensationally that of tuberculosis (in 1882). Koch was on his way from an obscure rural medical practice in Prussia to a prestigious state-financed laboratory in Berlin; Pasteur would soon become a French national hero. For many people, therefore, the new explanation of cholera was very convincing.

But many doubts remained among physicians and scientists, as well as among the general public. To some Koch's answer seemed too simple; could a disease with such devastating symptoms really be caused by a microscopic organism? Koch's germ might be a necessary component to a case of cholera, but was it a sufficient cause by itself? Didn't the entire environment, or perhaps the predisposition of the individual, play a role? Koch's arguments seemed to dismiss more general environmental causes, which might discount a whole world of sanitary improvements; they also denied that the moral behavior of populations (except in a very narrow and specific sense) had anything to do with the cholera pandemics. As such they countered some of the most deeply held beliefs about disease, and it is not surprising that the germ theory did not immediately sweep away all before it, despite the convincing evidence that supported it.

All through the period of the fifth pandemic such uncertainties remained; many of them centered around the arguments of Max von Pettenkofer, the preeminent public health authority in Germany and perhaps in the Western world. Some of those uncertainties related to political beliefs, as the next section ("Responses") shows.

And apart from the differences of scientific opinion symbolized by Koch and Pettenkofer, other understandings of cholera persisted in different populations. The will of God was still widely evoked, in 1884 in Naples, for example. Cholera was divine punishment for sin, and those who suffered from it were suspect, dangerous, and only got what they deserved. In several other places in the world, cholera was seen as a deliberate product of malign political power. In the Hijaz area of Muslim pilgrimage, some blamed the Western sanitary authorities for bringing the disease to Arabia. In some Russian communities, as well as in Naples and Marseille, popular riots against medical personnel and against state authority were inspired at least in part by the belief—or the fear—that governments were responsible for launching a deliberate attack on the poor by spreading cholera among them as discussed in the next section.

RESPONSES

Official Western responses to the fifth cholera pandemic extended the policies that Peter Baldwin calls *neocontagionism.* In general, that meant widespread inspections of travelers, disinfection of their belongings, and isolation of those

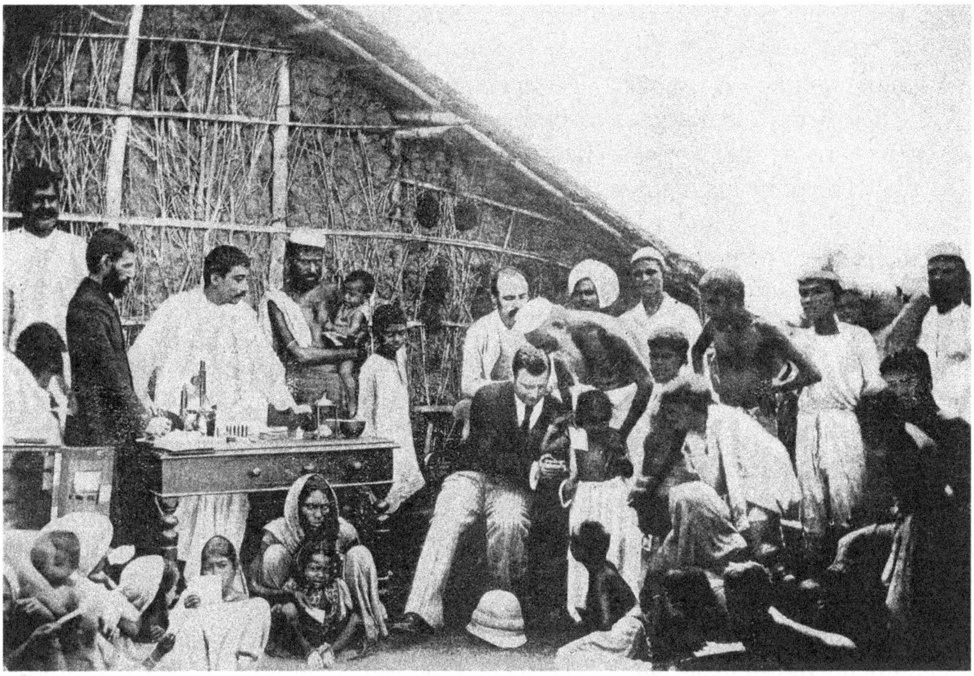

Waldemar Haffkine, the developer of a controversial cholera vaccine, inoculates a community in Calcutta (now Kolkata), India, in March 1894. (Wellcome Library)

who were judged to be sick. However, attempts to impose blanket quarantines on *all* travel or to create sanitary cordons that would bar *all* traffic were less popular.

At times the fear of cholera led to more comprehensive quarantines, as when Bristol (England) barred all traffic from Spain in 1885, or to attempts to maintain a sanitary cordon between one place and another, such as Marseille tried to impose between itself and neighboring Toulon in 1884. And while Britain, with a strong tradition emphasizing sanitation as the answer to disease, continued to invest heavily in infrastructure that generally improved the environment, by the 1890s British officials also increasingly recognized that individuals could carry disease, and so their regulations progressively called for inspections, reports to authorities, and isolation of the sick. Especially targeted were poor eastern European travelers (many of them Jews), singled out more as a result of cultural and political prejudices than because of any actual epidemic threat.

Koch's discovery of the bacterium apparently responsible for cholera changed these responses only gradually and only in degree. Not everyone accepted the notion that the germ was a *sufficient* cause of the disease (see the "How It Was Understood at the Time" section), and even if they agreed with Koch, the application of his theory simply "prompted a shift in the emphasis of an already existing neoquarantinist approach that dated back at least two decades" before Koch's discovery (Baldwin 1999, 165). Bacteriological testing, rather than symptoms, could now precisely identify a cholera victim and those so identified could be isolated.

The belief that people, and not their possessions, carried the bacterium gave the disinfection process a clearer focus. But inspection, notification of authorities, and isolation remained at the heart of official responses.

Koch's theory did not solve all problems with the identification of the sick, however. As early as 1885 it was realized that asymptomatic carriers of cholera existed: people who carried cholera germs but displayed no symptoms of disease. Should those people be isolated as well, when a bacteriological test revealed their apparent infection? The problem of the asymptomatic carrier complicated cholera policies in the 1880s and 1890s and would become particularly important in confrontations with typhoid fever.

Outside Europe, Western imperial powers applied variations of these policies in the areas they controlled or influenced. A quarantine station was placed in operation at Kamaran, off the coast of Yemen, in 1881, to supervise Muslim pilgrim traffic entering the Red Sea; the station detained and disinfected pilgrims. In India, in 1892, 200,000 pilgrims on their way to the Hindu shrine at Hardwar were barred from completing the journey by British fears of the spread of cholera. And by 1894 an international sanitary conference meeting in Paris laid down more stringent rules for the inspection of ships and pilgrims to Arabia: ships and their pilgrims should be inspected medically before their departure, physicians should accompany the voyage, and ships were required to provide at least minimum space and water supplies. All that represented considerable interference with both travel and free enterprise in the name of international public health. It also represented Western imperial arrogance.

Physicians continued to have ineffective responses to cases of cholera, however. The sadly counterproductive measures undertaken in the earlier cholera pandemics (symbolized by the use of such purgatives as calomel) were less common by the 1880s, but still had their advocates. Sir George Johnson, Queen Victoria's physician until his death in 1896, urged castor oil, another purgative.

But such therapies were apparently losing favor. In their place, some few physicians tried a reverse approach, attempting to rehydrate the body rather than purging it of fluids. Experiments with rehydration with intravenous infusions had begun earlier in the century and continued into the fifth pandemic. Another new medical response was the attempt to develop a preventive cholera vaccine, pioneered by Waldemar Haffkine, a disciple of Louis Pasteur. He announced that he had tried such a vaccine on himself and a few others in 1892, and then moved from Paris to Calcutta in 1893 to begin a large-scale cholera vaccination program in India. He claimed to have vaccinated over 40,000 people in India between 1893 and 1896. A variety of questions persisted about the vaccine's effectiveness. The Indian government was never entirely convinced of its wisdom, and its use was largely maintained for populations without a choice in the matter, such as soldiers and prison inmates.

As had been true in earlier cholera pandemics, many of the official state responses to the disease sparked varying levels of popular opposition and resistance. In some places (e.g., in Hamburg and Moscow in 1892), such opposition did not lead to violence and social turmoil, but in others it did. Two examples illustrate the different issues at stake that led to civil disorder.

Fifth Cholera Pandemic, 1881–1896

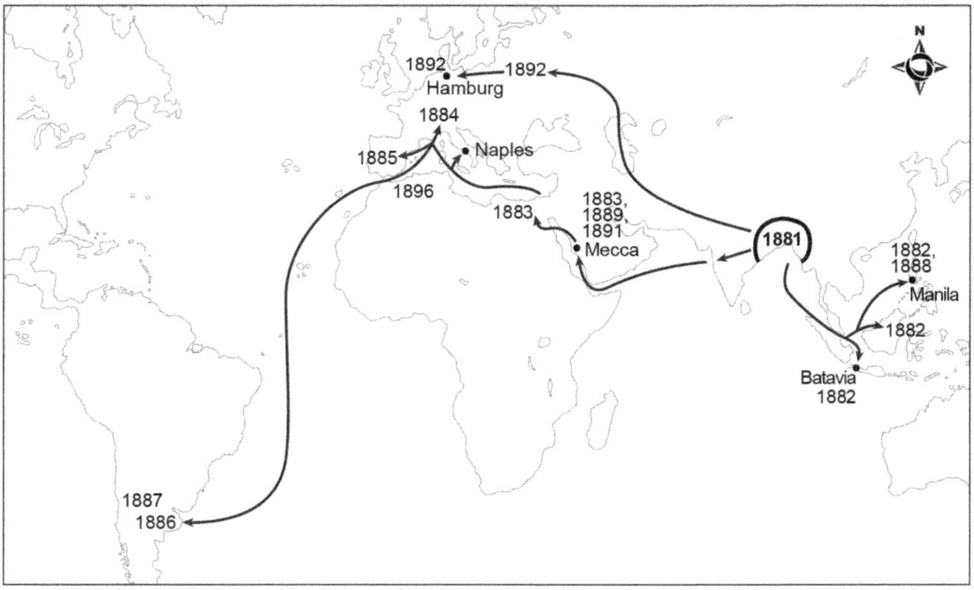

Cholera struck Naples with great violence in the late summer of 1884, and the epidemic rapidly peaked in September. In that month, the economic life of the city nearly came to a halt—businesses closed, unemployment soared, and as many as 150,000 people may have fled (including most of the upper and middle classes). In that atmosphere, panic swept through the city, and what a modern historian calls a "phobia of poisoning" seized the population (Snowden 1995, 138). Behind those fears, especially strong among the city's poor, lay both a long history of distrust of authority and a series of particular responses to the city's attempts to combat the epidemic.

The epidemic's toll was especially heavy in the poor sections of the city, one circumstance that suggested that the disease was a plot hatched by the city's governors to reduce the population of the poor. The city government, which had in effect denied the gravity of the epidemic in August, suddenly undertook a panoply of neocontagionist measures in September: disinfecting property and people, medical inspections, isolating the sick (including establishing special cholera hospitals). The very activity of a government that usually ignored the poor completely was suspicious, especially when that activity seemed like a military operation. Medical inspections, confiscations of property, and isolation of the sick were all compulsory.

The poor people of Naples resisted these measures in a variety of ways. Crowds continued to assemble for religious processions in defiance of bans on such gatherings; people ostentatiously defied municipal dietary advice and refused to report illness to authorities. Doctors, seen as the handmaidens of authority, were often greeted with hostility and violence when they came into the poorer quarters. The opening of two new cholera hospitals provoked what Snowden (1995, 147) calls "full-scale insurrections" on September 9 and September 14, as people took to the streets against the "poisoners" who would lock their families and friends away. It was largely the waning of the epidemic (see the "Unresolved Historical Issues" section) that made possible the restoration of order.

Significant disorder also accompanied the cholera epidemic in Russia in 1892. There too fear was the prevalent reaction of many people, and the neocontagionist attempts of authorities and their doctors were resisted by those who believed cholera to be a government plot. Mass government purchases of coffins seemed suspicious; bans on religious processions were resented; and as in Naples, compulsory medical inspections and the confiscation of property were backed by military force. So when cholera reached Astrakhan, a "frenzied mob" attacked medical personnel, burned down cholera barracks, and liberated their patients (Frieden 1977, 544). When a river steamer carrying migrant laborers reached Saratov, the laborers refused to submit to medical examinations and threatened to throw the captain in the Volga River if he obeyed a quarantine order. In the neighboring town of Khvalynsk a major riot included the murder of a physician, called a poisoner by the crowd. Some patients told another physician about rumors that an official "in leather gloves with an iron hook" carted drunks and other unfortunates to the cholera hospital where they would be brutally killed (Frieden 1977, 548).

Political and cultural resistance also greeted some Western imperial responses to cholera in Asia. The quarantine station established on the island of Kamaran off the coast of Yemen was widely resented by pilgrims in 1881 and in succeeding years, and many responded by taking advantage of their overwhelming numbers to avoid regulations, hide cholera cases from official eyes, and corrupt authorities. Widespread Indian protests at the 1892 closure of Hindu pilgrimage routes to Hardwar, while not accompanied by violence, were examples of the problems that led the government of British India to approach epidemic control very gingerly; Haffkine's cholera vaccine may not have been widely used because the Indian government feared violent resistance to any compulsory vaccination of the population.

UNRESOLVED HISTORICAL ISSUES

During the fifth cholera pandemic a new understanding of the cause of the disease was advanced: the germ theory, with the causative germ identified by Robert Koch in 1883. But while that explanation seemed increasingly convincing during the course of the pandemic, many doubts remained about it, doubts that would carry on into the sixth cholera pandemic starting in 1899 and lasting into the twentieth century.

One unresolved medical issue concerned a possible vaccine that would prevent cholera. One had been developed in 1892, but was it safe? And more important, the feasibility of a vaccine was keyed to acceptance of the idea that a microorganism was the necessary and sufficient cause of the disease, and that point remained in dispute. More generally, at the conclusion of the fifth pandemic it was still not certain whether human actions had anything to do with the pandemic's ebbing away. (That point remains something of an unsolved historical puzzle as well.)

Despite those uncertainties, it was more clearly understood in 1896 what measures might effectively stop a cholera epidemic. But the examples of violent (and passive) responses discussed in the last section illustrate a more important and unresolved issue: knowing what to do was one thing, and being able to do it was another. Systems of medical inspections, bacteriological tests, isolation hospitals, water purification, and sewage removal required two things, both clearly missing from 1884 Naples and 1892 Saratov. The first was a significant bureaucratic (and physical) infrastructure, which would certainly require heavy expense. The second was a level of acceptance by the populace of the wisdom, or necessity, of the inspections and isolation that interfered with personal liberties and traditional customs and of the higher taxes that would have to pay for those inspections, tests, and hospitals. The second point, an example of the perceived necessity of the *medicalization* (see Glossary) of a population, remained a slowly evolving feature of the twentieth century's responses to epidemics.

REFERENCES

Baldwin, Peter. *Contagion and the State in Europe, 1830–1930.* Cambridge: Cambridge University Press, 1999.

Frieden, Nancy M. "The Russian Cholera Epidemic of 1892–93 and Medical Professionalization." *Journal of Social History* 10 (1977): 538–559.

Snowden, Frank M. *Naples in the Time of Cholera, 1884–1911.* Cambridge: Cambridge University Press, 1995.

SUGGESTED ADDITIONAL READING

Abeyasekere, Susan. "Death and Disease in Nineteenth Century Batavia." In *Death and Disease in Southeast Asia: Explorations in Social, Medical, and Demographic History,* edited by Norman G. Owen, 189–209. Singapore: Oxford University Press, 1987.

Arnold, David. *Colonizing the Body: State Medicine and Epidemic Disease in Nineteenth-Century India.* Berkeley: University of California Press, 1993.

DeBevoise, Ken. *Agents of Apocalypse: Epidemic Disease in the Colonial Philippines.* Princeton, NJ: Princeton University Press, 1995.

Evans, Richard J. *Death in Hamburg: Society and Politics in the Cholera Years, 1830–1910.* Oxford: Oxford University Press, 1987. Reprint, Harmondsworth: Penguin, 1990.

Gardiner, Peter, and Mayling Oey. "Morbidity and Mortality in Java, 1880–1940: The Evidence of the Colonial Reports." In *Death and Disease in Southeast Asia: Explorations in Social, Medical, and Demographic History,* edited by Norman G. Owen, 70–90. Singapore: Oxford University Press, 1987.

Hamlin, Christopher. *Cholera: The Biography.* Oxford: Oxford University Press, 2009.

Howard-Jones, Norman. "Cholera Therapy in the Nineteenth Century." *Journal of the History of Medicine and Allied Sciences* 27 (1972): 373–395.

Kuhnke, LaVerne. *Lives at Risk: Public Health in Nineteenth-Century Egypt.* Berkeley: University of California Press, 1990.

Löwy, Ilana. "From Guinea Pigs to Man: The Development of Haffkine's Anticholera Vaccine." *Journal of the History of Medicine and Allied Sciences* 47 (1992): 270–309.

Maglen, Krista. *The English System: Quarantine, Immigration and the Making of a Port Sanitary Zone.* Manchester: Manchester University Press, 2014.

Mishra, Saurabh. "Incarceration and Resistance in a Red Sea Lazaretto, 1880–1930." In *Quarantine: Local and Global Histories*, edited by Alison Bashford, 54–65. London: Palgrave, 2016.

Pollitzer, R. *Cholera.* Geneva: World Health Organization, 1959.

Roff, William R. "Sanitation and Security: The Imperial Powers and the Nineteenth Century Hajj." *Arabian Studies* 6 (1982): 143–160.

29

Influenza Pandemic, 1889–1893

WHERE AND WHEN

In early October 1889, a wave of influenza began spreading from some of the central Asian regions of the then-Russian Empire, in modern Kyrgyzstan and Kazakhstan. It moved particularly rapidly to the west, where people infected by it traveled easily by rail and river, and in the last 10 days of October, influenza struck the cities of Moscow and St. Petersburg. From those cities, rail links quickly spread the pandemic to other major European capitals—Berlin, Vienna, Paris, all infected by mid-November—and those places in turn became centers for the further movement of the disease by railroad passengers. Almost all of Europe (except portions of northern Great Britain, Ireland, and Sardinia) experienced the influenza epidemic by the end of December 1889. By mid-December, steamship traffic had brought influenza across the Atlantic as well, as the northeastern United States received its first cases; the disease thereupon resumed its rail transit, reaching the upper Midwest in the first 10 days of January 1890.

This influenza pandemic dramatically illustrated the role of steamships (and their passengers and crew) in the diffusion of a disease. In December 1889, traffic across the Mediterranean carried influenza to Alexandria and Cairo. In January such diverse ports as Tunis, Cape Town, Buenos Aires, Tokyo, New Orleans, and San Francisco reported influenza; in February, Dakar, Algiers, Hong Kong, and Singapore; in March, Bombay. Influenza's reach into South America, Africa, and Asia was largely through seaports, in contrast with its spread along Europe and North America's dense rail networks. The disease's movement across thinly settled areas that lacked railroad tracks was much slower. For example, while it moved rapidly westward from its central Asian origins, moving eastward across Eurasia was much more problematic. Irkutsk, in Siberia, was affected by influenza on December 4, 1889, six weeks after Moscow; apparently the wave of influenza stopped there, for adjoining eastern Asia (Manchuria, Korea) only received the disease by sea, in the summer of 1890.

The pattern of influenza epidemics in 1889–1890 was similar almost everywhere. About two weeks after the first reported cases, incidence suddenly increased, remained very high for two or three weeks, and then declined, equally suddenly, in a further two weeks. The disease seemed to affect men and women, children and the aged, and all social classes indiscriminately.

Further spasms of this nearly worldwide pandemic recurred in 1891–1892 and 1892–1893, in some places inflicting even more serious morbidities and mortalities. Evidently the influenza virus had become embedded in some places, and epidemics resurged as a result. In some of these later reoccurrences, influenza began taking a higher death toll among the elderly.

World morbidity, or the rate of illness, was extraordinarily high between 1889 and 1893. Although precise figures will never be known (if only because many cases of influenza were never reported), it is a reasonable guess that between a third and a half of the world's population may have been ill with influenza at some time in those years. Although influenza was usually a mild infection whose mortality rate was very low, the vast numbers affected in this pandemic meant a large number of deaths. Often, influenza led to death when pneumonia joined it. David Patterson, a modern historian, has estimated that the 1889–1890 influenza pandemic killed between 270,000 and 360,000 people in Europe (Patterson 1986). Mark Honigsbaum, another modern authority, believes that perhaps 110,000 died from influenza in Great Britain alone between 1889 and 1892 (Honigsbaum 2014).

SIGNIFICANCE

The 1889–1893 pandemic was perhaps the first thoroughly documented attack of influenza, and it was the first one that was clearly worldwide in scope. It illustrated the new importance of the revolution in human transportation made possible by the railroad and the steamship. It also occurred when widespread telegraphy coincided with mass-circulation newspapers and rapidly increasing literacy rates to create much higher popular awareness—and fear—of the epidemic.

It also clearly illustrated, on a large scale, the characteristics of both earlier and later influenza epidemics: their very high morbidity rates, short duration, and relatively low mortality rates. The massive morbidity, however, made the 1889–1893 influenza the greatest single killer epidemic of the nineteenth century in Europe (although not in Asia, where cholera and plague epidemics took a higher toll). Finally, its sudden and unexpected appearance, and its very rapid spread, foreshadowed the even more serious influenza pandemic of 1918–1919.

BACKGROUND

Influenza is a term for a respiratory disease caused by a family of viruses with different subtypes. Its symptoms are similar to, but may be more severe than, those of the common cold. Its early history is not clear. Some references to diseases in twelfth-century Europe may have been to influenza, but that is not beyond doubt. Patterson (1986) places the earliest clear evidence for influenza in the late sixteenth century, but it is only in the eighteenth century that epidemics and pandemics of influenza can be identified, generally moving outward from a central

Asian base. Major influenza pandemics occurred in the 1830s and 1840s, but not again until 1889–1893, by which time changes in transportation led to a comprehensive worldwide pandemic. That pandemic also coincided with a period of rising Western concerns about perceived "national decline" and threats of lower-class unrest, as well as the tensions arising from the increasing pressure of Western imperial power on Africa and Asia.

HOW IT WAS UNDERSTOOD AT THE TIME

By 1889, Western medical opinion was being won over—although not completely—to the idea that microorganisms (bacteria, or germs) caused disease. So the 1889–1890 pandemic stimulated a search for its causative organism. An eminent German bacteriologist, Richard Friedrich Pfeiffer, claimed to have discovered such a bacillus in 1890, but his subsequent efforts to demonstrate the necessary connection between his bacillus and actual cases of influenza were not entirely convincing. For many, therefore, the cause of influenza remained unknown, although there was wide agreement that *some* microorganisms must be responsible. But regardless of the reliability of Pfeiffer's results, they successfully gave influenza a visual identity for the first time. And for many, Pfeiffer's bacillus was the answer, and those convictions were revived at the time of the 1918–1919 influenza pandemic.

It was also generally agreed that influenza was very contagious. Its spread along routes of human traffic clearly argued that infected people carried it and passed it to others through the air. The relatively mild character of its symptoms usually did not prevent people from traveling. Lending great weight to those convictions were the findings of the British researcher Henry Parsons, who carefully traced the pattern of reported cases as they followed lines of travel.

RESPONSES

The rapid movement of influenza, its immense morbidity, and the equally rapid decline of its incidence made public health measures difficult. Quarantines were not undertaken, and indeed the pandemic's speed and universality would have made them (especially by land) useless. Western physicians by the late nineteenth century had moved away from earlier humoral medicine, with its purgings and bleedings, but without a sure knowledge of the cause of influenza they had no clear remedy (or preventive advice) to offer, except response to symptoms such as fevers. Many cases of influenza were probably never reported, as sufferers brushed them aside as colds. Many people turned to popular or patent remedies.

UNRESOLVED HISTORICAL ISSUES

The relation of the influenzas of 1889–1893 and 1918–1919 is certainly an important one. Confidence in Pfeiffer's bacillus lingered in some minds from one pandemic to the next. More important: one of the distinguishing features of the

1918–1919 pandemic was its unexpected severity for young adults, ordinarily the least vulnerable age group in times of epidemic. Did people born before 1889—almost all of them over 30 in 1918—acquire some vital immunities from the earlier pandemic?

REFERENCES

Honigsbaum, Mark. *A History of the Great Influenza Pandemics: Death, Panic and Hysteria, 1830–1920.* London: I. B. Tauris, 2014.

Patterson, K. David. *Pandemic Influenza, 1700–1900: A Study in Historical Epidemiology.* Totowa, NJ: Rowman & Littlefield, 1986.

SUGGESTED ADDITIONAL READING

Crosby, Alfred W. *America's Forgotten Pandemic: The Influenza of 1918.* Cambridge: Cambridge University Press, 1989. (Orig. pub. 1976 as *Epidemic and Peace, 1918.* Westport, CT: Greenwood.)

30

Cholera Epidemic in Hamburg, 1892

WHEN AND WHERE

In August 1892, cholera broke out in the large north German port city of Hamburg. This epidemic was one of the fifth cholera pandemic's most serious appearances in Europe, for within a few weeks about 8,600 people in Hamburg had died.

In Germany fear of cholera was sparked by the disease's reappearance in the Russian Empire in July 1892. The Prussian border with Russia was closed. Although emigrant traffic from Russia to America continued, trains carrying emigrants through Germany were sealed. Despite such precautions, cholera made its appearance in Hamburg suddenly, when an apparent case of the disease was diagnosed on August 15. The bacillus then believed responsible for cholera was not found in that case, however, and so uncertainty lingered. A further case was diagnosed the following night (August 16–17), and although the bacillus was then found, the doctors who found it had no experience with cholera and so remained unsure of their findings. By August 19, the number of cases reached 31, but physicians remained reluctant to pronounce that cholera had in fact arrived.

Meanwhile physicians in the city of Altona, which immediately adjoined Hamburg to the west but was under another government (see the "Background" section), diagnosed cholera in the city's hospital on August 21. (The victim worked in Hamburg and had apparently contracted the disease there.) Still Hamburg physicians hesitated; the city's governing senate was only officially notified of cholera on August 23, and no public admission of cholera's presence was made until August 24. Nine crucial days had elapsed since the first case.

Those days of delay coincided with a serious heat wave that lowered the level of the Elbe River. (Hamburg is near the mouth of the Elbe.) Rising tides thus faced a weaker downstream river flow, and river water was pushed back upstream. Contaminated sewage reached the city's water supply as a result (see the "Background" section). By August 26, the number of cholera cases in Hamburg began to soar. Between that date and August 30, the city recorded over 900 new cases *every day*, while daily deaths soon thereafter regularly exceeded 400.

The epidemic only began easing in the last week of September. On October 10, only one new case was reported, and the epidemic was clearly over by mid-October. But by November 12, the total number of cholera cases in Hamburg had reached nearly 17,000, and about 8,600 people had died. (Hamburg's population in 1890 had been 623,000.) Of all deaths in Hamburg in September, 70% were caused by cholera. In many ways, the scale of the epidemic overwhelmed the city's efforts to contain it. Plans for disinfection failed; the city ambulance service proved completely inadequate; hospitals became enormously overcrowded (and no special cholera hospitals or wards existed when the epidemic began); and the disposal of the dead became a major problem, as it so often has been in epidemics throughout history.

Hamburg's government had failed in several important ways. As is discussed later (see the "Background," "How It Was Understood at the Time," and "Responses" sections), both government and physicians were reluctant to accept the germ theory of cholera that had been advanced in the 1880s. The dominant figure of germ theory, Robert Koch, had been dispatched from Berlin to Hamburg in the early stages of the epidemic, but his measures faced resistance there. And the Hamburg government permitted five ships carrying emigrants to the United States to leave the port between August 17 and September 1; all of the ships carried cholera as well as emigrants.

SIGNIFICANCE

The 1892 epidemic in Hamburg was a particularly well-documented case in the fifth cholera pandemic, as well as being the only major cholera epidemic of those years in Germany. The epidemic has provided important demographic data about the impact of a cholera attack, and that has contributed to a clearer understanding of other, earlier cholera epidemics in nineteenth-century Western cities. The Hamburg experience with cholera has been confirmed in some cities but not in others.

The Hamburg epidemic provided the first clear opportunity to apply the newly refined germ theory to a cholera outbreak. It also illustrated that in 1892 the germ theory had not yet won over all opinion, despite its apparent success in the eyes of later medical scientists. And the Hamburg cholera epidemic led directly to one of the most dramatic experiments in medical history (see the "Unresolved Historical Issues" section).

BACKGROUND

The political position of Hamburg played an important role in its particular response to the 1892 epidemic. Hamburg had for centuries governed itself as an independent city-state; when the German Empire was proclaimed in 1871 Hamburg was a part of it, but that empire was a federal political system and the separate states within it (including the city-state of Hamburg) retained some real powers over their internal affairs. Hamburg was governed by a legislature that represented adult citizens who possessed a certain amount of property, especially members of a mercantile business class. Some territory immediately adjoining Hamburg, including the city of Altona, was not within the city-state's boundaries—Altona was actually within the Kingdom of Prussia.

The interests of trade had long dominated the city's politics. Hamburg's leaders strongly upheld the ideology of nineteenth-century liberalism, which emphasized minimal government interference with economic freedom. Unlike many other places in Germany, the practices of medical police—an aggressive public health bureaucracy to supervise quarantines, isolation, sanitation, and the provision of nursing—had found little favor in Hamburg. The city government had established a Health Committee in 1818 and a Medical Board in 1870, but their powers remained merely advisory. While many of the governments of Europe mandated smallpox vaccinations of their populations early in the nineteenth century, Hamburg did so only in 1871, and only then after a very serious smallpox epidemic.

By 1892 Hamburg—and all of Europe—had been linked more tightly to distant places by a dense railroad network. That network had extended into Russia, so that when political moves (e.g., pogroms against the Jews) and economic events (a major famine in 1891 and 1892) in that country led to massive migration, those migrants could easily travel into and through Germany. In 1891 over 90,000 Russians moved through the two main German ports (Hamburg and Bremen) on their way across the sea. The Hamburg city government, together with steamship companies, welcomed the business, and erected shoddy barracks in the harbor districts to house the migrants while they waited for a ship. Sanitary conditions in the barracks were poor (sewage emptied directly into the Elbe).

Hamburg took its water from the Elbe, upstream from the city; in theory its sewage discharged into the river downstream. Hamburg remained, as did many other Western cities in the third quarter of the nineteenth century, vulnerable to outbreaks of waterborne diseases. A sand filtration system had been proposed for the city's water supply in the 1850s, but the city's property owners resisted both the taxes necessary to pay for it, and the acquisition of privately owned land that would be needed for more reservoirs. The filtration system was only approved in 1890, and at the time of the 1892 epidemic it was still under construction. When strong tides pushed river water upstream in August 1892, sewage was thus carried into the intakes of a water system that lacked adequate filters to purify the water.

Conclusive evidence linked the epidemic to the Hamburg water supply. Adjoining Altona, with a different water supply, remained almost entirely free of cholera. The experience of a particular apartment block in Hamburg illustrates the point. Although it was within the city limits of Hamburg, it happened to receive its water from Altona. The complex had 345 residents, and no cases of cholera (Evans 1990, 292).

HOW IT WAS UNDERSTOOD AT THE TIME

In 1892 the germ theory of cholera, as laid out by Robert Koch in the previous decade, had won wide and growing acceptance, but many doubts remained. Those doubts were especially strong in Hamburg, where political traditions opposed many of the measures that would follow from adopting germ theory. Germ theory called for aggressive state intervention—quarantines and isolation—to prevent the contagious movement of germs from one person to another. That intervention represented interference with individual freedom, especially individual freedom of trade.

If only for those political reasons, the arguments of Max von Pettenkofer, the Munich public health authority, enjoyed popularity in Hamburg. Pettenkofer believed that germs were an insufficient explanation for cholera; other, more general environmental factors also needed consideration. Pettenkofer emphasized the importance of personal hygiene and individual efforts to rectify the local environmental conditions that allowed the cholera germ (considered a seed) to take root and grow. That emphasis on personal responsibility was in harmony with Hamburg's political traditions of laissez-faire liberalism.

The official attitude of the Hamburg city government at the start of the epidemic reflected this reluctance to take state action. As discussed earlier, the government was slow to admit that a cholera epidemic had begun, or that it was serious; it feared disturbing the routine of the city, and especially of disrupting the trade on which the city lived.

RESPONSES

Many of the official responses to the epidemic were more-or-less forced on a reluctant city government by the authority of the imperial government based in Berlin, which was much more willing to take aggressive action. While the Hamburg authorities hesitated in the period between August 15 and August 24, other German governments, including the Kingdom of Prussia (the largest and most dominant member of the federation) began taking action. When Hamburg officially announced the presence of cholera on August 24, a network of quarantines was quickly set up by other German places that isolated Hamburg from contact. Those measures stayed in force for several months, seriously disrupting Hamburg's trade. Many of the trains that connected Hamburg with the rest of the country were cancelled.

On August 25, Robert Koch himself arrived in Hamburg, carrying authority from the imperial government to impose measures against cholera. Some of those measures attempted to intercept cholera germs in water and on food. Wagons were to circulate through the city carrying pure water, public boiling stations could kill germs in other water, public baths were closed, and the sale of raw fruit from barrows was prohibited. Disinfecting the dwellings of the sick, isolating the sick in cholera hospitals, closing schools, and banning dances and public meetings would all cut lines of contagion.

Not all these measures were enacted thoroughly or efficiently. The city government resisted some of them, and it had difficulty finding the labor force to implement others. Koch's determination to use evidence from bacteriological testing to identify cholera victims ran up against the fact that few technologists knew how to perform the tests. Ambulances to convey the sick to isolation were woefully inadequate; hospitals quickly became hopelessly overcrowded; schools were used as emergency cholera wards; some barrack-like hospitals were hurriedly thrown up; and a German army field hospital was dispatched. But many hospitals were of dubious benefit.

The disposal of the dead posed other problems for the city authorities. Some of the corpses were buried in mass graves that were sixty feet long, twelve feet wide, and only three-and-a-half feet deep.

Although public health measures against cholera were, therefore, somewhat focused by 1892, physicians could still offer little effective treatment for those who became ill. The positively dangerous practice of purging fluids from the body—that simply exaggerated what cholera was doing anyway—had become rare, but some doctors adopted a secret remedy that promised an anti-cholera bacterium and was in fact a purgative. Others still bled patients to adjust humoral balance. Some tried the newer therapy of intravenous saline injections, which at least attempted to return fluids to the body. Hot baths were a popular (and perhaps soothing) treatment. Many popular, commercial, or folk remedies existed as well, in a continuum with those prescribed by the orthodox physicians: patent medicines, disinfectants, camphor, warm cow-dung broth (noted by Evans 1990, 364), and electric shock therapy. But the sudden violence of cholera's onset meant that most patients simply suffered rapidly, to either die or recover without orthodox or unorthodox treatments.

The 1892 epidemic generated rumors, fear, and panic in Hamburg. Perhaps 40,000 people fled the city; one estimate had 12,000 leaving in two days (August 22 and 23), before the city government had even made a public admission that cholera was present. Most of those who fled were from the middle and upper classes; as has been true in many urban epidemics, people who could afford to leave, and/or who had someplace to go, were more likely to do so. The well-to-do who remained were also better able to isolate themselves safely in their homes, sending their servants out into the dangerous streets to get provisions.

And as had been true in earlier European cholera epidemics, the poorer sections of the city suffered a higher proportion of deaths. Contemporary beliefs continued to associate cholera with not only poverty but also with the reputed habits of the poor, especially their drunkenness. (Alcohol consumption did rise during the epidemic, fueling that perception.) Evans (1990) argues that the superior data available from 1892 Hamburg make possible some firmer statements about the actual connections between poverty and cholera, a subject of important historical speculation. The poor, according to Evans, were more likely to be stricken with cholera; death rates of those who contracted the disease were generally similar across social classes, but the poor were at much greater risk of infection.

The upper and middle classes were more likely to have fled, and more likely to preserve hygiene in their homes because they had servants to do the cleaning. Earlier typhoid fever epidemics had accustomed middle-class households to boiling their water. Meanwhile the poor lacked those advantages and were particularly at risk if they worked in or near the harbor (where polluted water was found), or in domestic service. Working-class women (many of them domestic servants) fared especially poorly.

Despite the ineffectiveness of the city government, the strong and sometimes unpopular measures imposed on it from without, and the affronts to dignity that the disease caused, little civil unrest shook Hamburg in 1892. The governing classes berated Koch, or the imperial chancellor Leo von Caprivi, or the Prussians from Berlin, but the population did not take to the streets or attack hospitals, as had happened in 1832 Manchester and Paris or 1884 Naples. For more discussion of both the impact of the epidemic on civil unrest (or its absence) in Hamburg, see the next section, "Unresolved Historical Issues."

UNRESOLVED HISTORICAL ISSUES

The installation of a sand-filtration water system did not prove to be a guarantee. In January 1893, Altona, which possessed such a system, suffered cholera cases while Hamburg was cholera-free. Other vulnerabilities evidently still existed; the practical technologies and skills involved in construction and installation might lag behind the demands of science.

One issue unresolved at the time of the epidemic was quickly settled. Whatever doubts persisted about Koch and his germ theory, the epidemic spurred the Hamburg authorities to quickly complete the sand-filtration water plant that had been so long delayed.

But in other ways, those doubts could not be stilled. In the immediate aftermath of the Hamburg cholera epidemic, the German government called a commission to investigate a proposed National Epidemics Law. Koch and his followers wanted the imperial German government empowered to establish quarantines and isolation procedures for the whole country; Pettenkofer, opposing those ideas, countered that local authorities should be left free to act against poor sanitation conditions.

The commission endorsed Koch's proposals, and Pettenkofer was then driven to a dramatic experiment to challenge the germ theory. Acquiring a sample of the *Vibrio cholera* bacilli that (according to Koch) caused cholera, he swallowed the sample on October 7, 1892. By October 9, he had experienced severe diarrhea but survived. One of his followers, Rudolf Emmerich, repeated the experiment before a crowd of witnesses on October 17; he too survived, after some severe digestive distress. Could the bacillus alone therefore be a sufficient explanation of cholera fatalities?

Pettenkofer, emboldened by the risky experiment, mobilized political resistance to the proposed Epidemics Law. Some German states (for instance, Pettenkofer's native Bavaria) were generally leery of granting centralizing power to Berlin anyway; others feared the power of government to intrude on personal liberty and family autonomy that quarantines and isolation might involve. Despite the experience of the Hamburg cholera epidemic, and the endorsement of the commission, in 1893 the Reichstag (the imperial legislature) turned down the law. Only in 1900, spurred by fear of the approaching plague pandemic (see volume 2, chapter 31), did the Reichstag agree to Koch's proposals.

The history of the well-documented 1892 Hamburg epidemic has raised some broad questions about the role of epidemics (especially cholera) in civil and political disturbances in the nineteenth century. The Hamburg population did not react violently to the epidemic or the measures taken against it by authorities. Did that mean that by the time of the fifth pandemic (of which the Hamburg epidemic was a part) European city populations had come to accept the necessity, or wisdom, of the medical and public health pressures on their habits? Had they become medicalized? Or does the apparent placidity of the Hamburg people reflect purely local circumstances rather than a general shift in behavior? Just a few years earlier (1884), after all, major disturbances had occurred in Naples. Or did protests and political action in response to epidemics simply take different forms? Instead of rioting about the disrespect shown to corpses in mass gravesites, did political action turn to more general calls for reform of a corrupt system?

REFERENCE

This chapter leans heavily on the following work, a thorough treatment of the Hamburg cholera epidemic:

Evans, Richard J. *Death in Hamburg: Society and Politics in the Cholera Years, 1830–1910.* Harmondsworth: Penguin, 1990. (Orig. pub. 1987. Oxford University Press.)

SUGGESTED ADDITIONAL READING

Evans, Richard J. "Epidemics and Revolutions: Cholera in Nineteenth-Century Europe." *Past and Present* 120 (1988): 123–146.

Hamlin, Christopher. *Cholera: The Biography.* Oxford: Oxford University Press, 2009.

Kudlick, Catherine J. *Cholera in Post-Revolutionary Paris: A Cultural History.* Berkeley: University of California Press, 1996.

Morris, R. J. *Cholera 1832: The Social Response to an Epidemic.* New York: Holmes and Meier, 1976.

Rosenberg, Charles E. *The Cholera Years: The United States in 1832, 1849, and 1866.* Chicago: University of Chicago Press, 1962.

Snowden, Frank M. 1995. *Naples in the Time of Cholera, 1884–1911.* Cambridge: Cambridge University Press.

31

Third Plague Pandemic, 1894–?

WHEN AND WHERE

The world's third pandemic of plague began in China in the mid-nineteenth century. After spreading slowly through that country for several decades, it reached the port cities of Canton (Guangzhou) and Hong Kong in 1894. From those points, sea transport rapidly carried plague to many points on different continents in the next few years and the pandemic became nearly worldwide. By 1912 the disease had been largely contained, but outbreaks continued to occur in Asia, Africa, and the United States throughout the twentieth century. A total of perhaps 15 million people died in the Third Plague Pandemic; and while most of those deaths occurred between 1894 and 1912, the potential for a revival of the pandemic still exists.

Bubonic plague began spreading in the southern Chinese province of Yunnan in the 1770s, originating in rodent populations in which the disease was enzootic. By about 1830 much of that province had been affected. At that point, the epidemic subsided, only to revive again in the 1850s. In that decade important rebellions shook China: the Taiping rebellion, in 1850–1851, contributed to a shift in river traffic routes between Yunnan and Canton; the Muslim rebellion in Yunnan itself led to massive troop movements and swarms of refugees between 1856 and 1873. Perhaps in part for those reasons, the path of plague out of Yunnan to the east was facilitated. Merchants converged on Beihai, on the south coast, and that city began experiencing annual plague epidemics in 1871.

Thus far, however, the movement of the disease had illustrated that its overland diffusion was slow: from western Yunnan to Beihai, about 600 miles in a century. But in 1885 a regular steamship service began between Beihai and Canton (about 300 direct-line miles apart). When bubonic plague broke out in Canton (and nearby Hong Kong) in 1894, the worldwide pandemic quickly followed. Between 50,000 and 100,000 people may have died of plague in each of those cities in 1894; both cities were major ports that traded widely with the rest of the world.

The rapid diffusion of the Third Plague Pandemic after 1894 bears some comparison with that of the Second Plague Pandemic, with Hong Kong/Canton taking the part played by Constantinople in 1347. The greater speed and immensely greater range of late-nineteenth-century steamship traffic meant a much wider geographic spread. Carried by overseas traffic, plague appeared in Bombay in 1896 and Calcutta in 1898; Japan, the Philippines, and Hawaii in 1899; and by 1900, in such distant ports as Sydney, San Francisco, Buenos Aires, and Glasgow. Cape Town was infected in 1901.

During the early stages of the pandemic, human understanding of the causes and epidemiology of plague were revolutionized, first by the discovery of the causative microorganism (*Yersinia pestis*) in 1894, and then by the gradual acceptance (between 1898 and 1908) of the role of rodents and insects in its spread (see the "Responses" section).

In most of those cities, the disease was contained, and neither a large death toll nor an epidemic that spread into the hinterland resulted. The tragic exceptions to that were China, Indonesia, and especially India, where between 1896 and 1921 perhaps 12 million people died of plague. The annual toll of the disease in India exceeded one million in 1904, 1905, and 1907.

And while the death tolls were not that high, the United States did experience the most dramatic plague visitations in its history. Bubonic plague arrived in Honolulu in November 1899 on ships from Hong Kong; the resulting epidemic, lasting through March 1900, led to 61 deaths. It also led to a serious disaster in the physical structure of the city and illustrated equally serious racial preconceptions of disease (see the "Responses" section). Plague then reached San Francisco in March 1900, alternately stimulating responses of hysteria and denial; the same racial conflicts and preconceptions played themselves out, more dramatically; when the epidemic was declared over, in 1904, 113 deaths had been officially reported. Plague returned to San Francisco in 1907, this time generating a different, but equally significant, set of responses (see the "Responses" section).

And while plague did not spread to people outside San Francisco on either occasion, it did establish itself as an enzootic disease among rodents in the western and southwestern United States. That enzootic reservoir, especially among ground squirrels and prairie dogs, persists to the present.

Subsequent sporadic outbreaks of plague did occur in the United States, notably in New Orleans in 1914 and 1919, Oakland in 1919, and Los Angeles in 1924. The last resulted in 36 deaths, 31 of them from the pneumonic form of plague.

The early stages of the Third Plague Pandemic reached Europe as well, although it did not establish itself there on a permanent basis as it has in the United States. Plague first appeared—taking 16 lives—in the Scottish port city of Glasgow in 1900. An outbreak in the English rural county of Suffolk in 1906 was not at first recognized as plague; only by 1910 were *Yersinia pestis* microorganisms found in the victims, and subsequent investigation revealed that an enzootic of plague had spread among local rodents. Between 10 and 20 deaths in the area, between 1906 and 1918, may have been due to plague. After 1918 plague disappeared from both the people of Suffolk, and the rodents. Elsewhere in Europe, Marseille (with much experience of plague in the Second Plague Pandemic) had an outbreak in 1930, while Paris, infected by rats off a steamer from India in 1917, had human cases of plague between that date and 1936.

In 1910 pneumonic plague appeared in the Chinese province of Manchuria. This epidemic did not originate in the Yunnan area nor did it reach Manchuria by sea. Instead it developed independently of the main Third Plague Pandemic among rodents of Mongolia, especially marmots. Between October 1910 and March 1911 perhaps 60,000 Manchurians succumbed.

For a variety of reasons (see the "Responses" and "Unresolved Historical Issues" sections) the Third Plague Pandemic diminished after about 1914, but sporadic outbreaks have persisted since, as some of the previously mentioned American and European examples illustrate. In the 1950s a sharp decline in plague cases occurred, falling from about 5,000 worldwide in 1953 to about 200 in 1959. But a dramatic surge in the 1960s, especially in Vietnam during the war there, took the number of worldwide cases over 4,000 every year between 1967 and 1971. In 1993 the number of worldwide cases was 2,065, including 191 deaths. And in the 1990s attention focused on the island of Madagascar, where antibiotic-resistant strains of *Yersinia pestis* had become enzootic in a population of rodents. That has resulted in a persistent threat of plague on the island, which manifested itself in 2017; by November of that year about 1,800 people had been infected and 127 had died.

Plague still has the power to frighten people in a way that few other diseases can do. In September 1994, an outbreak of pneumonic plague occurred in the Indian city of Surat, which (although the number of cases proved to be few) immediately created panic among travelers and was in the news around the world.

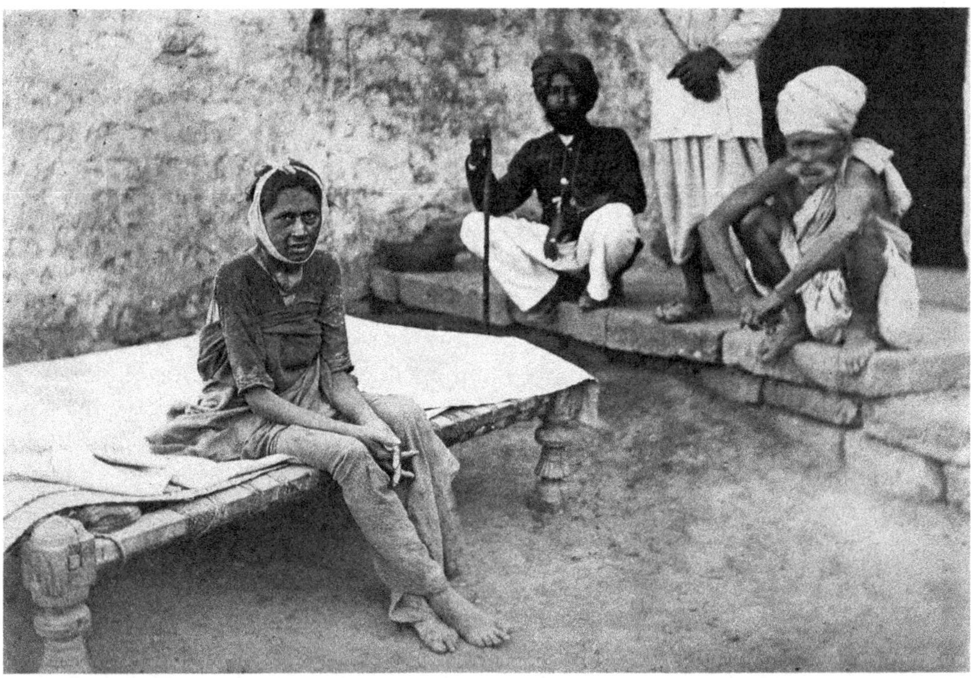

A female patient with bubonic plague in Karachi, a port city in what was then India (now Pakistan), 1897. The plague broke out in Bombay in 1896 and quickly spread to Karachi where a quarantine was established. (Wellcome Library)

SIGNIFICANCE

The Third Plague Pandemic quickly became a significant demographic event, especially in India between 1896 and 1914. Among twentieth-century pandemics, its worldwide death toll of about 15 million ranks with the most serious. It rivals the contemporary epidemics of AIDS, tuberculosis, and malaria, and it may trail only the catastrophic influenza pandemic of 1918–1919. In some places in the world its social and political importance was perhaps even greater. Especially in China and India, the experience of the disease, and different responses to it, focused tensions between the modern and the traditional, the rulers and the ruled. Dramatic confrontations between state medicine imposed from above and resistance to it from below resulted (see the "How It Was Understood at the Time" and "Responses" sections). And something of the same tensions played out in the United States as well, between different racial groups and between different levels of government.

In many areas of the world—not just in China and India where the mortality was highest—the pandemic led to improvements in sanitation and housing. In part the new understanding of the cause and epidemiology of plague inspired those improvements. The employment of those new conceptions contributed to halting the pandemic or preventing it from spreading further than it did. That success became a symbol of the power of twentieth-century biomedicine to resist epidemics, a confidence that crested in the mid-twentieth century.

And while the Third Plague Pandemic did not rival the second's mortality, it resulted in an even more widely diffused enzootic in rodent populations. Enzootic plague foci can now be found on several continents.

BACKGROUND

By the 1890s much of the world had passed under some degree of Western control, either in the form of direct political rule or indirect and informal economic influence. Even in places where Western control was largely informal (such as China), Western political and medical opinion often dictated official responses to the pandemic.

A dense network of oceanic trade knit the Western-dominated world together. Economies had become increasingly interdependent; steamship travel across the oceans had become frequent, reliable, and rapid. As had been true in the fourteenth century, ocean shipping remained the most efficient means of moving infected rodents, their fleas, and plague-infected humans, from one place to another. And shipping in the 1890s was a far more efficient conduit than it had been in the 1340s. Even when plague moved by land, those movements, though slower, usually followed trade paths. Some of that regional trade also reflected the pressure of the Western-dominated world market.

During the course of the Third Plague Pandemic, human interference with the physical environment increased. This at times meant ecological changes that affected plague's spread. Vietnam in the 1960s and early 1970s provides an example: the massive defoliation of the country that accompanied the war left dense bamboo thickets that turned out to be ideal habitats for plague-carrying rats.

By the 1890s international sanitary conferences (inspired earlier in the century by cholera) had become regular responses to epidemic threats, and they played a role in the plague pandemic as well. The quarantines decreed by earlier conferences remained a contentious subject, favored by most European states, resisted or resented by Ottoman Turkey and British India, and (therefore) by Britain itself. And also by the 1890s, Western scientific thought was placing increasing reliance on the general notion of a germ theory to explain disease. The rapid discovery of a germ for plague helped confirm that reliance.

HOW IT WAS UNDERSTOOD DURING THE PANDEMIC'S PEAK

Western scientific and medical opinion had long been convinced that plague was a *contagious* disease, but in some quarters those beliefs began to weaken in the nineteenth century. Most European governments still regarded such measures as quarantines of infected places, and isolation of infected persons, as the proper response to the threat of plague. But especially in Great Britain (which had not experienced plague since the seventeenth century), thoughts about disease increasingly reflected beliefs that sanitation held the key to health, and that diseases could best be countered by attacks on environmental pollutants.

As it happened, British authorities were the first Westerners to confront the Third Plague Pandemic, in their Chinese possession of Hong Kong (in 1894) and in India (in 1896). Their initial responses reflected that sanitationist view: the disease was a product of Chinese (or Indian) overcrowding, poverty, and general filth. But (also in 1894) two microbiologists, working in Hong Kong, identified a microorganism that they said was responsible for plague. Shibasaburo Kitasato and Alexandre Yersin had been trained, separately, by the founding giants of the germ theory: Kitasato by Robert Koch, and Yersin by Louis Pasteur. (At least for a time, their discovery confirmed the environmentalist view of British colonial physicians. The presence of the germ gave material meaning to filth, which was the home of the germ.)

The epidemiology of plague remained unclear, however; from where did the germ reach the body? Did it move from one person to another? In 1898 P. L. Simond, working in Bombay as part of a plague research commission, advanced the theory that the microorganism that infected rats was conveyed from one rat to another by fleas and might also be conveyed from rats to people by fleas. In the next ten years, that explanation was gradually accepted as experiments and observations strengthened it. Some of the earliest such evidence came from Sydney, from students of the 1900 plague epidemic there. W. Glen Liston, in Bombay, made crucial observations and experiments between 1903 and 1905, and by 1908 the Indian Plague Research Commission accepted the rat-flea connection.

Earlier in the nineteenth century, the Chinese (like many everyday Europeans, then and earlier) believed plague was the product of angry gods punishing human immorality. For Indians, plague was a new disease in 1896; neither traditional (Ayurvedic) medicine nor religious teaching had a body of ideas about it. For a variety of reasons (see the "Responses" section), many Indians became convinced that Europeans produced plague by spreading poison among the Indian population, and that view of the disease found echoes elsewhere in the world—including in the United States.

RESPONSES

Responses to the Third Plague Pandemic underwent some evolution between its first appearance in Canton and Hong Kong in 1894 and the pneumonic plague outbreak in Manchuria in 1910. Throughout, however, the hand of state medicine remained strong in different parts of the world, as political and medical authorities imposed drastic measures on populations that sometimes resisted (and modified) them.

The approaches of state medicine to plague in the 1890s first manifested themselves in British-ruled Hong Kong. A standing sanitary board had been established in that colony as early as 1883 with wide powers to inspect people and property, disinfect them, and isolate them to prevent the spread of infectious disease. This view—that disease was the product of filth—seemed to be confirmed by the 1894 plague epidemic, which concentrated its fury among the poorer (that is, thought to be filthier) Chinese sections of the colony. The sanitary board therefore moved to control the movements of the Chinese, disinfect or destroy the property of the sick, and isolate them.

But many Chinese disagreed with those measures and resisted their application. Landlords disliked state interference with their property; Chinese feared separation from their families; Chinese medical traditions did not consider diseases as contagions that could spread from one person to another, so why the isolation? And British attempts at control of movement had also to contend with the complex physical geography of the colony, a tangle of islands and inlets through which vital commerce flowed. In the face of both geographical complexity and Chinese opposition, the British authorities abandoned perhaps their most drastic scheme, which would have isolated plague victims on a ship away from the land, and agreed to use a plague hospital instead. Both in Hong Kong and in Canton (part of the Chinese Empire, still therefore theoretically independent of Western rule), Chinese leaders debated the wisdom of the British state medicine approach. Would Chinese adoption of such methods be a confession of national inferiority, and hence compromise Chinese sovereignty? Or was Western-style modernity necessary for maintaining national independence?

When plague reached Bombay in 1896, British colonial medical authorities there agreed with the 1894 Hong Kong approach, at least in principle. But the (British) Indian Medical Service had another tradition as well: a resistance to doctrines of contagion. British Indian opinion had resisted international calls for quarantines in response to earlier cholera pandemics, for India had itself been the object of such quarantines and its world trade could suffer accordingly. Perhaps motivated by such fears about damage to commerce, some Bombay authorities first reacted to plague by denying that the city was infected at all. (Other cities on other continents later would react to plague by denying it, too.)

Third Plague Pandemic, from ca. 1860 (in China) and Globally since 1894

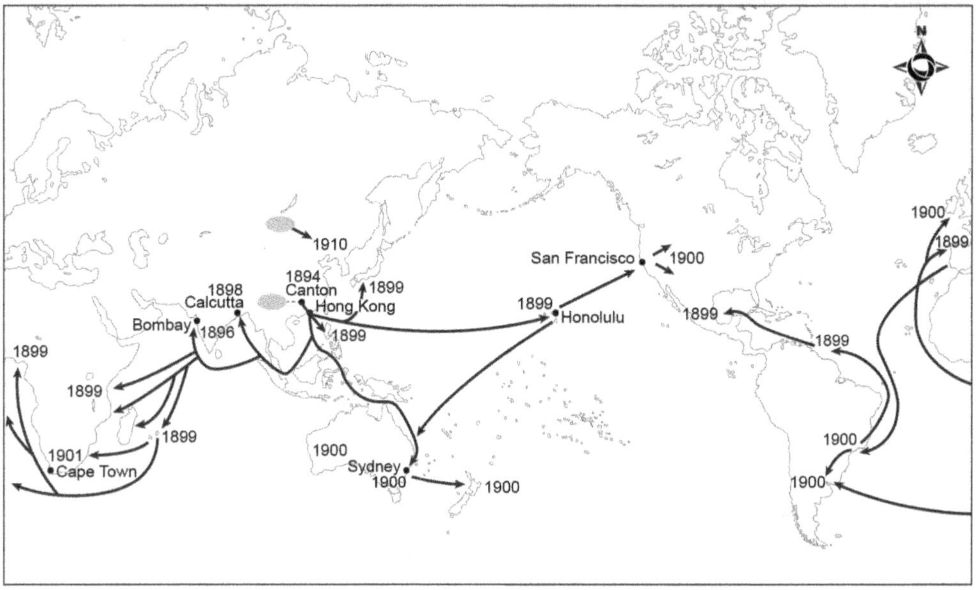

An International Sanitary Conference (meeting in Venice) reacted critically to such denials and imposed a quarantine on Indian goods. Fearful of the damage that would result to trade, the Indian and Bombay authorities reacted in turn. They began a vigorous program of identification, disinfection, and isolation. House searches rooted out plague victims, who were then isolated; their families were segregated from neighbors; and their property was disinfected or burned. Believing that plague germs might lurk on floors and spread to people with bare feet, such floors were treated with carbolic acid. (As Gregg [1985] notes, that action helped disperse rat populations more widely.) Internal quarantines within India attempted to seal off infected Bombay, and railroad passengers were monitored.

These policies stirred widespread Indian resentment and resistance for a number of reasons. No one wanted to be isolated in a hospital; many Indians resented such isolation because different castes were lumped together in the hospitals. Because symptoms of the body were important for a diagnosis of plague, bodies were subject to careful examination, which offended and shamed many Indian women. Even demands for blood samples (so that the plague germ might be discovered) were feared. And why, some Indians wondered, did so few Europeans contract plague? From that question, it was a short distance to an answer: plague was a poison spread by Europeans. What really happened when a blood sample was taken from you? Or when you were isolated in a hospital? The rules were widely evaded, while some Indians fled their homes. As early as October 1896, a riot occurred in Bombay, and it would be followed by others in the next several years, both in that city and elsewhere in India.

In 1898 and 1899, the Indian government found itself torn between conflicting pressures. From London, the British government demanded that the full resources of the Indian state be mobilized against plague; from the provinces of India itself came pleas for a more conciliatory policy that would defuse Indian objections. In part because the Indian state's resources were in fact limited but also in response to Indian objections, state medicine loosened its hold in those years. Inspections of houses and bodies were modified, and compulsory segregation and hospitalization diminished. Disinfections were performed in accord with Indian customs.

Two newer responses to plague also appeared, and they suggested that the stern state medicine approach might be unnecessary. In 1897 Waldemar Haffkine, a Russian-born physician in India, developed a plague vaccine. The vaccine slowly won supporters, although some in the British Indian medical establishment were leery of it and some Indians feared it as another European poison. By 1901, however, it had been widely administered in some areas of India, especially the northwest region called the Punjab. Suspicions of it persisted, however, fed by the deaths in 1902 of 19 villagers after they received vaccine that had been contaminated by tetanus.

The other new response focused official attention on rats, as conviction slowly grew that those animals were central links in the chain of infection. By 1908, earlier attempts to simply eradicate rats altogether had been abandoned in favor of controlling their access to human dwellings, an approach that had a better chance of success. It also eased the qualms that some Hindus felt about killing the animals.

When plague arrived in the United States, some of the same themes that had emerged in China and India repeated themselves: harsh state attempts at disinfection and isolation, popular resistance, racial stereotyping, and some denial that plague existed at all. The first American plague epidemic struck Honolulu, arriving on a ship from Hong Kong in November 1899. (Hawaii had just been annexed to the United States as a territory in the previous year.) When the disease was identified in the Chinese quarter of the city in December, the authorities decided that it was a Chinese problem. The Chinese quarter was therefore isolated by a cordon, and a program of disinfection and destruction of suspect property was begun. Unfortunately, the selective burning of such property got out of hand, and much of the Chinese quarter of Honolulu was destroyed by fire in January 1900.

Fear of plague preceded its arrival in San Francisco, where in 1899 Asian passengers traveling in the steerage quarters of ships were refused permission to land. The disease reached the city nevertheless, in March 1900. For the next several years, different elements of the population, and different arms of government, argued about what to do about it. Chinatown would be cordoned off; Chinese merchants and residents would object; courts would intervene to lift the cordon. Periods of massive disinfection involved the use of such corrosive materials as hydrochloric acid and sulfur-dioxide fumes. Chinese leaders debated whether to cooperate with the government or resist it. The governor of California called the report of plague in the city a scare, and many merchants and newspapers agreed with him, while doctors and the mayor pursued their zealous disinfection. Tensions between the white establishment of the city and the Chinese population rose. The Chinese of San Francisco, like the Indians of Bombay, feared that plague was a poison spread by whites. Perhaps the poison came with sulfur-dioxide fumes. So when attempts were made to introduce Haffkine's plague vaccine, many Chinese saw another possible poison and resisted it.

Cape Town, South Africa, where plague arrived in 1901, provides another example of responses guided by racial stereotypes. The health authorities of the city reacted to plague's arrival by moving about 6,000 black Africans to a new "native location" several miles outside Cape Town. A modern historian (Swanson 1977) has argued, persuasively, that this sanitary segregation grew out of the desire of employers to gain greater social control over their workforces, to which were added deep racial fears. The whites of Cape Town, by isolating the black Africans from themselves, increased their sense of personal safety—the plague epidemic simply provided an excuse for segregation. As Swanson puts it: "But 'the sanitation syndrome,' equating urban black settlement, labour and living conditions with threats to public health and security, became fixed in the official mind, buttressed a desire to achieve positive social controls, and confirmed or rationalized white race prejudice with a popular imagery of medical menace" (Swanson 1977, 410). It thus contributed to the emerging South African policy that would be called apartheid.

The responses to plague's return to San Francisco in 1907 illustrated the appeal of the new knowledge about the role of rats. Plague reappeared (in May 1907) when the effects of the great earthquake of April 1906 still dominated San Francisco life. The earthquake had created (in the words of a modern historian) a public health "disaster" (Craddock 2000, 147) with its disruption of water and sewer lines and overflowing latrines. Flies swarmed everywhere, and a surge in typhoid fever occurred. In this situation, rats ran riot, but curiously not much in Chinatown, which (despite the earthquake damage) benefited from the drastic clean-up of the earlier plague epidemic. When plague cases began in May 1907—spreading through the summer and into 1908—very few Chinese were affected. (The final death toll was 103, almost all white.)

Instead of turning on the Chinese residents, the city health officials now turned on the rats. Bounties were paid for dead rats. More important, new construction (or reconstruction, underway because of the earthquake) secured buildings from rats: concrete replaced wood, buildings were raised above the ground, and rat-friendly structures (notably wooden decks and chicken coops) were torn down. The plague epidemic therefore reinforced the urge to rebuild San Francisco as a modern city.

As chapter 35 will show, the Chinese government, under the pressures of foreign rivalry in Manchuria and the arguments of the influential physician Wu Lien-Teh, undertook a thorough program of cordons around infected areas, inspections, disinfections, and isolation of victims. Transients (and the poor more generally) were under suspicion. In Los Angeles in 1924, authorities followed this Manchurian approach, as well as embarking on a San Francisco-style assault on rats. Denial was still alive as well; the epidemic was called "malignant pneumonia" in the newspapers (Gregg 1985, 43).

All the responses to the Third Plague Pandemic discussed so far were preventive ones. Most were in the realms of isolation, public health, and sanitation, and most were extensions of practices that had been developed centuries earlier, during the Second Plague Pandemic. But the new understanding of the cause and epidemiology of plague resulted in new preventive approaches as well. The first of these was Haffkine's vaccine. The second was rat control. The conviction that rats spread the disease focused previously broad environmental sanitation measures on a more manageable (and more cost-effective) target.

In the later stages of the pandemic, some formidable new weapons against plague emerged from laboratories. Some of these refined attacks on the vectors, the rat and the flea. The development of the revolutionary insecticide called DDT, first deployed in World War II, made an impact on fleas (although its effect on malaria-bearing mosquitoes was more important). And the powerful rat poison called warfarin, when it was introduced in 1948, probably had a role in the sharp reduction of worldwide plague incidence in the 1950s.

Therapeutic responses to plague lagged behind the preventive ones. Haffkine's vaccine, and variations of it, proved to have some therapeutic (as well as preventive) effect on plague; its application reduced mortality rates among the infected. But the striking therapeutic responses came in the 1930s and 1940s. First, the application of the sulfa drugs (in 1938) reduced mortality rates for bubonic plague from about 50% to about 10%. Then antibiotics appeared, and although the first one (penicillin) had little effect on plague, its successors, especially streptomycin (1944) and tetracycline (1948), proved enormously effective. In Pune (India) in 1948 the use of antibiotics cut mortality rates from bubonic plague from 58% to 4%. If plague could be diagnosed in time, it could be cured.

UNRESOLVED HISTORICAL ISSUES

One of the same questions about the Second Plague Pandemic—"why did it diminish?"—might be asked of the Third Plague Pandemic as well, but the answer is clear: human intervention meant attacks on both the vectors of plague (rodents and insects) and then (with antibiotics) *Yersinia pestis* itself. Attacks on the vectors stopped a 1945 plague outbreak in Peru in four days. Antibiotics have reduced the mortality rate in plague epidemics from the 50% range that characterized the Second Plague Pandemic to less than 10%.

But doubts about the importance or even the role of *Yersinia pestis* persisted among some historians and biological scientists alike. By the early 2000s, such questions were largely settled by the evidence of molecular biology. The analysis of DNA extracted from remaining soft tissue of suspected plague victims has led to firm conviction that *Yersinia pestis* was the culprit. Other uncertainties, however, remain about the complex of relationships between microorganisms, vectors, and hosts. *Yersinia pestis* can survive for long periods, often underground. There it may infect colonies of a wide variety of burrowing mammals (certainly not only rats), more-or-less resistant to it, that are called "maintenance hosts." It may also reach more plague-susceptible animals that then become "amplifying hosts" that may then intersect with humans. As this chapter has shown, enzootic plague colonies of animals exist widely in the world.

Yersinia pestis may also have evolved in another way, one that poses real menace. The two greatest contemporary epidemic killers—tuberculosis and malaria—have developed increasing resistance to the drugs used to fight them. In 1997 antibiotic-resistant strains of plague were discovered in Madagascar (Dennis and Hughes 1997, 702–704).

REFERENCES

Craddock, Susan. *City of Plagues: Disease, Poverty, and Deviance in San Francisco.* Minneapolis: University of Minnesota Press, 2000.

Dennis, David T., and James M. Hughes. "Multidrug Resistance in Plague." *New England Journal of Medicine* 337 (1997): 702–704.

Gregg, Charles T. *Plague: An Ancient Disease in the Twentieth Century.* Rev. ed. Albuquerque: University of New Mexico Press, 1985.

Swanson, Maynard W. "The Sanitation Syndrome: Bubonic Plague and Urban Native Policy in the Cape Colony, 1900–1909." *Journal of African History* 18 (1977): 387–410.

SUGGESTED ADDITIONAL READING

Arnold, David. *Colonizing the Body: State Medicine and Epidemic Disease in Nineteenth-Century India.* Berkeley: University of California Press, 1993.

Benedict, Carol. *Bubonic Plague in Nineteenth-Century China.* Palo Alto, CA: Stanford University Press, 1996.

Bolton, J. L. "Looking for *Yersinia pestis:* Scientists, Historians and the Black Death." In *The Fifteenth Century XII: Society in an Age of Plague*, edited by Linda Clark and Carole Rawcliffe, 15–37. Woodbridge: Boydell, 2013.

Carmichael, Ann G. "Plague Persistence in Western Europe: A Hypothesis." *The Medieval Globe* 1 (2014): 157–191.

Chase, Marilyn. *The Barbary Plague: The Black Death in Victorian San Francisco.* New York: Random House, 2003.

Curson, Peter, and Kevin McCracken. *Plague in Sydney: The Anatomy of an Epidemic.* Kensington: New South Wales University Press, n.d.

Drancourt, Michel, and Didier Raoult. "Past Plague." In *Paleomicrobiology: Past Human Infections*, edited by Raoult and Drancourt, 145–159. Berlin: Springer, 2008.

Echenberg, Myron. *Plague Ports: The Global Urban Impact of Bubonic Plague, 1894–1901.* New York: New York University Press, 2007.

Klein, Ira. "Death in India, 1871–1921." *Journal of Asian Studies* 32 (1973): 639–659.

Klein, Ira. "Plague, Policy and Popular Unrest in British India." *Modern Asian Studies* 22 (1988): 723–755.

Mohr, James C. *Plague and Fire: Battling Black Death and the 1900 Burning of Honolulu's Chinatown.* New York: Oxford University Press, 2005.

Morelli, Giovanna, Yajun Song, Camila J. Mazzoni, Mark Eppinger, Philippe Roumagnac, David M. Wagner, Mirjam Feldkamp, et al. "*Yersinia pestis* Genome Sequencing Identifies Patterns of Global Phylogenetic Diversity." *Nature Genetics* 42 (2010): 1140–1145.

Peckham, Robert. *Epidemics in Modern Asia.* Cambridge: Cambridge University Press, 2016.

Risse, Guenter B. *Plague, Fear, and Politics in San Francisco's Chinatown.* Baltimore, MD: Johns Hopkins University Press, 2012.

Shah, Nayan. *Contagious Divides: Epidemics and Race in San Francisco's Chinatown.* Berkeley: University of California Press, 2001.

32

Sixth Cholera Pandemic, 1899–1923

WHEN AND WHERE

The sixth worldwide cholera pandemic began in 1899, as earlier ones had, in the Indian province of Bengal where the disease had long been endemic. As cholera spread outward from that historic center, it may have merged with other, lesser centers of infection where it had also become endemic; for that reason, the chronological division between the fifth and sixth pandemics may not be precise. In 1899 cholera again began spreading across the Indian subcontinent, west toward Bombay and Madras, and northwest to the Punjab.

In 1900 cholera accounted for about 10% of all deaths in India, an indication of the severity of this spreading pandemic. By 1901 Southeast Asia was affected, as epidemic cholera carried by sea from Indian ports reached Burma, Singapore, and Java. In 1902 the same ocean tentacles stretched both further east (to China and then the Philippines) and west (to Arabia and the Muslim pilgrim sites of the Hijaz, and eventually to Egypt). Although the toll in Arabia was much less than that inflicted in the 1890s, a very serious cholera epidemic shook the Philippines where the disease accounted for a frightening 31% of all deaths in 1902.

Persia (now Iran) began experiencing cholera deaths in 1903, and in 1904 the disease disrupted Persian society significantly. Perhaps 13,000 cholera deaths occurred in Tehran in a few months, and other Persian cities suffered proportionally similar mortality. In the same year (1904) cholera reached into Russian areas bordering the Caspian Sea, as it had done repeatedly in the nineteenth-century pandemics; from Astrakhan cholera cases spread into Russia, and by 1905 some reports of cholera came from the Austro-Hungarian Empire.

The spread of the pandemic seems to have halted between 1905 and 1909, but serious death tolls persisted in places where it was established. India suffered a particular spike in cholera deaths in 1906, for example. But then in the course of 1909 and 1910 cholera surged through Java (where 60,000 cholera deaths occurred in those years) and Russia (causing about 100,000 deaths between May and December 1910). Cholera also reached western Europe in 1910, as an epidemic tongue reached out across the Adriatic Sea from the Balkans to Italy.

Sixth Cholera Pandemic, 1899–1923

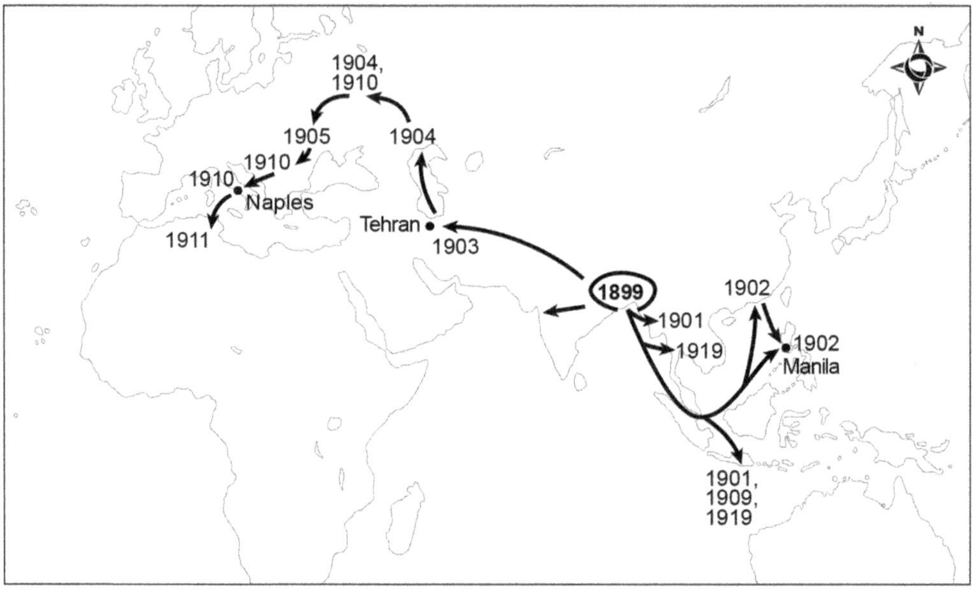

Within Italy, cholera especially attacked the city of Naples, where rural people gathered from southern Italy to begin their emigration to—especially—the United States and Argentina. Cholera apparently came with them in 1910, and between then and 1912 the disease claimed perhaps 18,000 Italian lives, most of them in 1911. From Italy, cholera was carried across the Atlantic, as a few cases reached New York on emigrant ships in 1911. The disease was, however, contained and did not spread further in the United States. A cholera epidemic in Tripoli at the end of 1911 was blamed on native beggars by the Italian authorities occupying the territory, but Italian troops may equally well have brought it there.

The chaos of World War I, and the Russian Revolution with its ensuing civil war that lasted until 1921, created conditions ideal for the continuance of the sixth cholera pandemic, and so the disease flourished, especially in Russia and the war fronts of eastern and southeastern Europe, until the early 1920s. And in Asia some further outbreaks crippled Java and Thailand in 1919; cholera claimed 13,000 lives in Bangkok in that year.

By the early 1920s, world societies began to get cholera epidemics under control. When the sixth pandemic came to an end is in dispute; a conventional date argued by Pollitzer (1959) is 1923. But as many as 34,000 people may have died of cholera in China in 1932.

SIGNIFICANCE

The sixth cholera pandemic took a very high death toll, mostly in Asia. Although the total number of deaths remains unknown, Indian figures give some notion of its severity. In the two decades between 1900 and 1920, perhaps eight million Indians died of cholera, about four million in each decade. But the nearly simultaneous appearance of plague in India diverted attention from cholera, despite its ravages. (As a measure of the decline of the sixth pandemic, the Indian cholera death toll in the 1920s was "only" about 2.2 million.)

The pandemic also occurred in the shadow of more dramatic events, especially World War I and the great influenza pandemic of 1918–1919. Millions died of cholera early in the twentieth century, but millions more died of influenza within a much shorter period. And as was true of the influenza pandemic, cholera's impact was greatest in Asia, where it attracted less attention from Western scholars and public opinion than it deserved.

The sixth cholera pandemic also occurred at a time when a widespread consensus had developed about the cause of the disease. Some governments at least thought, therefore, that they could take actions that would stop an epidemic. An important gap remained, however, between the theoretical powers of authorities over an epidemic's spread, and the political realities that both interfered with those actions and diverted them from appropriate paths. The sixth cholera pandemic is therefore an excellent example of the ways in which social and political forces, as well as medical and scientific ones, affect the history of an epidemic. (See especially the "Responses" section later.)

BACKGROUND

The sixth cholera pandemic began in areas of Asia that had (at different points in the nineteenth century) fallen under the domination of Western colonial powers. Something of the strengths and weaknesses of Western colonial rule that formed the political background for the pandemic is illustrated by examples that follow, but it is generally true that the sixth pandemic occurred at a time punctuated by occasional resistance to that colonial rule. That resistance, and the often-brutal Western response to it, led to periods of social and political turmoil in which epidemic diseases such as cholera could flourish.

By the early twentieth century, the provision of clean water supplies and the removal of sewage had transformed most of the cities of western Europe and North America. Partly for that reason, cholera from the sixth pandemic made little headway in those places, although Italy was a notable exception.

Earlier cholera pandemics (and particularly their perceived relation to the movement of Muslim and Hindu pilgrims) had spurred the creation of an international system of disease control, and in the early stages of the sixth pandemic that system had been formalized by the Paris Convention of 1903. That international agreement, signed by 24 nations, committed each nation to notify the world when cholera or plague was present, and to publicize the measures it took against the disease. The signatories also agreed on steps that should be taken in response to a notice of cholera elsewhere: ships from the infected country would be quarantined on arrival, the crew and the steerage passengers (that is, people not from the upper and middle classes) would be isolated for five days while they underwent bacteriological examinations, decks were washed down, and cargo could not be unloaded until the health of the ship was confirmed. Captains and owners of ships were to ensure that medical records of their voyages were kept, and that suspicious cases of sickness on board be isolated and their possessions disinfected.

The imposition of these measures (or the threat of their imposition) at different points in the sixth cholera pandemic influenced some of the political responses to it.

HOW IT WAS UNDERSTOOD AT THE TIME

By the first decade of the twentieth century, Western physicians and public health professionals had largely accepted the notion that cholera was caused by the microorganism called *Vibrio cholerae*, discovered by Robert Koch in the early 1880s; further, that people ingested this organism with their food and drink, that it could linger in foods, and that it most often was found in water contaminated by sewage. The germ theory had, therefore, displaced earlier less focused beliefs in general environmental pollution.

Many people still associated cholera with outsiders and their habits, however. Those outsiders varied from one part of the world to another. Italians in 1910 blamed the cholera epidemic on Jews and especially on gypsies, claiming that poison began with those groups. The British in India continued to associate cholera with the dirty natives (as the British conceived them) as did the Americans in the Philippines. Meanwhile different Asian peoples (e.g., Filipinos and Persians) saw cholera as the occasion for Western power to assert itself over their lives. And some pious Muslims (and perhaps Christians as well) still regarded cholera as a product of God's will.

RESPONSES

Some generalizations about different levels of response to the sixth pandemic emerge from three case studies of the epidemic's progress: in the Philippines in 1902, in Persia in 1904, and in Italy in 1910. (A further example may be found in volume 2, chapter 36.)

Philippines

In the Philippines, cases of cholera first appeared in the Manila Bay area in March 1902, probably conveyed there with trade from south China. The disease arrived during a tense period in the history of the Philippines. Formerly a Spanish colonial possession, the islands had been taken over by the United States as a result of the Spanish-American War of 1898. The Americans inherited not only a new colonial possession but an insurrection, begun by Filipinos against Spanish rule in 1896 and continued against the Americans. By 1901 that insurrection had largely died down, with the capture of its leader Emilio Aguinaldo; fighting actually ceased in early 1902, about the time that cholera arrived. The United States therefore still had a heavy military presence in the Philippines, and furthermore it had been engaged in campaigns against another epidemic, plague, which had arrived in the midst of the rebellion.

In that situation, the response of the American rulers was predictably militaristic and heavy-handed. Infected quarters were burned down, a system of passes restricted the movement of people and goods, and families of the stricken were isolated in reconcentration zones already in place as a response to the insurrection; the cholera victims, therefore, joined the rebels. But when the rebellion was declared over, the zones were abolished and the ex-rebels—and the cholera families—were permitted to move away. The destruction of the dwellings of the afflicted continued, however. Were homes being burned to halt cholera contagion or as punishment for rebellion?

These measures, especially the isolation of victims and their families, inspired fear in a population that was uncertain of the intentions of its new rulers. Some fled; many others attempted to hide cholera cases from the authorities. Flight and concealment alike contributed to maintaining, and further spreading, the epidemic. The indiscriminate attempt to stamp out the disease by isolating victims and contacts, and destroying their possessions, was unsuccessful. Cholera persisted in the Philippines well into 1903, and only officially ended in 1904. Although the total mortality remains uncertain, the epidemic took a heavy toll over the entire archipelago. Capiz City, on Panay, may have been typical; its population fell from about 25,000 before the epidemic to less than 20,000 after it.

Persia

Cholera began to strike in Persia in December 1903, probably brought into the country by groups of religious pilgrims. By the turn of the century, Persia, a theoretically independent monarchy, had fallen under increasing British (from the south and the Persian Gulf) and Russian (from the north) influence. As an aspect of that influence, European powers had claimed power over some of the administration of public health measures in the country. (When plague reached Bushire in 1899, for example, the British Resident [a diplomatic representative] in that city imposed a quarantine.) By 1903 some of those foreign public health administrators were not British but Belgian, the result of a compromise designed to soothe Russian fears of British domination of Persia. The foreign officials responded to the cholera outbreak by attempting to stop pilgrim traffic (a special Western fear since at least the fourth cholera pandemic) and establishing quarantine camps on the borders of the country. These measures failed and angered many segments of Persian opinion. As had happened in the Philippines, people fleeing the stern countermeasures contributed to the spread of the disease.

By late June 1904, about 200 people were dying in Tehran every day. Officials tried to hide the magnitude of the epidemic from the ruling shah, Muzaffar al-Din, but he noticed that his diet had been changed by his servants. It was then decided that he should take refuge in the mountains (as his father had done in the cholera epidemic of 1892); his court set out with a retinue of 2,000, but cholera struck them while they were in transit. Panic overcame the shah, who wished to set off for Russia in a car (in 1904!); his advisers convinced him that doing so might cost him his throne, and he returned to Tehran. He remained in seclusion there for two months, until mid-September 1904, while his government came to a near-halt.

Pushed by Western officials determined to halt a contagious disease, Persian communities destroyed the properties of the stricken and undertook the rapid (and unceremonious) disposal of the dead. Such actions furthered embittered the poor, who both lost their possessions and saw their deceased loved ones denied their burial customs. A large number of people fled, both in the cities such as Tehran, and in villages where cholera seemed to threaten. In one bizarre case, a gang of thieves arrived in a village and pretended to be stricken by cholera. When the villagers fled, the thieves looted the abandoned place and left.

While no reliable mortality figures exist for the Persian cholera epidemic of 1904, several estimates from different communities suggest that perhaps 5% of the population perished—for example, 13,000 in Tehran, a city of about 250,000 (many of whom had fled, so the mortality among those who remained was obviously higher). The Persian experience, then, mirrors the Philippine experience in some important ways, although the mortality may have been lower. In both cases, a foreign power responded with harsh measures of isolation, quarantine, restricted movement, and seizure of property believed infected; in both cases many fled, if not from the disease, then from the harshness of official response; and in both cases flight contributed to the further diffusion of the epidemic.

Italy

The experience of Italy in 1910 differed in some ways from the two previous examples, but popular reactions seemed similar. Cholera reached southern Italy in the summer of 1910, probably brought to the district of Apulia by fishermen who ventured widely over the Mediterranean. The prefect of the province of Bari, responding to the widespread fear that cholera would affect trade and tourism, urged the Italian government to conceal the presence of cholera, referring instead to an outbreak of meningitis. That fiction could not be maintained very successfully, but the government in Rome attempted to stamp cholera out before the world noticed. On August 10, the state fastened a heavy regulatory hand on the region of Apulia: all cholera victims were to be isolated in a separate facility, their families interred in a camp, and their personal effects burned.

These drastic measures sparked widespread evasion and significant popular resistance, which was countered in turn by more repressive power. Stories spread that blamed gypsies for poisoning people with cholera, and the Italian government in effect endorsed such legends. The notion that poisoners were afoot simply added to popular panic and anger. In the face of escalating popular uproar in Apulia, in which serious threats of revolution seemed to grow, the government abruptly shifted gears, giving up its attempts to make war on cholera on September 3. Rather than attempting to quarantine and isolate whole populations, it turned instead to the much more focused bacteriological approach, appealing to the population for cooperation in laboratory testing that would clearly identify the disease. That approach at least calmed the popular uproar and prevented revolutionary agitation from affecting Naples, the largest city of southern Italy and the port from which massive emigration from Italy to the Americas was then underway. Concern with cholera would bring that emigration traffic to a halt.

Cholera arrived in Naples nevertheless, and then returned much more seriously in 1911. The number of cholera deaths in Naples in 1910 may have been as high as 700, and it would be much higher in 1911. But the Italian government launched an elaborate campaign to conceal the severity of the epidemic from the world, in part because of its fears of stirring up the kind of revolutionary turmoil that greeted it in Apulia in 1910, and in part to protect important economic interests.

Popular reaction to cholera measures in Italy, therefore, shared some things with those of Persia and the Philippines: fear of isolation, resentment at the destruction of personal property, and a conviction that cholera was a poison spread by an "other." In the colonial Philippines and quasi-colonial Persia, the "other" was an occupying foreign power; in Italy the "other" was a marginalized minority. Philippine and Persian resistance to cholera measures limited their effectiveness, and other colonial peoples might exercise such power even more clearly. When in 1905 the Indian state of Bombay proposed to control cholera's spread by regulating Hindu pilgrim traffic, the central governing authorities of British India forbade it, reminding the city of the dangers of popular resistance to such measures. And as we have seen, Italian resistance caused the authorities to change policies dramatically.

Medical responses to cholera evolved in two important directions, one in respect to prevention, the other to therapy. Waldemar Haffkine, a Russian-born bacteriologist working in India, had produced a cholera vaccine in the 1890s. Through much of the sixth pandemic, however, its use remained controversial and so it was largely experimental. In India, where the need for such a vaccine was clearly the greatest, fears of popular reactions to the application of such a foreign substance, by a process that invaded the body in an intrusive way, remained strong. Its application was therefore, according to David Arnold, "confined mainly to soldiers, prisoners, and tea-estate workers" (Arnold 1993, 197). By World War I, however, the German army was inoculating its millions of soldiers.

Through the nineteenth century, therapy for cholera victims had followed a path memorably called by the historian Norman Howard-Jones "a form of benevolent homicide" (Howard-Jones 1972, 373). The conviction that cholera should be combated by massive purgings of the fluids of the body, using such substances as calomel, lingered through the century; such treatment simply magnified the drastic dehydration of the system caused by the cholera infection. The countering approach, injecting infusions of liquid, had also been tried by an experimental minority. Then between 1906 and 1909, the British physician Leonard Rogers, working in Calcutta, perfected techniques of rehydration that when applied reduced cholera mortality dramatically. Through the nineteenth-century pandemics, roughly half of those who became ill with cholera died, usually very quickly and in great agony. Rogers's techniques reduced that mortality rate from 50% to less than 20%.

UNRESOLVED HISTORICAL ISSUES

The sixth cholera pandemic illustrated two general, and different, approaches to the control of such an epidemic: the broad-scale environmental and the bacteriological. The first relied on a variety of sanitation and disinfection measures, together with heavy control of population movement; the second on laboratory testing of samples and then action as needed, on a much narrower front, to isolate those with the disease. Tension remained between those responses throughout the sixth pandemic.

The success of the bacteriological approach depended (as it still does) on a variety of preconditions, many of which were only partially fulfilled in the early twentieth century. Among those are adequate and accurate laboratory testing facilities and trained personnel, a society with the wealth to sustain such facilities, and a level of acceptance by the population that will assure cooperation—that is, the "medicalization" of the population. In many twentieth-century (and early twenty-first century) societies, those conditions remain unfulfilled, and so cholera has revived in the years since 1961.

During the sixth pandemic, the Haffkine vaccine and the methods of rehydration had only begun to win acceptance; between them they would later dramatically reduce both the incidence of cholera and its mortality.

REFERENCES

Arnold, David. *Colonizing the Body: State Medicine and Epidemic Disease in Nineteenth-Century India.* Berkeley: University of California Press, 1993.

Howard-Jones, Norman. "Cholera Therapy in the Nineteenth Century." *Journal of the History of Medicine and Allied Sciences* 27 (1972): 373–395.

Pollitzer, Robert. *Cholera.* Geneva: World Health Organization, 1959.

SUGGESTED ADDITIONAL READING

Bashford, Alison, ed. *Quarantine: Local and Global Histories.* London: Palgrave Macmillan, 2016.

Bourdelais, Patrice. "Cholera: A Victory for Medicine?" In *The Decline of Mortality in Europe*, edited by R. Schofield, D. Reher, and A. Bideau, 118–130. Oxford: Clarendon, 1991.

Burrell, R. M. "The 1904 Epidemic of Cholera in Persia: Some Aspects of Qātār Society." *Bulletin of the School of Oriental and African Studies* 51 (1988): 258–270.

DeBevoise, Ken. *Agents of Apocalypse: Epidemic Disease in the Colonial Philippines.* Princeton, NJ: Princeton University Press, 1995.

Gardiner, Peter, and Mayling Oey. "Morbidity and Mortality in Java, 1880–1940: The Evidence of the Colonial Reports." In *Death and Disease in Southeast Asia: Explorations in Social, Medical and Demographic History*, edited by Norman G. Owen, 70–90. Singapore: Oxford University Press, 1987.

Hamlin, Christopher. *Cholera: The Biography.* Oxford: Oxford University Press, 2009.

Kuhnke, LaVerne. *Lives at Risk: Public Health in Nineteenth-Century Egypt.* Berkeley: University of California Press, 1990.

MacPherson, Kerrie L. "Cholera in China, 1820–1930: An Aspect of the Internationalization of Infectious Disease." In *Sediments of Time: Environment and Society in Chinese History*, edited by Mark Elvin and Lin Ts'ui-jung, 487–519. Cambridge: Cambridge University Press, 1998.

Roff, William R. "Sanitation and Security: The Imperial Powers and the Nineteenth Century Hajj." *Arabian Studies* 6 (1982): 143–160.

Snowden, Frank M. *Naples in the Time of Cholera, 1884–1911.* Cambridge: Cambridge University Press, 1995.

Terwiel, B. J. "Asiatic Cholera in Siam: Its First Occurrence and the 1820 Epidemic." In *Death and Disease in Southeast Asia: Explorations in Social, Medical and Demographic History*, edited by Norman G. Owen, 142–161. Singapore: Oxford University Press, 1987.

33

Sleeping Sickness in East Central Africa, 1900–1905

WHEN AND WHERE

Sleeping sickness, also called African trypanosomiasis, has been a serious endemic disease in areas of west and central Africa for many centuries. In the years between 1900 and 1905, an explosive epidemic of sleeping sickness ravaged portions of east central Africa, especially along the shores of Lake Victoria, in territories that then belonged to the British and German Empires and the so-called Congo Free State (actually under the personal rule of Leopold II of Belgium). The epidemic was first noticed in February 1901 in the town of Kampala (the capital of modern Uganda), although it had certainly begun earlier. It centered in the territory called Busoga, along the northeastern shore of Lake Victoria; it spread from there to other points along the shore of the lake, and down the valley of the Albert Nile that flows out of Lake Victoria.

The total death toll cannot now be known, but mortality was very heavy. One well-informed contemporary estimated that in the Busoga region 200,000 people—two-thirds of the total population—had succumbed to sleeping sickness by 1905. A telling example of the epidemic's mortality: before the disease set in, a local chief had under his command 17,000 soldiers; by 1920 his territory included only 120 taxpayers. And in the years immediately following the Lake Victoria epidemic, sleeping sickness claimed huge death tolls in adjacent parts of Africa. Perhaps 500,000 people died in the upper reaches of the Congo River basin, for example.

SIGNIFICANCE

The magnitude of this epidemic, and the high rate of mortality among those stricken, make it one of the great epidemics of African history. The sleeping sickness epidemic of the early twentieth century also claims significance as a turning point both in the development of tropical medicine, and in the complex interactions of Western imperial rule and African health. The epidemic stimulated the rapid discovery of the causative organism of sleeping sickness and the route of transmission to humans, and those discoveries represented some of the great triumphs of modern biomedicine. But that new understanding of the disease led to overly simple attempts to eradicate it by the colonial authorities, attempts that overlooked the ways in which colonial rule had disrupted African ecologies and thus contributed to the epidemic and to the persistence of sleeping sickness in many parts of Africa.

BACKGROUND

Sleeping sickness, or African trypanosomiasis, results from the body becoming infected by a parasitic microorganism, one of several members of the family of such organisms called *Trypanosoma.* Different trypanosomes are found in a number of animal species, including cattle, some antelopes and monkeys, and humans. They are carried from the bloodstream of one animal to another by the bites of the tsetse fly, an insect common in particular areas of Africa, especially in zones where open grassy plains (savannas) meet woodlands. Those areas, especially in western Africa, had long been the centers of endemic sleeping sickness, the symptoms of which had been known to Europeans from their first contacts with western African people. Europeans gave the disease a variety of names, including African lethargy and sleepy distemper. (A related trypanosome also carried a disease that affected domestic cattle, called *nagana*, or livestock trypanosomiasis.)

Many of the peoples of western Africa had long experience with trypanosomiasis, in both its human and cattle manifestations. They had evolved methods of avoiding tsetse flies (if only because both humans and cattle suffered from the pain of their bites) and so kept the disease at bay. They moved cattle at night, when the flies were inactive. They isolated people infected by the disease. They created areas of cultivation in which the forest cover of the flies was removed, while other areas were left wooded and set aside for wild animals; the flies feasted on the wild animals and did not enter the cultivated zones.

The movements of large groups of people always meant the possibility of transferring the disease to new areas previously uninfected, and in the nineteenth century a number of such movements occurred in Africa, for a variety of reasons. Shifting military and political power accounted for some migrations, as (for example) when the Turko-Egyptian control of Sudan was challenged by the forces of the Sudanese leader Muhammed Ahmed (called "The Mahdi") and his followers in the 1880s and 1890s. International trade increasingly drew interior African kingdoms into its orbit; apart from the continuing traffic in slaves, the demand for such commodities as palm oil (from west Africa) and ivory meant in turn a sizable number of people were conscripted as porters carrying those goods moved through and out of Africa. Then in the years after about 1880, European states rapidly laid formal claim to the map of Africa, bringing it under direct imperial rule. A more systematic exploitation of African resources followed. King Leopold II of Belgium pursued a particularly single-minded course in the Congo Free State, demanding labor services from the population for the extraction of ivory and rubber. The British and German rulers of the lands around Lake Victoria began extending plantation agriculture to produce coffee and cotton, especially after a railroad (1901) connected the lake's shores with Mombasa, on the Indian Ocean.

By about 1900, therefore, major disturbances were occurring in the pattern of settlement in Africa. A high demand for wage labor put people on the move, to work on plantations run by European settlers, on railroad and road construction, in mines, and as porters. Planters cleared lands for cultivation. The territories of Africa claimed by European empires often had little relation to historical ethnic regions, or even to natural geographical boundaries; people were therefore sundered from those ethnically closest to them, and thrown together with strangers. All this meant major disruption of the total ecology of the continent.

And in 1889 a devastating epidemic of the cattle disease rinderpest began, which in about 10 years may have killed an astonishing 95% of Africa's cattle. The death of cattle meant that many pasture lands quickly reverted to bush in which tsetse flies spread, greatly increasing the chances of trypanosome infections for people.

HOW IT WAS UNDERSTOOD AT THE TIME

The symptoms of sleeping sickness had long been familiar, although one version of the disease, more chronic than acute, went through a series of stages. A period of headaches, fever, and nausea might later be succeeded by neurological

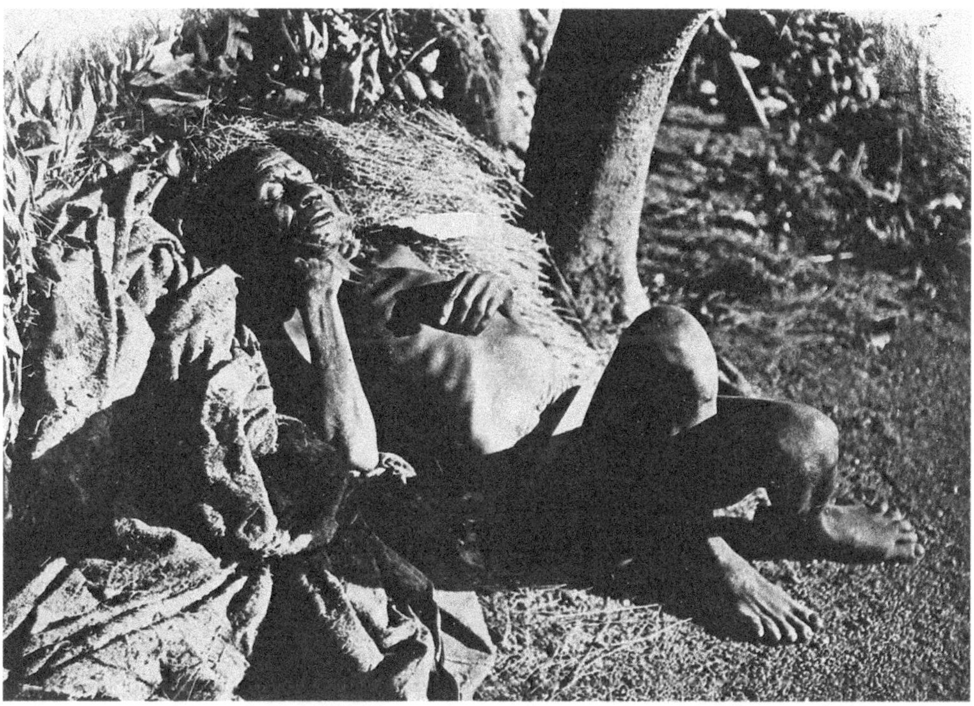

A man in the last stages of sleeping sickness, Buruma Island, Uganda, 1902. He was carried out of his hut, photographed, and carried back in again, during which time he merely opened his eyes before relapsing into deep sleep. (Wellcome Library)

symptoms, including the sleepiness that gave the disease its name. When the disease reached those later stages mortality rates were very high.

When two British doctors, the brothers Albert and J. H. Cook, encountered the cases in February 1901 that would be seen as the opening of the epidemic, the field of tropical medicine was a new and exciting one, especially because of its application of the germ theory and its recent discovery of the role of insects in the transmission of malaria and yellow fever. Patrick Manson, one of the pioneers of tropical medicine, had suggested that sleeping sickness was a filariasis disease, caused by a microscopic worm. Could an insect vector be found for sleeping sickness as well?

The news that sleeping sickness had apparently begun along the shores of Lake Victoria alarmed both the British government and Belgium's King Leopold. The British Foreign Office commissioned a team from the recently organized London School of Tropical Medicine to investigate, and in 1902 this group announced that trypanosomes had been found in Busoga cases. Another British commission, led by David Bruce (who had earlier discovered the parasite responsible for *nagana*, the sleeping sickness that affected cattle) arrived in 1903, and by August of that year Bruce had convincingly shown that a certain parasite (*Trypanosoma brucei*, later shown to have two different variants, *T. b. rhodesiense* and *T. b. gambiense*) caused sleeping sickness, and that tsetse flies carried the parasite to humans.

At least on one level the cause of sleeping sickness had been unraveled, in what would be hailed as another of the great triumphs of tropical biomedicine. On its basis, European colonial powers undertook a number of responses to sleeping sickness. Later scholars have realized that those responses were flawed (see the "Responses" and "Unresolved Historical Issues" sections).

Some questions remained in contemporary understanding of sleeping sickness. One of the other European investigators who came to the shores of Lake Victoria in the wake of the epidemic was Robert Koch, the famous German microbiologist. In 1906 he found a number of boatmen plying the lake who were both apparently healthy and infected with the sleeping sickness–inducing trypanosomes. A few years later British investigators confirmed Koch's findings. The existence of healthy carriers posed a problem for the accepted belief that infection by the trypanosome caused sleeping sickness.

RESPONSES

Convinced that (1) the epidemic of sleeping sickness was a recent importation to eastern Africa and (2) trypanosomes carried by tsetse flies caused it, the colonial powers proposed two different solutions. British authorities argued that the epidemic had been spread to the shores of Lake Victoria by people on the move: perhaps the Sudanese soldiers involved in murky lakeside struggles between British and German agents in the early 1890s; perhaps Africans moving more freely as a consequence of European pacification of African territory. The answer to sleeping sickness was, therefore, the control of population movements and the isolation of people from tsetse-infected regions. Sir Hesketh Bell, the British Commissioner in Uganda, ordered a massive evacuation of people from the shores of

Lake Victoria in 1906–1907 in an attempt to break the links between people and tsetse flies. The British continued to follow that approach in subsequent decades. And as British researchers had dominated the first phases of emergent tropical medicine, their ideas had carried weight with their international colleagues.

The other approach—an attempt to eradicate the trypanosome itself—was more favored in French, and to a certain extent, Belgian territories. Koch had urged the adoption of a specific medicine, atoxyl, which he thought a valuable cure for those infected by trypanosomes. In French and Belgian colonies, therefore, sleeping sickness was treated as a medical problem, with a medical solution. (Atoxyl, and some other antitrypanosome drugs developed in subsequent decades, had a beneficial effect in some cases and could lead to fatal side effects in others.)

Both the British and the Franco-Belgian approaches meant very significant imperial interference in the lives of Africans. In one case, people might be sweepingly moved from their homes and resettled on new lands; in the other, the colonial government created a substantial public health bureaucracy to test the population's blood and administer injections. That bureaucracy became a symbol both of an empire's paternal medical care of its people, and of its interfering power over their lives. Among both European colonizers and Africans such policies sparked debate about the desirability or necessity of forcible or even punitive detention, debates that might spill over into passive or even active resistance. And to a large extent the policies depended on metropolitan "experts" without regard to the opinions of local colonial medical practitioners, let alone the opinions of Africans themselves.

UNRESOLVED HISTORICAL ISSUES

Historical views of the causes of this epidemic have changed considerably since the 1960s. Up to that point, the explanation that colonial officials had accepted on the heels of the epidemic held the field. According to that view, African trypanosomiasis, long an endemic disease in western Africa, spread relatively suddenly to east central Africa at the end of the nineteenth century, triggering an unexpectedly serious epidemic. The movement of native Africans, perhaps in the wake of wars, perhaps in response to new employment opportunities in mines and plantations, and in any case eased by the better order and governance brought by European rule, carried the disease into new territory. Once the disease arrived in eastern and central Africa, European colonial powers, acting on newly gained scientific understanding, undertook measures to control its spread and eradicate it.

Since the 1960s, a different interpretation has entered the historical picture. It grants at least partial truth to the old view, but insists on the importance of a broader disease ecology. The presence of healthy carriers in eastern Africa at the time of the epidemic suggests that sleeping sickness may have been long endemic there as well, and if so that the importation theory may be wrong. While the movement of Africans undoubtedly played a role in the spread of the epidemic, equally important may have been the changes wrought in the environment by the new pressures of plantation agriculture and other Western-backed economic initiatives, changes that altered the long balance between humans and tsetse flies that African peoples had evolved. In some more indirect way, therefore, the intrusion of Western imperial power into Africa had a disastrous effect on the relations of people and diseases. And why do some people infected by trypanosomes develop sleeping sickness while others do not? Do levels of nutritional health or stress matter? If so, many of the labor practices engaged in by colonial entrepreneurs certainly worsened the standards of living of laborers, and perhaps therefore made them more susceptible to diseases.

What is at stake, therefore, in these two different explanations of the 1901–1905 sleeping sickness epidemic is two different views of the nature and effects of Western imperial power, one positive, the other negative.

REFERENCE

Ford, John. *The Role of the Trypanosomiases in African Ecology: A Study of the Tsetse Fly Problem.* Oxford: Clarendon, 1971.

SUGGESTED ADDITIONAL READING

Hoppe, Kirk Arden. *Lords of the Fly: Sleeping Sickness Control in British East Africa, 1900–1960.* Westport, CT: Praeger, 2003.

Lyons, Maryinez. *The Colonial Disease: A Social History of Sleeping Sickness in Northern Zaire, 1900–1940.* Cambridge: Cambridge University Press, 1992.

McKelvey, John J. *Man against Tsetse: Struggle for Africa.* Ithaca, NY: Cornell University Press, 1973.

Neill, Deborah J. *Networks in Tropical Medicine: Internationalism, Colonialism, and the Rise of a Medical Specialty, 1890–1930.* Stanford, CA: Stanford University Press, 2012.

Prins, Gwyn. "But What Was the Disease? The Present State of Health and Healing in African Studies." *Past and Present* 124 (1989): 157–179.

34

Typhoid Mary's "Epidemics," 1906–1915

WHEN AND WHERE

In the summer of 1906, six cases of typhoid fever occurred in the same household in Oyster Bay, New York. In 1907 these cases were linked to one person, Mary Mallon, a cook who had worked in the household. When Mallon's presence was traced to 22 (perhaps 26) other typhoid fever cases in seven different households, she was confined to an island isolation hospital in New York by public health authorities in March 1907.

Her detention became an important legal issue (as discussed later); she appealed, protesting innocence of wrongdoing, and in February 1910 she was released. The terms of her release included her promise to stop working as a cook. Nevertheless, she eventually began such work again. After 25 typhoid fever cases occurred in a maternity hospital where she was employed, she was again confined to the island isolation facility in March 1915 and remained there until her death in 1938.

The epidemics directly and clearly associated with Mary Mallon, therefore, amounted to perhaps about 50 cases of typhoid fever, three of which proved fatal.

SIGNIFICANCE

"Typhoid Mary," according to *The New Shorter Oxford English Dictionary*, has become a phrase meaning "a person who transmits a disease widely without showing its symptoms," and (figuratively) "a transmitter of undesirable opinions, sentiments, etc." Its usage comes from the popular furor around the case of Mary Mallon. The epidemics (if indeed the word can be applied at all) for which she was responsible were, as the prior paragraphs show, minor. Their significance stems not from their slight morbidity and mortality, but first from the symbolic associations that made Mary Mallon (renamed *Typhoid Mary*) part of American popular culture. Since she first came to public attention, many different understandings have been projected on her, her name, and the supposed results of her life for her society. Those understandings have illustrated the continuing importance of gender, ethnicity, and class in American history, for those categories help explain why this one person was singled out when others might have been. (See the "How It Was Understood at the Time" and "Unresolved Historical Issues" sections)

On another level, Mary Mallon was the first "identified, charted, and reported" (Leavitt 1996, 14) healthy typhoid fever carrier in North America. As such her case had some significance in the history of the medical understanding of disease. More important, her case raised significant questions about the relations between scientific evidence, public health, state power, and the rights of individuals in a free society, questions that remain unsettling. What legal power should be granted to bacteriology (or other scientific, analytic approaches) to explain and identify disease? How far does the authority of the state, acting in the name of public health, extend in the regulation of the lives of individuals and the limitation of their freedoms?

BACKGROUND

Typhoid fever was a serious disease in the urban communities of the nineteenth-century Western world. Since the 1840s, some students of the disease, notably the Englishman William Budd, had argued that it passed to people through water supplies. While no consensus agreed about that, such arguments supported the more general nineteenth-century campaign (especially strong in Great Britain) to expel filth from the environment. This gospel of sanitation was applied to the provision of clean water supplies and the separation of water from sewage, and such campaigns began to reduce typhoid rates in some cities by the 1870s.

Then in the years after 1880 the causative organism of typhoid fever, *Salmonella typhi*, was identified, and that organism began to be traced from excretions of typhoid sufferers into water supplies. From that point onward, the story of typhoid fever seemed one of the early triumphs of the germ theory and of the new science of bacteriology, although its ravages had already begun to decline because of sanitation improvements undertaken not in response to germs but to more general filth.

The enthusiasm for the germ theory that grew through the period from 1880 to 1900 (and thereafter) had two effects important for Mary Mallon's case. If diseases were produced by specific microorganisms (germs), attention shifted to the *individuals* who carried or were infected by them, and away from the more general filth of an environment for which *society* as a whole might be responsible. And if disease was defined as infection by a microorganism, then bacteriology, laboratory testing, would determine who was diseased.

Despite the new understanding of typhoid fever (and the rigorous policing of water supplies), local outbreaks of typhoid fever continued, and that fact encouraged speculation about the existence of healthy carriers, people whose digestive systems carried (and emitted) *Salmonella typhi* without themselves manifesting any signs of the disease. The possibility of a healthy or asymptomatic carrier of a disease had been raised in the 1880s, first about diphtheria. Robert Koch, the German pioneer of bacteriology, had extended the healthy carrier idea first to cholera (in the early 1890s) and then to typhoid fever, between 1900 and 1902. Several such typhoid carriers had been identified in Europe between those dates and Mallon's case in 1907; George Soper, the American epidemiological investigator who discovered Mary Mallon, was familiar with the European accounts.

HOW IT WAS UNDERSTOOD AT THE TIME

By 1907 general agreement existed that typhoid fever resulted from an infection of the digestive system by *Salmonella typhi.* To prevent its spread, water supplies (the most common route of transmission of the germ) should be purified, and typhoid sufferers should be isolated so that food consumed by others would not be infected by their presence. What should be done about the asymptomatic carrier was not at all clear, however, as the case of Mary Mallon would illustrate.

RESPONSES

As the brief narrative earlier ("When and Where") shows, the response to "Typhoid Mary's Epidemics" involved a thorough reliance on laboratory testing

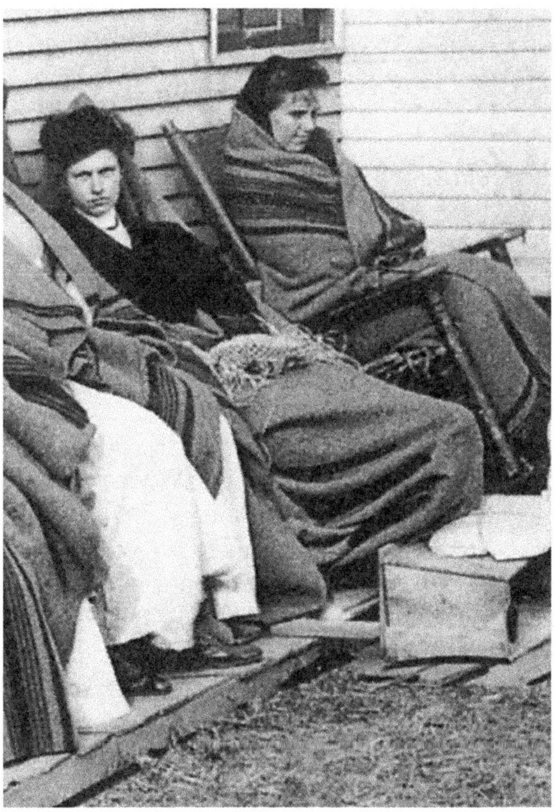

Mary Mallon, in the dark dress and looking at the camera, during one of her confinements in an isolation hospital. (Science History Images/Alamy Stock Photo)

and bacteriological evidence to identify the cause of the outbreaks of the disease, and then on the coercive power of the state to compel the isolation of that cause.

After the Oyster Bay outbreak in 1906 (6 cases in a household of 11), the owner of the property commissioned an investigation by George Soper, an engineer who had researched other typhoid epidemics from the standpoints of sanitation and epidemiology. Soper decided that the household's cook (at the time of the outbreak), Mary Mallon, might be a healthy carrier, although such a phenomenon had been little documented (and only in Europe). When Soper traced her previous employments, he discovered that typhoid fever cases had followed her from job to job.

Soper found Mallon in New York City, told her his beliefs, and tried to convince her that she was a danger to others. Mallon—understandably—denied that she was ill and refused to cooperate. Ultimately, Soper convinced the New York City Department of Health that Mallon should be taken (forcibly if necessary, which it proved to be) to a hospital where samples of her blood and excreta could be taken and examined. When those samples showed that Mallon harbored *Salmonella typhi*, she was ordered confined in a cottage on a New York island used as an isolation hospital.

In 1910 Mallon, who had continuously protested her confinement and gained the support of some lawyers, was released. But a further outbreak of typhoid in a hospital where she worked led to her re-isolation in 1915.

UNRESOLVED HISTORICAL ISSUES

Mary Mallon's case focused attention on some issues that the new science of bacteriology had brought forward. Some of those issues were not satisfactorily or clearly resolved at the time, and some remain contentious to this day.

The healthy carrier, a new concept, posed some of those issues. How were such people to be discovered in the first place? Should investigators trace all the contacts of typhoid victims? Concentrate on epidemic locales and trace those in contact with those places? Subject all food handlers to bacteriological examination? Each of those approaches would affront the privacy of individuals, and some of them would require considerable public expense.

Once a healthy carrier was found, what action should the state take? Could public health rely on the findings of microbiology? What if some bacteriologists disagreed about a particular case? Mallon's body carried *Salmonella typhi* only intermittently, and so judging her dangerous to the public depended on when the test was made; her appeals against confinement included testimony from some scientists who argued that she wasn't infected.

The germ theory created a new definition of sickness, one in which disease was now identified by the presence of a microorganism in the body. The arbiters of disease were thus microbiologists working in a laboratory. Many physicians, who had previously possessed the power to identify disease by an examination of clinical symptoms of a patient, resisted this intrusion. Just when was a person sick? Mary Mallon claimed that she was perfectly healthy, and clinical examinations agreed. What then constituted typhoid fever: infection by a microorganism or clinical symptoms?

Mallon's case did not set a clear precedent. Many other asymptomatic carriers of typhoid fever were later discovered who were *not* confined to isolation quarters. Some of them were, like Mallon, food handlers; for example, Frederick Moersch, a confectioner, was linked to a typhoid outbreak involving 59 people in 1915, but he was not isolated. By 1938, the year of Mallon's death (in isolation), 349 asymptomatic carriers of typhoid fever were registered in New York City alone, and only Mallon was confined.

Why then was Mallon singled out? Judith Walzer Leavitt, the historian whose sensitive study of the subject is the basis of this chapter, argues that a complex of social conceptions made Mallon suspicious. She was a single woman, a domestic servant, and an immigrant from Ireland. In all of those ways, Leavitt believes, Mallon did not meet the expectations of middle-class femininity and behavior. At times, she lived with a man who was not her husband. According to a popular stereotype, Irish people had hot tempers. Certainly Mallon furiously resisted authority, whether of Soper or of the city health department; Mallon, a working-class Irishwoman, had a different (and much more suspicious) understanding of authority, whether political or medical. She persistently denied that she was sick. American public opinion in the late nineteenth and early twentieth centuries, already fearful of the menace that immigrants posed to public health, found in her life and behavior confirmation of its prejudices.

Why did Mallon return to cooking for a living, after her promise (on her first release in 1910) not to do so? Was she simply willfully ignorant, or even (as later historical representations of her implied) actively malicious, a cook who killed? Or had the authorities that imposed the prohibition on her taken away her only skill, leaving her with no practical way of surviving? Other, later, asymptomatic carriers were sometimes retrained for other careers, but no such offer was made to Mallon.

Historical interpretations of Typhoid Mary have evolved. For many years, she was seen as a person who obstructed the path of scientific medicine, and her detention was seen as necessary. But as faith in the powers of scientific biomedicine began to falter in the last quarter of the twentieth century, the unresolved questions about the necessity, justice, and effectiveness of Mallon's isolation have revived. Those questions, about the proper relation between the demands of public health and the rights of the individual, and about the relation between scientific beliefs and legal proceedings, remain alive with continuing epidemics. (See, e.g., volume 2, chapter 41, on the contemporary HIV/AIDS pandemic.)

REFERENCES

Readers interested in "Typhoid Mary" should consult one book before they read anything else on the subject:

Leavitt, Judith Walzer. *Typhoid Mary: Captive to the Public's Health.* Boston: Beacon Press, 1996.

SUGGESTED ADDITIONAL READING

Hardy, Anne. *Salmonella Infections, Networks of Knowledge, and Public Health in Britain, 1880–1975.* Oxford: Oxford University Press, 2015.

Kraut, Alan M. *Silent Travelers: Germs, Genes, and the "Immigrant Menace."* New York: Basic, 1994.

Leavitt, Judith Walzer. "'Typhoid Mary' Strikes Back: Bacteriological Theory and Practice in Early Twentieth-Century Public Health." *Isis* 83 (1992): 608–629.

Markel, Howard. *Quarantine! East European Jewish Immigrants and the New York City Epidemics of 1892.* Baltimore, MD: Johns Hopkins University Press, 1997.

35

Pneumonic Plague Epidemic in Manchuria, 1910–1911

WHEN AND WHERE

What soon was diagnosed as a pneumonic plague epidemic first appeared in the city of Manchouli in late October 1910. That city lay on the Amur River, the border between Russia's far eastern provinces and the faltering Chinese Empire, and was the point at which Russia's Trans-Siberian Railway crossed the border. Deaths began in that city on October 28. Proceeding rapidly along railway lines, plague reached the Russian-dominated city of Harbin on November 8; from Harbin the epidemic trail followed other rail connections into the important Chinese-controlled city of Mukden (by January 2, 1911) and Changchun (January 3). The epidemic from that point followed a largely southwestern path in the direction of China proper. Although some cases were reported within 12 miles of Beijing by mid-January, by March 1911 the Manchurian epidemic had apparently ended.

Manchuria had become a zone of conflict between the ambitions of Russia and Japan, made even more complex by the continuing interests of other Western powers that had established extraterritorial power in nineteenth-century China. The railways that figured so largely in the course of the epidemic had been developed by either Russia, Japan, or China itself. So that—for instance—the plague's onward path to the south when it reached Mukden would follow either a Japanese line to Darien (Dalian) or a Chinese line into China proper. Japanese measures to protect their vital seaport at Darien in effect diverted the epidemic on to the Chinese line.

In addition to following rail lines, the epidemic was concentrated in the cities along those routes, although it originated outside settlements. Railways not only conveyed the plague but also the use of infected stationary rail cars as places in which people were isolated magnified the death toll, as well as concentrating it in the cities. The epidemic in effect followed a rolling pattern, bringing waves of first increasing and then decreasing mortality; Manchouli's epidemic had largely abated when Harbin's began, for example.

Estimates of total mortality range between about 45,000 and 60,000. As in the history of (untreated) pneumonic plague, mortality of those infected may have exceeded 90%.

SIGNIFICANCE

This epidemic occurred during a time of heightened international interest in Manchuria, interest that had become a major power competition. A war between Russia and Japan had left Russia determined to hold the position in Manchuria that remained to it and victorious Japan ambitious for more. Both therefore willingly employed their resources to respond to the threat of plague, with differing results as will shortly emerge. When the consequences of losing a war with Japan in 1894–1895 and the international response to the so-called Boxer Rebellion of 1900–1901 left the Qing dynasty tottering, China was left open to the influence of modern Western medicine, especially as presented by the influential Wu Lien-Teh, in response to the plague epidemic. Wu's name subsequently became renowned in plague literature, as well as in (incomplete) Western understandings of Chinese medical traditions.

BACKGROUND

As a consequence of the Boxer Rebellion, in 1901 Russia occupied much of the Chinese province of Manchuria. In Russian history, this occurred in a period of rapid industrialization, accompanied by a great extension of railways; the Trans-Siberian Railway, begun in 1891, had received Chinese permission to run through northern Manchuria to Vladivostok in 1896. Harbin, along the railway line, developed as a Russian city in the years after 1897; by 1910 it had 44,000 people of "European" origin.

Tensions between Japan and Russia, largely over Manchuria, had resulted in a war between February 1904 and September 1905, in which Japan was victorious. A conference mediated by the U.S. president Theodore Roosevelt ended the war, with Japan now in control of the formerly Russian-controlled ports of Port Arthur and Darien, the latter the terminus of the railway running south from Mukden. Russia remained dominant on the line through Harbin to Vladivostok.

These Manchurian zones of rivalry reflected larger international geopolitics that had seen the ancient Chinese Empire conceding zones of "extraterritoriality" within its borders to Western powers. That process had begun in 1842 at the conclusion of the "Opium War," when the victorious British imposed on China the Treaty of Nanking, which both ceded Hong Kong to Britain and created other "extraterritorial" zones in Chinese ports. Other European states—France, Germany, Russia—followed, wresting similar concessions from China, as the century went on. This process resulted in tension within China, between a conservative impulse to reassert traditional Chinese traditions and a reformist zeal to adopt "modern" Western ways. Those modern ways included medical beliefs, which became crucial in responses to the plague epidemic.

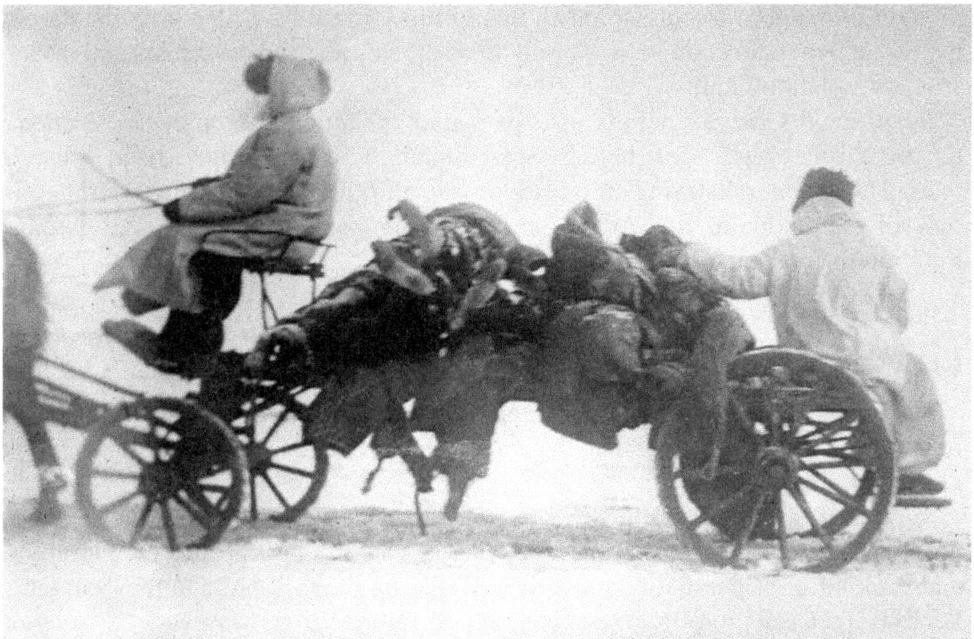

Removing bodies during the pneumonic plague epidemic in Manchuria, a province of China, c. 1910. (Library of Congress)

One of the exported resources of the areas of Mongolia and adjoining Manchuria was the fur of the burrowing rodent called the tarbagan (or marmot), valued for its similarity to sable. Western demand for the fur escalated in the late nineteenth century, spurred by the growing commercial power of aniline dye manufacturers whose products could further aid the marketing of tarbagan fur as "sable." That in turn led to poverty-stricken transients, enthusiastic about possible rewards, joining the experienced local trappers of tarbagans in Mongolia and Manchuria. And those newcomers became important conduits for the plague epidemic, for the tarbagan population of Mongolia had been infected with *Yersinia pestis* that might be transmitted to humans by insects.

A final background circumstance: bubonic plague was almost endemic in the Amur Valley and neighboring areas of eastern Asia. The experienced trappers of tarbagans suspected those rodents as its home and acted accordingly.

HOW IT WAS UNDERSTOOD AT THE TIME

This epidemic occurred at a time when Western beliefs about plague were rapidly evolving. The identification of a possible causative microorganism, conveyed from rodents to humans by insects, had shifted the focus on responses from sanitation to the control of contagious infection. At the same time, thinking about "plague" remained largely focused (as it had for centuries) on *bubonic* plague, with little attention to its pneumonic cousin. Such beliefs therefore led to the eradication of rodents and insects, and to the isolation of both those infected and those thought in danger of being so. Such quarantines might be a response dictated by persistent beliefs in contagion, as well as by the impulse to bar rodents and insects from an isolation facility.

Traditional Chinese beliefs also persisted, although the epidemic occurred during a time when such beliefs came under increasing attack from Western ones. Those general strains on tradition were amplified both by the sheer magnitude of the epidemic, and by the specific response to it by influential Chinese individuals.

RESPONSES

A variety of responses occurred across the conflicted territory of Manchuria, reflecting the different Russian, Japanese, and residual Chinese dominance of a particular area.

In and around Harbin, in the Russian/European area of settlement, Russian military authorities, business interests, and physicians concentrated on quarantine and the control of population movement, isolating the infected and their contacts. Lacking real isolation quarters, they settled on sealed railway cars as isolation sites. In the persistent belief that rodents and insects were responsible, rat eradication played a role; however, the sealed cars confined the pneumonic plague victims together with their contacts, allowing the cars to become death traps. The official response also included actions to prevent the epidemic from proceeding east along the railway that led to Vladivostok, thus halting that traffic—an action that was in conflict with the demands of commerce, and so the prohibition could only be imperfectly enforced.

Harbin also included a substantial Chinese settlement in which the influence of the imperial Chinese state still predominated. There Wu Lien-Teh, an ethnic Chinese physician educated in the West, was early convinced that pneumonic plague was the cause; when performing an autopsy on a plague victim he discovered *Yersinia pestis* in the lungs, leading him to argue that the attention to rats and fleas was misguided. He urged the wholesale cremation of the deceased, which affronted traditional burial customs. Wu's Western approach pleased modernizing Chinese opinion (as well as Europeans and Americans on the scene), but rival Chinese explanations of cause contested it. Did smoking inferior grades of opium, the only sort which the poorer Chinese could afford, cause plague? Did paper money, unless it were sterilized, spread the disease?

Mukden was the most important Manchurian city of traditional imperial Chinese rule, and although that remained true in 1910, Western diplomats, businessmen, and missionaries had gained influence as well. Chinese medical authorities responded to the appearance of plague by employing cordons of police, medics, and disinfection workers to impose quarantines and isolation on those thought dangerous. Especially suspect were transients such as those on their way home for the Chinese New Year, who had gathered in ramshackle inns and hostels near the railway station. In those sites, as well as in the poorer quarters of the city, the epidemic was most serious and the anti-plague workers there suffered particularly high mortality. Attempting to prevent the epidemic from spreading to the south—in the direction of Peking—the Chinese government closed that railway line (to Newchwang) that it controlled.

Japan controlled another railway leading south from Mukden, one that reached the vital ports of Dalian and Port Arthur that had been wrested from Russia in the 1904–1905 war. The Japanese response to the epidemic was efficient and ruthless. The swift blocking of the railway diverted possibly plague-infected Chinese transients from Mukden to the Newchwang route; trains on the Dalian route were inspected, sanitary cordons were established along the line, and some Chinese travelers were detained and isolated while en route. These measures certainly contributed to the very low plague mortality in Dalian and Port Arthur.

Alarmed alike by the frightening mortality and growing Russian and Japanese influence in Manchuria, the diplomats of the United States, joined by their German, French, and British colleagues, suggested to the Chinese Viceroy in Mukden that he summon an international plague conference. (Such conferences had become a repeated response to epidemic threats to Europe, especially those posed by cholera, since 1849.) Fearing international interference with their respective positions in Manchuria, the Russian and Japanese governments only hesitantly participated. After a period of negotiation, the Chinese Viceroy convened the conference in Mukden in April 1911. Wu Lien-Teh chaired the conference, which contained a series of scientific papers summarizing the contemporary understandings of plague; in attendance were 33 delegates representing 11 countries. This meeting marked the first appearance on the international stage of a Chinese state in the midst of coming to terms with what was seen as "modernity."

UNRESOLVED HISTORICAL ISSUES

The general issue of "what ended the plague," discussed previously in this volume, may be raised here as well. Between the appearance of bubonic plague in Hong Kong in 1894 and 1911, a major shift had occurred in understanding of the disease, an understanding that in Manchuria was applied to pneumonic plague as well. Did the combination of isolation, quarantine, and rapid cremation of the dead suffice to stamp out the disease? Did the microorganism not survive in cold weather? Did the waning of the traffic accompanying the Chinese New Year play a role? Did the recourse to fireworks represent simply an example of ancient Chinese superstition, or might it have incidentally disinfected *Yersinia*-laden air?

Did the epidemic contribute to the subsequent Japanese vision of their continuing role in Manchuria, bringing order and health to a dangerously corrupt environment? Did it, that is to say, form a link in a causative chain between 1911, 1931–1932 (when Japan occupied Manchuria and converted it to the puppet state of Manchukuo), and 1937 (when the Sino-Japanese War began the Asian phase of World War II)?

How much did the epidemic contribute to the fashioning of a modern Chinese system of public health, and to the Chinese acceptance of the very conception of the reality of infectious disease?

SUGGESTED ADDITIONAL READING

Gamsa, Mark. "The Epidemic of Pneumonic Plague in Manchuria, 1910–1911." *Past and Present* 190 (2006): 147–183.

Lei, Sean Hsiang-lin. "Sovereignty and the Microscope: Constituting Notifiable Infectious Disease and Containing the Manchurian Plague." In *Health and Hygiene in Chinese East Asia: Politics and Publics in the Long Twentieth Century*, edited by Angela Ki Che Leung and Charlotte Furth, 73–106. Durham, NC: Duke University Press, 2010.

Peckham, Robert. *Epidemics in Modern Asia.* Cambridge: Cambridge University Press, 2016.

Rogaski, Ruth. "Vampires in Plagueland: The Multiple Meanings of *Weisheng* in Manchuria." In *Health and Hygiene in Chinese East Asia*, edited by Angela Ki Che Leung and Charlotte Furth, 132–159. Durham, NC: Duke University Press, 2010.

Summers, William C. *The Great Manchurian Plague of 1910–1911: The Geopolitics of an Epidemic Disease.* New Haven, CT: Yale University Press, 2012.

36

Cholera Epidemic in Naples, 1910–1911

WHEN AND WHERE

One of the most dramatic outbreaks of cholera in the twentieth century occurred in Naples, Italy, in 1910 and 1911. Cholera struck southern Italy in the summer of 1910, and by August it reached Naples, the largest city of the region. A heavy series of rainstorms in the third week of September contributed to favorable conditions for the disease's spread, by washing dirt (including garbage) into wells and cisterns. Government authorities were loath to admit cholera's presence (see the "Significance" and "Responses" sections); they did so on September 25 but still minimized the risks and then (prematurely) declared the end of the epidemic on October 30.

In fact, this 1910 epidemic had been a serious one, which may have caused about 700 deaths. And far from being over by October 30, a chain of cholera infection persisted in Naples through the winter of 1910–1911. Nevertheless, the government again proclaimed that Naples was free of cholera on February 26, 1911, although the number of cases accelerated in the following months. By the second week of May 1911, the epidemic had become grave and remained so until at least September. Both the municipal government of Naples and the government of Italy made increasingly determined (and complex) attempts to conceal the facts about it, attempts that were largely successful. By the end of August, the authorities were admitting that some cholera had been present, but they continued to downplay its extent.

The modern historian Frank Snowden, who has uncovered the story of the epidemic, estimates that perhaps 2,600 people died of cholera in Naples between May and September 1911. The toll was proportionately highest in the poor quarters of the city, areas where the poor had settled relatively recently after earlier epidemics had led to the clearance of older slums. Snowden also estimates the death toll from cholera in Italy in 1911 as at least 16,000, and perhaps higher.

SIGNIFICANCE

The Naples cholera epidemic of 1910–1911 was the last major outbreak of cholera in Western Europe. But its real significance derives from the remarkable efforts of the Italian (and Naples) governments to deny its existence, efforts that were so successful that historians neglected it for much of the twentieth century, asserting that cholera had ceased to be a problem in Europe after the 1890s. Economic and political pressures drove the Italian and city governments, and so the epidemic is a particularly vivid example of how those factors influence reactions to epidemic disease.

The epidemic (and its subsequent history) also illustrates the ability of modern government authorities to shape the understanding of an epidemic catastrophe for later generations.

BACKGROUND

Some understanding of the political and economic situations of Italy in general, and of Naples in particular, clarifies the responses of the authorities to the 1910–1911 cholera epidemic.

The economy of Naples depended very heavily on its position as the principal port of embarkation for the massive emigration underway from southern Italy to (especially) the United States and Argentina in the early twentieth century. Between 1906 and 1915, perhaps 3.5 million Italians emigrated, many of them through the port of Naples; in 1908 alone 787,000 passengers passed through the port. The city derived huge economic benefits from the services and goods it provided to both the ships and the emigrants. Lodging-house keepers were a numerous and influential economic interest. Any disruption of the emigrant traffic would work real hardship on the city; word of a cholera epidemic might lead other countries (such as the United States and Argentina) to forbid migration to their shores from an infected port, and thus bring the emigrant traffic to a complete halt. In addition, the city leaders hoped to attract outside investment both for business and for capital improvements; fear of cholera might frighten such investment away.

Meanwhile, in 1910 and 1911, a tense political situation existed in Italy, as groups on the left (socialists and radicals) confronted the governing coalitions of Catholic and liberal parties, hoping to seize on any evidence of incompetence or scandal to gain power. The dominant parties feared violent revolution; in 1900 an anarchist had assassinated the king. The 1910 epidemic in southern Italy, and the government's initially heavy-handed response to it, had provoked serious violence, especially in Taranto between December 30 and January 10. In 1911 the authorities hoped to avoid an even greater uproar by suppressing the news of an epidemic altogether.

The Italian government also wished to present a happy and successful face to the world in 1911, the fiftieth anniversary of the foundation of the united Kingdom of Italy. The nation hoped to put itself forward as a modern, prosperous, and progressive society, which of course would include a model system of public health.

Any consideration of the background of the 1910–1911 cholera epidemic in Naples should also remember that the city had suffered an important cholera epidemic in 1884, and that major civil disturbances had resulted from the attempts to bring that epidemic under control. In 1910 the authorities wished to avoid a repetition of that earlier experience.

HOW IT WAS UNDERSTOOD AT THE TIME

By 1910 most educated Italian opinion accepted the central role of germs (*Vibrio cholerae*) as the cause of cholera. They therefore (at least in principle) agreed with a variety of public health measures designed to prevent the passage of the germs from a cholera sufferer to others. As the next section suggests, however, much room for argument remained about the practical application of those measures.

RESPONSES

The official responses to the Naples cholera epidemic of 1910–1911 had two aspects. City and national authorities took a number of steps that might generally be called public health responses. But those measures were overlain by government attempts to minimize the epidemic in the public mind and even to deny its existence.

When cholera reached Naples in August 1910, the Italian government was already taking extensive actions against the disease in other parts of central Italy, and those actions had stimulated widespread (and noisy) popular resistance. With that turmoil in mind, the Naples city government delayed admitting that cholera had arrived, while it quietly began its public health responses. It hired extra doctors, nurses, laboratory technicians, and grave diggers; it began surveillance of railroad passengers arriving in Naples from infected rural areas, without imposing a noticeable quarantine on such travelers, and it enlisted physicians, priests, teachers, landlords, and employers as informers to identify cholera victims. Once identified, cholera victims were quietly isolated (and their relatives might be isolated as well) and their property was disinfected. The city authorities also inspected food markets and urged the population to beware of fresh fruits and vegetables (the likely bearers of the bacterium). Emigrants arriving for the ships in the harbor were moved directly from the railroad station to carefully segregated quarters. Such measures were said to be precautionary, not a response to an epidemic already in progress.

By October 30, 1910, the city proclaimed that the danger had passed, although it clearly had not. Snowden remarks that "the logic of their reasoning was that a little cholera was less harmful than a major depression" (Snowden 1995, 286). The prime minister of Italy, Luigi Luzzatti, was less sure that cholera had disappeared. He proposed that emigrants while in transit be housed in a government hostel on the outskirts of the city until their health was assured. He thus hoped both to preserve the vital emigrant business and reassure the suspicious American and Argentine authorities that cholera would not be carried across the sea.

This central government proposal met furious resistance in Naples. Boardinghouse owners staged a demonstration; the city government denied that the cholera infection was present and instead denounced talk of cholera as a plot of foreigners, socialists, and northern Italians to sabotage the prosperity of the city; the city council went so far as to call on Neapolitans to prepare for an armed insurrection. In the face of this reaction in February 1911, Luzzatti closed the hostel and agreed that Naples was cholera-free. Shortly thereafter his government fell from power, to be replaced by one led by the veteran politician Giovanni Giolitti.

But by the second week of May, cholera had reached serious levels, and the epidemic raged from that time until at least September. The governments of Italy and the city of Naples were now in accord: the prosperity of the city and prestige of the country demanded that the epidemic be denied. Order in Naples must be maintained at all costs. Some deaths were admitted but were blamed on gastroenteritis. The Italian government's Department of Public Health took charge from the city authorities; while some of the public health measures applied in 1910 were revived, an atmosphere of secrecy surrounded them. Actions that might attract public attention (such as soup kitchens for the poor) were avoided.

A remarkable conspiracy of silence enveloped the epidemic. Neither the Italian parliament nor the Naples city council discussed it. Hospital and cemetery records for the summer months of 1911 made no mention of causes of death, and the records of the hospital for infectious diseases kept (or least preserved) no patient records between May and November 1911. Medical journals were also silent. This cover-up relied on the self-interest of many Italians and on appeals to patriotism; but some journalists were also bribed, the police seized some pamphlets, and some people were threatened with prosecution if they publicized the epidemic.

International opinion posed other problems. Publicity would lead to a collapse of trade generally (and of the emigrant traffic especially); it might also lead to massive internal disorder that would discredit the country. The Italian leaders quietly urged other states (particularly the United States) that only subversives and revolutionaries would benefit from news of a cholera epidemic. And although the U.S. Public Health Service had a medical officer in Naples who knew that cholera was present, from June 1911 through 1912, no U.S. official mentioned the Naples epidemic. Argentina was threatened with diplomatic and trade reprisals if it attempted any quarantine of Italian traffic.

By August 1911, the Italian government became more forthright, perhaps pushed by the inevitable news leaks and coverage of the epidemic in foreign newspapers. (In Thomas Mann's novella *Death in Venice*, the protagonist tries to learn the facts: "Obsessed with obtaining reliable news about the status and progress of the disease, he went to the city's cafés and plowed through all the German newspapers, which had been missing from the hotel lobby during the past few days" [Mann 1998, 347].) The Vatican newspaper began attacking the Italian government's cover-up; socialist and radical journalists did likewise. The government now took the position that some cholera deaths had indeed occurred, but that the toll was slight.

The government also established some official mortality and morbidity figures for the epidemic that seriously underestimated the likely actual toll. Ultimately, those government figures claimed that about 6,100 people had died in Italy of cholera in 1911; over 800 of those deaths were said to have occurred in the province of Naples. As Snowden's careful reconstruction shows, those figures emerged from a number of statistical tricks; for example, cholera deaths were only confirmed by bacteriological analysis, when many others certainly occurred without any postmortem analysis of that kind possible. Snowden believes the true Italian toll in 1911 was at least 16,000, and in Naples, at least 2,600.

Apart from denying that cholera existed, medical practitioners responded to the disease in several ways. For many, despite their allegiance to the germ theory, cholera was still to be fought by a purging of the toxins of the body. The persistent failure of such therapies led many people to seek alternative and unorthodox cures, as they had done in earlier cholera pandemics.

Some physicians knew of the rehydration techniques developed in India by Leonard Rogers, and they pressed the Italian government to invite Rogers to Italy. Doing so, the government feared, would admit the seriousness of the epidemic. Eventually Rogers was allowed to practice his methods in Palermo, but only for three weeks; he was not permitted to proceed to Naples.

UNRESOLVED HISTORICAL ISSUES

The Naples cholera epidemic of 1910–1911, while it extracted fewer lives than the epidemic of 1884, was in many ways comparable to it in severity. Yet the reaction of the Neapolitan population was strikingly different. In 1884 riots greeted official attempts at isolation and disinfection; in 1911 the population meekly collaborated in a denial that the epidemic even existed. Frank Snowden hypothesizes that by 1911 the people had become more "medicalized," more willing to accept what public health measures the government took (however quietly the government acted); he also suggests that the Roman Catholic Church in Italy had become more accepting of the dictates of public health, and less insistent that religion had an answer to cholera that might differ from that of science or the state. Or did the government's cover-up of the epidemic work so well that the population genuinely did not notice the disease in their midst?

The true mortality and morbidity of the epidemic may never be precisely known. Snowden based his estimates on a very careful examination of different evidence that survives, and either directly or indirectly contradicts the official figures; readers interested in the evidence should consult his book (Snowden 1995, especially chapter 7 "Concealment and Crisis: 1911," 297–359).

Until Snowden unearthed that evidence, the magnitude of the 1910–1911 cholera epidemic in Naples passed largely unnoticed in historical writing. Robert Pollitzer, in his authoritative survey of cholera undertaken for the World Health Organization in 1959, seemed to accept the official Italian statistics and claimed that in 1911 "cholera became manifest in all parts of Italy, including Sicily, but assumed serious proportions in only a few of the numerous affected localities" (Pollitzer 1959, 43). Richard Evans, in an influential article published in 1988, asserted that the sixth pandemic "had virtually no impact on western Europe" and that after the Hamburg cholera epidemic of 1892 "the age of epidemics in western Europe was largely over" (Evans 1988, 125, 146). Those examples, chosen from the work of eminent scholars, simply illustrate how effective over time the Italian government's concealment of the epidemic proved to be.

REFERENCES AND SUGGESTED ADDITIONAL READING

Evans, Richard J. "Epidemics and Revolutions: Cholera in Nineteenth-Century Europe." *Past and Present* 120 (1988): 125, 146.

Hamlin, Christopher. *Cholera: The Biography.* Oxford: Oxford University Press, 2009.

Mann, Thomas. *Death in Venice and Other Tales.* New York: Viking, 1998. (Orig. pub. 1913 in German.)

Pollitzer, R. *Cholera.* Geneva: World Health Organization, 1959.

This chapter is based largely on the following book, which should be consulted by readers who wish to know more about the subject:

Snowden, Frank M. *Naples in the Time of Cholera, 1884–1911.* Cambridge: Cambridge University Press, 1995.

See also "Suggested Additional Reading" in volume 2, chapter 32 "Sixth Cholera Pandemic, 1899–1923."

37

Poliomyelitis in the United States, 1916

WHERE AND WHEN

In the summer of 1916, a major epidemic of poliomyelitis occurred in the United States, especially in the northeastern states. Its most dramatic appearance was in and around New York City, the largest city in the country and the one that dominated media images. Between June and October of 1916, about 27,000 Americans were stricken by the disease, and of them 6,000 died. New York suffered 8,900 of those cases and 2,400 deaths. Most of those victims in New York City were young children.

SIGNIFICANCE

This epidemic's historical significance stems more from its impression on medical and popular opinions than from its demographic impact. It may be called the world's first major poliomyelitis epidemic, and it came at a time when Western medical science had made strong, and widely accepted, claims of mastery of disease. Those claims led to responses that historian John Paul regards as the "high-water mark in attempts at enforcement of isolation and quarantine measures" (Paul 1971, 148). The epidemic spread despite those efforts. Medicine's relative powerlessness in the face of the 1916 epidemic was therefore particularly disturbing, and the reactions (medical, political, and popular) of Americans revealed important social and intellectual prejudices and tensions. The 1916 epidemic initiated a period of 40 years when American obsession with poliomyelitis made it the shock disease of the age, the one around which fear gathered and against which a new scale of private philanthropy was mobilized in the search for remedies or preventive vaccines.

BACKGROUND

Poliomyelitis—also called polio or infantile paralysis—began to appear in the consciousness of Europeans and North Americans in the late nineteenth century, beginning with isolated outbreaks in rural towns in Norway, Sweden, France, and the New England states. The first city to experience an epidemic was Stockholm, the Swedish capital, where 44 cases were reported in 1887. In 1905, Sweden reported over 1,000 cases of poliomyelitis, and in 1907 New York experienced its first polio epidemic. Other American cities (Cincinnati in 1911 and Buffalo in 1912) were affected as well.

Later in the twentieth century, it came to be understood that the virus responsible for poliomyelitis has a very long history as a common childhood infection. In earlier centuries, large numbers of people were infected early in their lives, and in most cases those infections resulted in simple mild fevers or perhaps no symptoms at all. Occasionally more serious symptoms, including stiffness, muscle weakness, or even paralysis that crippled limbs, resulted, but people did not associate those symptoms with a common childhood fever. That is, poliomyelitis was not a separately understood disease. Most children were infected early and harmlessly, and so enjoyed immunity from later attacks that might have been more serious. Its epidemic appearance in the late nineteenth century, we now believe, was an unintended byproduct of improved sanitation in "advanced" countries of North America and Europe, where children were raised in relatively germ-free surroundings and thus only contracted the poliomyelitis virus after infancy, when they might have been more susceptible to serious symptoms.

HOW IT WAS UNDERSTOOD AT THE TIME

The disease manifested itself most dramatically when its initial fever was joined by stiff neck and back muscles and then a spreading paralysis that might lead to permanent crippling or, in the worst case, interference with the muscular ability to breathe and hence death by asphyxiation. In 1916 several aspects of its cause and course were being debated. It had been associated with germs, and those germs had supposedly been transmitted from one laboratory animal to another. No one had as yet seen the germs, since they were too small for the microscopes then used; they were therefore examples of what was called a *filterable* virus that could pass through the filters designed to stop bacteria. Whether polio was contagious, and if so what the mode of contagion was, remained uncertain.

These epidemics occurred at a time when several different explanations of the cause of disease had gained scientific popularity. One was the belief that diseases flourished in dirty environments, and so the solution to disease was to be found in a broad effort to clean up environments. From the mid-nineteenth century, these attempts came especially to focus on providing clean water supplies and removing sewage. In some ways competing with that broad environmentalism was the more recent conviction that microorganisms—germs—caused disease. The believers in the germ theory had less interest in a general clean-up and more in identifying the microorganism that caused a disease and in isolating those individuals who were infected with those germs. In fact, both popular and more professional medical opinions often acted on some combination of these beliefs, both of which represented different strands of modern science at the time.

The approaches taken to poliomyelitis in 1916 illustrate the ways in which those beliefs were entangled. The equation of dirt with danger was, especially in the United States, connected with social and political attitudes toward different ethnic and racial groups. In the cities of the northeastern United States that meant the very large communities of recent immigrants from southern and eastern Europe: Italians, Slavs, and Eastern European Jews, among others. Americans from earlier migrations feared these newcomers in a variety of ways, and in 1916 those fears focused on the supposed relation between the immigrants, their dirt, and the poliomyelitis epidemic. Did the germ of polio flourish in the congested quarters of Manhattan's Lower East Side? That's what many influential New Yorkers believed.

But the disease was as likely to be found in more prosperous districts, and dirty-immigrant theorists had to find ways in which the germ was conveyed out of its slummy home. Did servants and tradespeople carry it with them by day when they came to work with their betters? Possibly. But another then-exciting idea about the transmission of disease offered a way to combine the germ and filth theories. In the last decade of the nineteenth century and the first decade of the twentieth, the links between diseases and their transmission by insects had been convincingly shown, first for malaria and yellow fever (transmitted by mosquitoes), more recently for plague (transmitted by fleas). In the enthusiasm for discovering insect transmitters, the housefly became a favorite suspect for such different diseases as diphtheria and typhoid fever, and now for poliomyelitis. The housefly was present everywhere, clustering on foods and especially on the 2.5 million pounds of horse dung that landed on the streets of New York every day (Flink 1978, 34). The housefly, it was believed, carried the germs of polio from the filth of the immigrant quarters to the leafy suburbs.

RESPONSES

In 1916 American city governments and their public health officials reacted to the epidemic in ways that reflected their beliefs in dirt and germs as a cause, and the housefly as an agent of transmission. The germ theory supported fears of contagion, and so one important response was to isolate the sick from the healthy. Many healthy New Yorkers (as well as Philadelphians and other American city dwellers) left the city in the summer of 1916, seeking the healthier air of the seashore or the Adirondack, Catskill, or Pocono Mountains. Fearing that poorer immigrants might infect them there, the wealthy sponsors of charities that funded fresh-air vacations for the poor stopped such events in the summer of the epidemic. Children were urged to avoid crowded places, especially beaches and pools, and that particular fear conditioned American family behavior until the 1950s. The states that surrounded New York—New Jersey, Connecticut, Pennsylvania—began inspecting New Yorkers who crossed their borders, denying admission to those who seemed ill. In response, New York (and other cities) began issuing health passes certifying the bearer's good health.

Public health authorities quarantined individual dwellings, placing frightening placards outside the homes of sick people. They also attempted to isolate all the sick within special wards of hospitals. In New York, if a home could provide a separate toilet, a separate eating place, and a private nurse for the sick member of the family, the sufferer could remain at home; otherwise, the authorities insisted on the patient's removal to an isolation hospital. Only the well-to-do could meet those conditions; the poor immigrant families could not. The fear of immigrant quarters also showed itself in attempts to regulate or prevent ethnic feast days and festivals, which would be accompanied by contagious crowds. Such measures generated considerable resentment and resistance from within the immigrant communities, meaning that their application was never complete or effective. The general concern with the dangers of crowd contagion also led to a two-week delay in the opening of New York schools in September.

Fears of germs coexisted with fears of dirt, and so authorities flushed streets, arrested those who broke sanitary regulations, and encouraged the private use of disinfectants and soaps. Such measures were especially directed, again, at the immigrant quarters of cities, where particular efforts at sanitary education were pursued: clean hands, clean toilet habits, cover open foods, and avoid such likely contagious behavior as kissing. Screens and fly swatters were insisted upon.

The epidemic in New York City peaked in August; between the middle of that month and its end, the number of cases fell from over 1,200 to 500, and by the end of October, the number had dropped to less than 50. Many unresolved questions remained about the disease, and those difficulties meant that it was hard to see the waning of the epidemic as a triumph of scientific medicine. The pattern of the epidemic's spread remained unexplained, despite the ease with which it was blamed on the housefly. Likewise in doubt was the path of infection within the body. Physicians (and the public) remained uncertain about how to diagnose the disease and even more uncertain about an appropriate therapy for it.

UNRESOLVED HISTORICAL ISSUES

The disease's spread in 1916 certainly contradicted any belief that it affected only the dirty immigrant populations. Its victims included the daughter-in-law of the eminent American Ambassador to France, Walter Hines Page. Meanwhile African Americans, perhaps the lowest group on the U.S. socioeconomic pole, were little affected by polio, and Manhattan, the most crowded place, had a lower infection (and mortality) rate than some rural (and presumably more salubrious) settlements.

Did the germ reach the body through the nasal passages, as the leading American expert, Simon Flexner, argued? Or was its path through the digestive tract? Was poliomyelitis primarily a disease of the nervous system, or were the nerves only affected in some cases? How was the disease defined and diagnosed? Was it defined from its symptoms, so that polio meant stiff neck and back muscles and the onset of paralysis? Or from an examination by a pathologist of damage to organs? Or from the presence in the body of the germs, even if no symptoms manifested themselves? This epidemic occurred at a time when considerable tension could exist between private physicians, who upheld the virtues of clinical diagnoses of individual patients whose peculiarities they knew well, and laboratory scientists, who relied on impersonal blood testing or pathology reports. Those professional rivalries contributed to the diagnostic uncertainty.

Perhaps most important to the public was the general ineffectiveness of the therapies offered for poliomyelitis. Some of those therapies represented older medical traditions, while others reflected fashionably modern ideas. If polio was a disease that entered the body through the digestive tract and affected all the body's systems, could its germs be drained out by bleeding? Could the irritation of the affected muscles be countered by another irritant, such as a hot plaster on the skin? If germs caused the disease, could some magic bullet be found that would kill the germs, in the way that the recently developed arsphenamine attacked the microorganisms that caused syphilis? How could the symptoms—fever, aches, paralysis—best be relieved? Especially appealing was the promise of an anti-polio serum, along the lines of the serum recently employed against another serious childhood scourge, diphtheria. In 1916 several researchers experimented with such sera in the struggle with poliomyelitis. None of these therapies proved very effective.

AFTERMATH

The 1916 epidemic began a period of over 40 years when poliomyelitis was never far from the center of American concerns about disease. In the subsequent decades, the association of immigrant filth with polio lost strength, especially after the eminent political leader Franklin D. Roosevelt fell ill with the disease in 1921, a case that clearly showed that the disease did not respect rank and wealth. But the fears of contagion, if anything, increased, especially the fears of places such as public beaches and pools where crowds of children gathered. By the 1930s, a major fund-raising organization had developed, and the activities of that National Foundation for Infantile Paralysis, the first great twentieth-century philanthropy that targeted a specific disease, raised new questions about the relation between publicity, fund-raising, the popular conceptions of a disease, and scientific research.

REFERENCES

Flink, James J. *The Car Culture.* Cambridge, MA: MIT Press, 1978.

Paul, John R. *A History of Poliomyelitis.* New Haven, CT: Yale University Press, 1971.

SUGGESTED ADDITIONAL READING

Oshinsky, David M. *Polio: An American Story.* New York: Oxford University Press, 2005.

Rogers, Naomi. *Dirt and Disease: Polio before FDR.* New Brunswick, NJ: Rutgers University Press, 1992.

38

Influenza Pandemic, 1918–1919

WHEN AND WHERE

The most widespread disease event in human history, an influenza pandemic, occurred between the spring of 1918 and the early months of 1919. It is now thought that at least 50 million people died in this pandemic, perhaps 18 or 20 million in India alone; the death toll in the United States may have been 675,000 (or 550,000 more than normal for the period). And staggering as those numbers were, the number of the sick was far higher. As many as 25 or 30 million Americans—over 25% of the population—suffered from influenza in those months, and although only the roughest estimates are possible, that proportion may have been true of nearly all the inhabited areas of the earth. When historical evidence is more complete, the modern estimate of 50 million deaths may prove a serious understatement; the toll might have reached as high as 100 million.

This pandemic swept through the world in three waves, of which the second was much the most serious. The first, beginning in March 1918, has most often been traced to Kansas, in the central United States; by April it had turned up in western Europe (where its appearance may have followed the arrival of American troops joining the war) and China as well, and then rapidly to India in May, northern Europe, Australia, and Southeast Asia in June. (The appearance of influenza in Spain in that spring may explain why the pandemic sometimes was called Spanish influenza, although no clear evidence exists that the pandemic began there; word of the disease there spread because Spain, not involved in the then-raging World War I, did not feel compelled to hide influenza's ravages from enemies.) Although this first wave was overshadowed by the next, it may have arrived at a crucial point in the military history of the war. In the spring of 1918, the German military leaders, hoping to seize a favorable moment between the collapse of their Russian enemies to the east and the buildup of American forces in the west, began a major offensive on the western front. The Germans were unable to achieve the breakthrough they desired, however, in part because "in June influenza laid low nearly half a million German soldiers whose resistance, depressed by poor diet, was far lower than that of the well-fed Allied troops in the trenches opposite"

(Keegan 2000, 408). By July 1918, this German offensive was over, while the first wave of influenza abated.

In August 1918, a new wave began as influenza reappeared in France, and then rapidly moved by sea across the Atlantic (striking first Boston in the United States) and down the west coast of Africa (where Freetown, in Sierra Leone, was first hit). In September, the disease spread across the United States from east to west and began fanning out across Europe and west Africa. By October, most of Europe had been affected, as had most of south and Southeast Asia; in November, influenza reached such far corners as the interior of Siberia and the islands of the Pacific. By January 1919, when Australia was reinfected in this second wave, very few inhabited places on earth remained untouched: isolated northern portions of Iceland and the islands of American Samoa.

Influenza shares many of the symptoms of the common cold: a cough, headache, fever, congested nose, general aches. The 1918 pandemic caused all those things, but it very often also resulted in lung complications and some form of pneumonia, and those problems contributed to the higher number of serious or fatal cases. The onset of the disease was very rapid, both for individuals and for entire communities; an epidemic wave in a given city might last three or four weeks, while most individuals recovered within a few days—unless pneumonic complications set in.

In the United States, the second wave moved generally westward from its original foothold in New England. Thus, the peak period of mortality in Boston was the first week of October 1918; in Philadelphia, Baltimore, and Washington, the third week; in New York and Chicago, the fourth week; in St. Louis, San Francisco, and Los Angeles, the first week of November. The epidemic caused 33,400 deaths in New York, 15,800 in Philadelphia, and 14,000 in Chicago. These represented mortality rates of between 5.2 (Chicago) and 9.3 (Philadelphia) per 1,000 population. For the United States as a whole, the mortality rate was comparable to Chicago's. In Europe, the second wave similarly fanned out from France, moving south and north into the Mediterranean lands, southern Scandinavia, and Great Britain in September, then eastward to Germany, eastern Europe, and Russia in October. In most of Europe, mortality rates were similar to those in the United States; in London 23,000 died, and the mortality rate in Great Britain has been estimated at 4.9 per 1,000 population. Some cities with environments likely to favor respiratory complaints experienced higher death rates: smoke-choked industrial Pittsburgh in the United States, for example. Mortality rates in parts of Asia and Africa were much higher, as will be discussed shortly.

Although the geographical origins of the pandemic have been controversial (see the "Unresolved Historical Issues" section), sea transportation accounted for some of its spread in both its first and second waves. The first wave apparently landed in India from a ship docking in Bombay on May 29; the second wave was carried from Europe to west Africa by sea, first reaching Freetown on August 31, and then proceeding down the coast: Accra on September 2, Lagos on September 14. Especially important were the shipborne cases that reached isolated Pacific islands: Guam on October 26, Western Samoa on November 7, Tahiti on November 16. In such isolated islands, influenza apparently found virgin soil conditions, and a very high rate of mortality resulted. Of the 36,000 people of Western Samoa, 8,500 died in the epidemic, or about 230 per 1,000 population; over 1,000 Tongans of a population of not more than 15,000 perished. Even more dramatic mortality rates struck isolated settlements in Alaska that depended on sea transportation to the outside world; the village of Wales, for example, lost 170 people out of 310.

One of the most striking features about this pandemic was its severity for young adults, those people most often best able to resist epidemics. Mortalities in many epidemics may be graphed as a U or reverse bell curve, with mortalities highest for the very young and the very old. The 1918 pandemic often resembled a W, with a frightening spike for those between the ages of 18 and 35. Reasons for that peculiarity remain unsettled (see the "Unresolved Historical Issues" section).

The people of Asia and Africa were at greater risk of death in the pandemic. Its second wave spread across India from west to east, peaking in Bombay in October, in central and northern India in November, and in Bengal in December; the peak mortality in Assam and Burma, east of Bengal, occurred in November, illustrating the disease's movement there by sea. Mortality rates for the subcontinent as a whole may have been as high as 60 deaths per 1,000 population, 12 times the European and North American figures. Within India, Hindus of low caste suffered much higher mortalities than those of high caste, illustrating the vulnerabilities of poor populations everywhere. Poor nutrition and an inability to find even basic nursing care weakened the poor person's ability to resist bacterial infections that often accompanied influenza, while in 1918 India the failure of expected monsoon rains led to crop failure and yet more inadequate nutrition. Some parts of Asia and Africa—for example, the Belgian Congo, Ghana, and the Netherlands East Indies—suffered similarly catastrophic mortality rates. In India, says the historian I. D. Mills, "rivers became clogged with corpses because firewood available was insufficient for the cremation of Hindus" (Mills 1986, 35–36).

The third wave of the great pandemic was a relatively minor echo of the second. In the United States, influenza deaths, on the decline in many places from late November through December, rose again in late January and February, but in no cases did they reach the levels of the fall of 1918. Influenza also reached Australia again in January; an Australian quarantine kept the second wave away.

SIGNIFICANCE

In sheer magnitude, the influenza pandemic of 1918–1919 stands as one of the great disease events of world history. At the time, it became a frustrating rebuke to the new confidence of Western biomedicine, and it has been frequently cited since as illustrating the possibility of another great influenza pandemic. Influenza scares in the late twentieth and early twenty-first centuries invariably call the 1918–1919 experience to mind.

But at the same time, much of the significance accorded to lesser epidemic catastrophes cannot be found here. The impact of the pandemic seemed very transient, quickly passing away. The reasons for its apparent insignificance are discussed in "Unresolved Historical Issues."

BACKGROUND

The 1918 influenza pandemic began during World War I, and its second wave roughly coincided with the war's end: November 11, 1918. The conditions of that great war certainly facilitated the spread of epidemic disease in many ways. In Europe especially the war brought armies of unprecedented size together, making contagion easy. Other large masses of people were transported across the oceans to take part, as soldiers or as laborers, in the European fighting: Americans after 1917 when the United States entered the war, various imperial peoples (Indians, Australians, Africans from British and French colonies, and others) from the war's early days. Ocean transport itself, in large and crowded steamships, was an obvious opportunity for contagion. The demand of the combatants for vital raw material resources promoted a vigorous ocean trade between Europe and the rest of the world. In all the belligerent states, the need to maintain patriotic zeal in a war marked by seemingly endless bloody stalemates led to regular rallies, speeches, and parades, all of which gathered still more people in contagious crowds. War fronts themselves became centers of other epidemic infections, notably typhus and tuberculosis, further weakening the affected populations. The war also had drained professional medical services—doctors and nurses—away from their ordinary tasks, leaving the civilian population more vulnerable. And by 1918 Russia's government (including its public health infrastructure) had dissolved in revolution, which would in November engulf Germany and the Austro-Hungarian lands as well.

More generally, conditions favoring the spread of disease across the world had developed by the early twentieth century. The world's population was larger and more urban; the large American cities, for example, contained very crowded tenements in which infections easily spread. A network of economic and political relationships, with Europe at its center, had connected all the continents; World War I was simply another stage in an accelerating time of materials and people moving to and from Europe and elsewhere. Particularly significant for the spread of epidemics were the steamship and the railroad. Steamships reduced trans-Atlantic crossings from weeks to days; railroads reduced land journeys from days to hours. The spread of the second wave of the 1918 pandemic illustrated the importance of such transportation. Influenza moved rapidly down the west coast of Africa by sea, while its progress into the interior of Africa was much slower—except in those places, such as South Africa, where rail lines led inland. India, carpeted with a dense network of railroads, suffered swiftly and catastrophically from influenza.

All these circumstances, especially those of the war, may have helped spread disease, or worsen its effects. But we must remember that the influenza pandemic struck almost everywhere, including places (Western Samoa, distant Alaska) as far from the zones of fighting as can be imagined.

The 1918 event was not, of course, the first influenza pandemic. Waves of influenza had repeatedly swept over large areas of the world in the past. The most recent one had been in 1889–1890; its spread, too, had been facilitated by the modern transportation links powered by steam. Questions remain about a possible

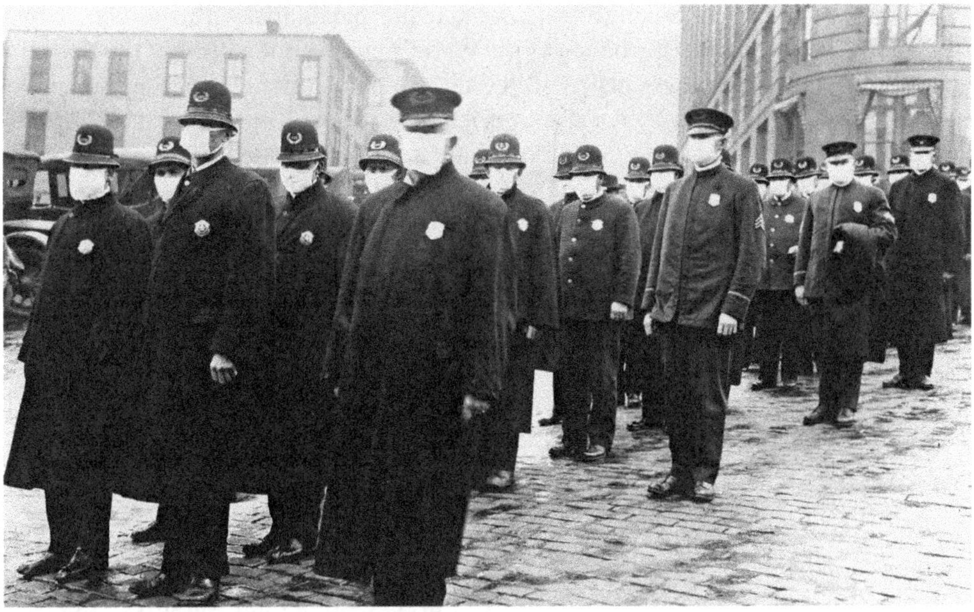

Members of the Seattle police force wear protective face masks during the influenza pandemic of 1918. The wearing of face masks was controversial in many cities. (National Archives)

connection between exposure to influenza in that pandemic and immunity from influenza in 1918.

HOW IT WAS UNDERSTOOD AT THE TIME

The 1918 influenza pandemic arrived at a time when the confidence of Western medicine in its therapeutic powers had reached new heights. The germ theory seemed to answer questions about the cause of disease. The principle of vaccination had been extended beyond its original application to smallpox and to other diseases. A specific chemical agent had been applied as a magic bullet against syphilis. Surely a germ of influenza could be found, a remedy could cure it, and a vaccine could prevent it. A candidate influenza germ had already been found, called Pfeiffer's bacillus, named for the eminent German bacteriologist Richard Pfeiffer who announced its discovery in 1892.

Not everyone agreed that Pfeiffer's bacillus was responsible, however, and in 1918 the evidence remained mixed. Partisans for and against the bacillus argued throughout the 1918 pandemic, but most authorities did agree that *some* microorganism, a germ or a virus, caused influenza. (In fact, Pfeiffer's bacillus had nothing to do with influenza; an influenza virus was first discovered in 1933.)

In practice, most authorities also assumed that influenza was contagious. Especially in France, physicians warned about contagious places of a localized miasma that should be avoided. That explanation showed that the belief in environmental causes still existed, even though it might also recognize a role for germs. Many thinkers also—not surprisingly—associated the pandemic with the war, which they saw as a massive disturbance of the world's environment. Might the dreadful poison gas that the belligerents spewed on European battlefields or the vast explosions of ceaseless artillery give rise to infectious vapors (or even germs)? In some way, was influenza nature's (or God's) angry reaction to the disturbance of the environment?

War propaganda also entered into the understanding of the pandemic. Was the enemy responsible for the disease? The widespread belief that the pandemic began in China (see "Unresolved Historical Issues") may have begun with German propaganda that blamed the epidemic on Chinese laborers employed by the Allied Powers.

RESPONSES

The influenza pandemic struck very quickly, and (especially as the seriousness of the second wave became apparent) governments in Europe and North America felt pressured to do *something* about it. The urgency of a total war already existed and magnified demands for action against the disease. The most frequent actions were taken against possible contagion: schools, churches, and theaters were ordered to close down. Some markets and taverns were also affected by government-ordered closures. In the United States, the wearing of gauze masks that covered the mouth became a symbol of official policy, as cities demanded their people don such masks in public places.

Some of these measures met varying degrees of resistance from the public. In San Francisco wearing masks became a civic joke for some, while others protested the mask rule as an infringement of civil liberty. The California State Board of Health gave those protestors ammunition, claiming that the masks were ineffective anyway and so not necessary; the city government disagreed. When the Pennsylvania State Board of Health ordered taverns closed, the mayor of Pittsburgh denounced the idea. In London the requirement that movie theaters be regularly ventilated led the theater owners to complain that the supposed immorality of the movies was responsible for such an unfair restriction; why, they asked, were not equally crowded trains ventilated as well?

Other government actions attacked supposed sources (or residences) of germs. Some communities organized fumigation spraying of things and places, a practice that had been employed against the mosquito-borne diseases yellow fever and malaria. Campaigns against public spitting (a serious problem in an age of chewing tobacco) were reinforced; they too had already been put in place by antituberculosis movements, as had attempts to control dust in public.

Governments also had to deal with a rapid collapse of necessary public services, at least in the three or four weeks when an epidemic was at its peak. Labor was already at a premium in those countries at war, for the military services demanded millions of conscripts. The epidemic therefore further seriously reduced the already thin number of garbage collectors, morticians, and gravediggers, at a time when the demands for the services of the latter two, for example, rose dramatically. City governments had varying success in organizing the continuance of such services.

One frequent government response to epidemics had been quarantines. Influenza simply moved too rapidly and universally for them to be effective, and most authorities realized that. In the United States, military bases (which had been some of the original focal points of the epidemic) were quarantined, but they remained special cases. Elsewhere in the world, quarantines only enjoyed success where geographic isolation was easily reinforced. The first wave of influenza reached Australia, but not the second, apparently because the Australian government operated an effective quarantine. The city of Fairbanks, in Alaska, kept influenza out; so too did the American islands of Samoa.

The vigorous (if not very effective) government responses in Europe and North America were not repeated elsewhere. Much of Asia and Africa was under the control of European imperial powers, and the colonial governments on the spot had seen whatever resources they had stripped away by the demands of war. Even if the will to take action against influenza had been there, the money usually was not.

Medical professionals in both Europe and North America approached the pandemic with confidence, but their measures were largely pointless. A variety of vaccines and antitoxins were prepared, some with great fanfare, but none with any effect. Doctors urged the liberal application of antiseptic substances to persons and places. Many more traditional therapies were still tried, especially the arsenic compounds that had been popular for ailments since the sixteenth century, and the quinine that worked so well against malaria. Their use reflected the conviction that chemical remedies could be found, a belief that had gained strength after Paul Ehrlich's development of a specific chemically prepared remedy for syphilis in the years shortly before the war.

The best actions that the healing professions could take in 1918, however, related more to easing the pain of the sufferers, not curing or preventing the disease. For that reason, nurses actually played a more important role than did physicians, and the shortages of nurses stood as real handicaps to meaningful responses to the epidemic. The needs of war called nurses into military duty, away from the homeland cities. And those nurses who remained (whether in London, Berlin, New York, or Calcutta) were further reduced by illness or death in the same pandemic that called for their services.

Popular responses in Europe and North America suggested that by 1918 populations had accepted and perhaps even internalized the dictates of modern biomedicine. There was widespread participation in the routines of fumigation and antiseptic sprays; crusades against spitting were led by members of the public; those who refused to wear gauze masks might be criticized by others. Such preventive medical suggestions as the inhalation of eucalyptus vapor became popular. But, at the same time, others refused to take the epidemic seriously, ridiculing the gauze masks and other required precautions. In Pittsburgh, schools remained open but authorities ruled that a child who sneezed should be sent home. Children began taking pepper to school to induce sneezing. And in the midst of general acceptance of medical dictates, an unknown number of people still turned to religion for succor. Drinking water in which were soaked bits of paper containing written extracts from the Koran, reported as a remedy in Nigeria, was perhaps an extreme example, but one that probably reflected some worldwide religious convictions about the pandemic.

In some places in the world (Nigeria, again, for example) some people responded to the epidemic by attempting flight from it. But generally, influenza spread so rapidly throughout the globe that flight was not feasible; no place was safe. That speed also meant that little sense of siege could develop in stricken communities; by the time people seriously resented wearing gauze masks, the danger had passed. The epidemic's reach was so universal that finding scapegoats among marginal minorities was unrealistic. Especially in those countries involved in the world war, reactions to the war situation overshadowed concerns about the epidemic.

UNRESOLVED HISTORICAL ISSUES

Questions persisted about different aspects of this pandemic after it passed, and some of those questions remain unresolved.

What caused the pandemic? At the time medical science searched for a germ, and different candidates were proposed, notably Pfeiffer's bacillus. No such answer proved satisfactory. In the 1920s, researchers isolated the first of the so-called filterable viruses, submicroscopic organisms that could pass through a filter that stopped bacteria; in 1933 an influenza virus was so isolated. But the 1918 influenza virus evidently had different effects from that of 1933; was it a different organism? The search for the 1918 virus gained ground in the 1990s, when samples of it began to be recovered from frozen corpses in Alaska, and from British and American pathology archives. In 2005, the U.S. Centers for Disease Control and Prevention announced the reconstruction of the virus, a bird disease that jumped directly to humans.

Where did it originate? Many historical accounts have argued that the 1918 pandemic began in the United States and spread initially to Europe with American troops crossing the Atlantic to join the war. In 1918 many associated the pandemic with the disturbances of the environment caused by the war, but its nearly simultaneous appearance in regions of the world far from the fighting fronts argued against that theory. Subsequently, the possibility that the virus spread to humans from another species has been considered, with swine and birds thought most likely. The major swine flu scare in the United States in 1976 stimulated interest in such possibilities, but their connection to the 1918 pandemic remains uncertain. Many influenza pandemics have seemingly originated in southern China. If the 1918 pandemic did not have much effect on the south Chinese population, would that suggest that the disease was already at home there? Unfortunately, the extent of the 1918 influenza in south China remains in dispute. Still another possibility: the 1918 influenza was not new in 1918, but had already been infecting people in the several years earlier. Bronchitis was widespread in 1917; was it an earlier wave of the 1918 flu?

Why was the 1918 influenza so lethal, relative to other, earlier influenza pandemics such as that of 1889? Was its virus simply genetically different in important ways? Was much of the world's population virgin soil for it, differing only in degree from the terrible experiences of the western Samoans? More specific: why were young adults affected so seriously? Part of the answer to that puzzle might lie in the 1889 pandemic. Were those exposed to it more resistant to the 1918 disease? If so, those over the age of 29 should have suffered less. Certainly those over 40 seemed to have suffered lower mortality rates than those in their twenties, but what about those in their thirties? In addition to those complications, some evidence calls into question the generally accepted vulnerability of young adults. In the Netherlands East Indies (Indonesia), the 1.5 million deaths seem to have been equally concentrated among the young, the old, and those in the middle.

Historians have also attempted to find correlations between vulnerability to influenza and such variables as class, race, gender, and ethnicity. Of these, class and gender seem most likely. Women generally suffered higher mortalities, perhaps because pregnant women were especially vulnerable, perhaps because women (as the primary caregivers themselves) were less likely to receive nursing care when they fell ill. Arguments linking influenza mortality to race and class in the United States have been inconclusive. African Americans suffered low mortality, American Indians high mortality, yet both were economically poor groups. In India, however, evidence that connects the disease to class and caste is clearer: the lower classes and castes suffered disproportionately. And everywhere, rural and urban locations seem to have been at equal risk.

Questions also remain about the larger social and political effects of the pandemic. In many places, especially in the West, those effects seem to have been surprisingly slight. In Africa and Asia, however, the higher levels of mortality had correspondingly longer-lasting consequences. In Nigeria, for example, the 1918 death toll was high enough to create a serious labor shortage that in turn affected food production levels. The British colonial authorities turned to another crop, cassava, whose cultivation required less labor, and hence changed both agricultural patterns and human diets. In India mortality in 1918 was so high that a steep drop in the birth rate followed in 1919, perhaps because of a large number of deaths in the population of young (potentially childbearing) adults, perhaps because high levels of sickness led to decreases in the rates of coition and marriage. The decrease in the growth of population was temporary, but decreased agricultural productivity rippled through the Indian economy in the following decades.

Alfred Crosby (1976) correctly called 1918 "America's Forgotten Pandemic." Why was it subsequently so neglected? It occurred during a huge war, one that was then simply called the Great War or the World War, one that dwarfed all previous conflicts. The war dominated the news of the time; the war accustomed people in the Western world to horrific rates of death among healthy young males. In addition, influenza—unlike some earlier great epidemics—did not create vivid images. Its symptoms shaded into the familiar ones of the common cold or the grippe. Deaths from influenza-related pneumonia were painful enough, but left no victims suddenly and shamefully collapsed in the street in their own excrement, as cholera had done. Those who recovered from influenza (and most did) were not disabled or disfigured as the victims of smallpox were. Those permanently disabled in the 1920s and 1930s were those with war wounds, not those recuperating from influenza. Few lasting economic, social, political, or intellectual effects could be traced to the 1918 pandemic. And a very important factor: the 1918 pandemic was also forgotten in the West because so many of its millions of victims were in Asia and Africa, perhaps 20 million in India alone. Many individual families in North America and Europe experienced the tragedy of the 1918 pandemic, but their numbers were vastly exceeded in places that were invisible to Western eyes.

Another circumstance, however, has recalled 1918–1919 to the Western (and American) mind: the prospect of another influenza pandemic, stirred by recurrent waves of new influenzas arising in Asia. Fears have been stoked by the widening understanding of the rapid mutations that influenza viruses undergo, and hence the difficulty of staying abreast of them with effective vaccines. (See volume 2, chapter 46.)

REFERENCES

Crosby, Alfred W. *Epidemic and Peace, 1918.* Westport, CT: Greenwood Press, 1976. (Now available as *America's Forgotten Pandemic: The Influenza of 1918.* Cambridge: Cambridge University Press, 1989.)

Keegan, John. *The First World War.* New York: Vintage, 2000.

Mills, I. D. "The 1918–1919 Influenza Pandemic—The Indian Experience." *Indian Economic and Social History Review* 23 (1986): 1–40.

SUGGESTED ADDITIONAL READING

Brown, Colin. "The Influenza Pandemic of 1918 in Indonesia." In *Death and Disease in Southeast Asia: Explorations in Social, Medical and Demographic History*, edited by Norman G. Owen, 235–256. Singapore: Oxford University Press, 1987.

Fanning, Patricia J. *Influenza and Inequality: One Town's Tragic Response to the Great Epidemic of 1918.* Amherst: University of Massachusetts Press, 2010.

Hildreth, Martha L. "The Influenza Epidemic of 1918–1919 in France: Contemporary Concepts of Aetiology, Therapy, and Prevention." *Social History of Medicine* 4 (1991): 278–294.

Honigsbaum, Mark. *A History of the Great Influenza Pandemics: Death, Panic and Hysteria, 1830–1920.* London: I. B. Tauris, 2014.

Johnson, Niall P. A. S., and Juergen Mueller. "Updating the Accounts: Global Mortality of the 1918–1920 'Spanish' Influenza Pandemic." *Bulletin of the History of Medicine* 76 (2002): 105–110.

Kolata, Gina. *Flu: The Story of the Great Influenza Pandemic of 1918 and the Search for the Virus That Caused It.* New York: Farrar, Straus and Giroux, 1999.

McLane, Ryan. "Influenza and Quarantine in Samoa." In *Quarantine: Local and Global Histories*, edited by Alison Bashford, 136–153. London: Palgrave, 2016.

Ohadike, Don C. "Diffusion and Physiological Responses to the Influenza Pandemic of 1918–1919 in Nigeria." *Social Science and Medicine* 32 (1991): 1393–1399.

Patterson, K. David. "The Influenza Epidemic of 1918–1919 in the Gold Coast." *Journal of African History* 24 (1983): 485–502.

Patterson, K. David, and Gerald F. Pyle. "The Geography and Mortality of the 1918 Influenza Epidemic." *Bulletin of the History of Medicine* 65 (1991): 4–21.

Phillips, Howard, and David Killingray, eds. *The Spanish Influenza Pandemic of 1918–1919: New Perspectives.* London: Routledge, 2003.

Porras Gallo, M. Isabel, and Ryan A. Davis. *The Spanish Influenza Pandemic of 1918–1919: Perspectives from the Iberian Peninsula and the Americas.* Rochester, NY: Rochester University Press, 2014.

Rice, Geoffrey W. *Black November: The 1918 Influenza Pandemic in New Zealand.* 2nd ed. Christchurch: Canterbury University Press, 2005.

Tomkins, Sandra M. "Colonial Administration in British Africa during the Influenza Epidemic of 1918–19." *Canadian Journal of African Studies* 28 (1994): 60–83.

Tomkins, Sandra M. "The Failure of Expertise: Public Health Policy in Britain during the 1918–19 Influenza Epidemic." *Social History of Medicine* 5 (1992): 435–454.

39

Poliomyelitis in the United States, 1945–1955

WHEN AND WHERE

In 1952 new cases of poliomyelitis in the United States numbered about 58,000. That number had been rising since before 1946, when 35,000 new cases appeared. Between World War I and World War II, the incidence of American poliomyelitis had generally been below 10,000 per year; in what had been the great previous epidemic year, 1916, the cases numbered about 27,000. The years between about 1945 and 1955 were therefore an unusual period of epidemic poliomyelitis in the United States, and that period is made more dramatic by the precipitous decline in the disease that followed. By the years between 1961 and 1965, new poliomyelitis cases averaged only 570 per year, a decline largely explained by the development of preventive vaccines.

While the number of people affected by poliomyelitis in the epidemic was substantial, other factors also contributed to the sense of fear that the epidemic engendered. Other diseases struck far more people, but most Americans of the period between 1945 and 1955 regarded poliomyelitis as *the* epidemic of the time. And the sudden conquest of it, involving a scientific triumph, was a correspondingly dramatic outcome.

Poliomyelitis really only came on the world stage in the twentieth century, although it had a long history as a widespread and usually not very serious childhood infection. Epidemics of the early twentieth century, especially that of 1916, involved the paralytic crippling of many of its victims, most of whom were young children. (In the 1916 New York epidemic, 95% of the cases occurred in children under age 10.) The disease was therefore also frequently called infantile paralysis. But in the 1930s, 1940s, and 1950s, its incidence progressively spread out over other age groups; in 1947 only 52% of New York City cases were under age 10, and 10% were adults. In its epidemic period, the disease was less clearly infantile paralysis, for all ages now seemed at risk. But the heart-rending spectacle of the crippled child also remained important in the public conception of the disease's terrors.

Poliomyelitis did not occur uniformly across the United States during the period between 1945 and 1955. Earlier in the century, it had been sporadically epidemic in particular places (e.g., New York in 1916 and Los Angeles in 1934), and while the overall incidence rose steeply that remained true in 1945–1955 as well. Thus, for example, the city of Rockford, Illinois, suffered 321 cases in 1945, in a population of about 85,000. For the United States as a whole, the incidence of poliomyelitis per 100,000 population per year never exceeded 40; the 1945 Rockford number was 378.

And while attention focused on the U.S. experience in the years after World War II, poliomyelitis rates then rose in Europe as well. Great Britain had never suffered more than about 1,500 cases per year before the war, but the number reached over 7,700 by 1947. In 1952 Copenhagen endured an incidence of 238 poliomyelitis cases per 100,000 population, a very serious epidemic indeed.

SIGNIFICANCE

The sudden end of the U.S. poliomyelitis epidemic stood as perhaps the most dramatic success against disease achieved by modern biomedicine. The epidemic thus has a significant place in the annals of disease in part because of its demise (see the "Responses" section).

Epidemic is, as the preface to this book argues, an imprecise word. At least to the general public, outbreaks of disease are called epidemics not only when their incidence rises above its normal rate but also when they catch public attention for some less quantifiable cause. In the United States in the first 60 years of the twentieth century, fear of poliomyelitis sometimes resulted in public hysteria, and that fact alone confers further significance on this epidemic. It was significant in part because people *called* it a significant epidemic. The pictures of the victims of the disease contributed to that perception: children struck down by crippling paralysis, sometimes fatally, before their promise could be fulfilled. Those pictures were more painful because the epidemic occurred at a time when public confidence in the powers of scientific biomedicine had reached new heights. Surely a cure must be just around the corner. When efforts to find the cure seemed to fail, dashed hopes led to greater hysteria.

A relatively new social phenomenon—a privately funded philanthropic pressure group—generated some of the pictures of the popular epidemic of poliomyelitis. The National Foundation for Infantile Paralysis (begun in 1938) played important roles in both the construction of the epidemic in public opinion and in the direction of the research mustered against it. The roles thus pioneered by the foundation would become part of Western, and especially American, responses to later epidemics and indeed to other social crises.

Finally, the development and deployment of successful preventive vaccines would stand as a case study of difficult questions for the relationship among science, medicine, society, and ethical standards (see the "Unresolved Historical Issues" section).

BACKGROUND

The rise of poliomyelitis in the United States (and in the Western world generally) was paradoxically related to improvements in public health, and especially to improvements in sanitation. Apparently, poliomyelitis, an infection caused by a virus, has long been found in human populations, and before the twentieth century probably was a common and not very serious childhood disease. It was not identified as a separate disease, however; for most children its symptoms included only a mild fever and (if the nervous system was affected at all) some minor aches and pains. Occasionally more permanent muscle weakness or even paralysis resulted, but those cases were not associated with the widespread minor fevers of childhood, which had many and largely undifferentiated causes.

What changed that picture was the growing emphasis on sanitation, stemming first from a general conviction (first gaining great strength in the eighteenth century) that diseases had their origins in impure environments, and then from the growing appeal of the germ theory at the end of the nineteenth century. To prevent disease, eliminate germs. The United States, Canada, and the countries of northern Europe took the lead in the sanitation crusades of the late nineteenth and early twentieth centuries, and it was in those countries that poliomyelitis first appeared as a crippling, even fatal, disease. The first identifiable epidemics of poliomyelitis struck Norway, Sweden, and the United States in the late nineteenth century. Scholars of the disease now believe that successful sanitation systems prevented the widespread infections in young children that would prevent later, more serious, cases; the result was the inadvertent creation of a virgin soil population for the poliomyelitis virus.

A revealing study in the 1950s showed an inverse relationship between infant mortality rates and the incidence of paralytic poliomyelitis; places with high infant mortality rates (e.g., Egypt, Algeria, and Mexico) had minimal rates of poliomyelitis, while places with low infant mortality rates (e.g., Sweden, Australia, and the United States) had high incidences of poliomyelitis. A graph illustrating the contrasts is in Paul's work (1971, 367). Widespread infections (of many kinds) in infancy both resulted in high mortality and in immunity for the survivors; the sanitary regimens of the West preserved far more infants, but left them more vulnerable to later poliomyelitis infections.

American perceptions of the disease changed considerably between the first major epidemic in 1916 and the post–World War II epidemic. In 1916 poliomyelitis was associated with the dirt of the lower orders, especially of recent immigrants (see volume 2, chapter 37). The pattern of infection in that epidemic often did not support that class-based association and that contributed to weakening belief in it. The infection of a prominent American political figure, Franklin D. Roosevelt, with poliomyelitis in 1921 also suggested that the disease could afflict the affluent. It was therefore perhaps more respectable, but at the same time more generally threatening; it could not be contained safely in urban slums.

The National Foundation for Infantile Paralysis, founded in 1938, was intimately associated with Roosevelt, who had been elected president of the United States in 1932. (Roosevelt had established a private foundation in 1927 to support a mineral spring spa in Warm Springs, Georgia, as a therapeutic place for poliomyelitis victims; that foundation evolved into the National Foundation for Infantile Paralysis.) The foundation's leaders, especially Basil O'Connor, quickly proved masters of public relations and fundraising. Their campaigns, especially the March of Dimes and the annual polio poster child, focused the attention of the country on the disease, its tragic but gallant victims, and the hope that science, properly mobilized, would find a cure. Poliomyelitis became a widespread popular concern in large part due to the foundation's efforts.

Perhaps because it was now such a general concern, poliomyelitis now inspired somewhat different fears than those of 1916. Any place where crowds gathered in the summer now seemed dangerous, not just the teeming quarters of immigrant groups. Public bathing places—swimming pools, lakes in parks—inspired particular dread for the parents of American children in the 1930s, 1940s, and early 1950s.

The 1945–1955 epidemic also played on a stage set by the events of World War II. Epidemics among troop detachments (e.g., in the Mediterranean and in the Philippines) illustrated that infantile paralysis did not confine itself to infants. More important, the combatants in the war had massively mobilized science against their enemies. Radar, the insecticide DDT, penicillin, the guided missile, and the atomic bomb all appeared during the war. Penicillin quickly mastered venereal diseases (and others); surely poliomyelitis could be mastered as well, and the National Foundation in effect declared war on it.

HOW IT WAS UNDERSTOOD AT THE TIME

Since the work of Karl Landsteiner in 1908–1909, it had been generally agreed that a virus caused poliomyelitis and that the virus spread the disease contagiously from one person to another. Less clear were the precise identification and description of the virus, and its pathway into the body. Was it passed through the respiratory system, entering the body through the nasal passages? Or was it swallowed with food, such as contaminated milk? Was the public habit of spitting dangerous? Did insects, especially flies, play a role? Once in the body, did it settle in the nervous system, as its paralytic symptoms suggested? Or was its first target the digestive system, with the nerves only reached in some cases later? The long-dominant figure in American thinking about poliomyelitis, Simon Flexner (1863–1946), was convinced that the nerves were the first and principal target of the virus.

By the 1930s, however, the consensus view had moved away from Flexner, and the digestive system seemed the most likely answer. If so, a preventive vaccine might be easier to develop, especially because it might be more safely tested; some preparation of a modified or weakened virus would form the basis of such a vaccine, but if the nerves were its first destination any vaccine, however attenuated, carried the risk of immediate paralysis for those on whom it was tested. The odds were improved if the nerves were only secondarily the targets of the virus.

(Belief that poliomyelitis was caused by a virus led to emphasis on preventive vaccines, not on curative agents such as antibiotics. Penicillin, and other later antibiotics, had proved effective as cures for bacterial diseases, but not for viral ones.)

In the years after 1945, research into possible vaccines followed one of two different paths. Some hoped to develop a vaccine from an attenuated or weakened polio virus, while others looked to a vaccine from an inactive or killed virus.

The more general public understanding of poliomyelitis focused not on its biology, but on its pathological symptoms. Infantile paralysis was still a popular term for it, despite the shifting of the ages afflicted by it; *paralysis* especially was a focus, with the images of crutches and braces, orthopedic beds to enforce immobility, and the Drinker respirators (iron lungs) that enabled paralyzed torsos to breathe as described in the next section.

RESPONSES

Many of the responses to the 1945–1955 epidemic continued those followed in the 1920s and 1930s. Because attempts at the cure of poliomyelitis had been consistently disappointing, most responses focused on therapy that would ease symptoms, and perhaps reverse some paralysis. Two schools of thought, almost diametrically opposed, existed about such therapy. One approach, the more dominant one in the United States, urged the immobility of the stricken limbs, in effect arguing that rest might restore some function. Advocates of this method placed arms and legs in plaster casts and confined patients in complicated beds. Generally, this approach was favored by the National Foundation for Infantile Paralysis, which devoted some of the funds it raised to supplying such gear. The Drinker respirator, or iron lung, a device that encased the body in a metal tube within which pressure alternated, was developed in 1929 to assist breathing by weakened chest muscles; the National Foundation for Infantile Paralysis also promoted and funded the supply of these machines.

An alternate method, which emphasized the stimulation of afflicted muscles with exercise, was especially promoted by the Australian nurse Elizabeth Kenny, who had many followers in the United States. She established a clinic in Minneapolis that applied her approach. Relations between the National Foundation for Infantile Paralysis and Kenny were tense; the poliomyelitis epidemic seemed to generate rivalries, perhaps because American society's obsession with the disease magnified the stakes.

The National Foundation for Infantile Paralysis had also decided to support the basic research that might lead to a vaccine, as well as to provide respirators and other therapeutic machinery. The foundation, appealing for funds from the public, felt pressured to hold out the promise of a cure as soon as possible. Those contributing to the March of Dimes (given a new symbolic twist when the image of Roosevelt was put on the 10-cent coin after his death in 1945) wanted to hear that the end of poliomyelitis was near.

In the late 1940s and early 1950s, a number of different research teams worked on potential vaccines. Hilary Koprowski, working for a pharmaceutical company, revealed in 1951 that he had tried a vaccine on a small group of volunteers. In the next year Jonas Salk of the University of Pittsburgh began trials of a vaccine, prepared from a *killed,* inactive virus; some of Salk's subjects were from a home for crippled children, and others were adult residents of a state school for the mentally retarded. Salk announced in 1953 that his vaccine had been successful. The year 1952 had been the worst of the epidemic so far, and 1953 promised to be even worse. In that situation the National Foundation for Infantile Paralysis decided to throw its resources behind a massive trial of Salk's vaccine, in effect gambling on a quick and dramatic victory. In the spring of 1954, the foundation arranged for

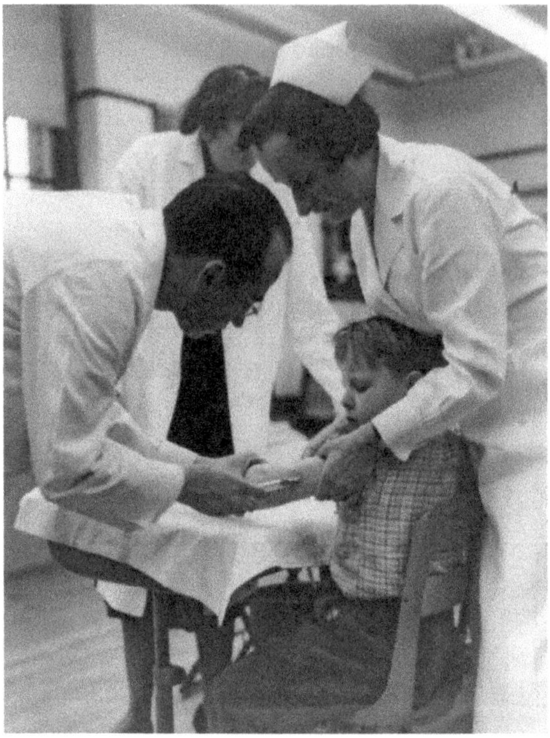

Dr. Jonas Salk, who developed a pioneering polio vaccine, inoculates a child at an elementary school in 1954. (Library of Congress)

1.8 million American children, mostly between the ages of six and nine, to take part in a test of the Salk vaccine. Some would receive the vaccine, some would receive a placebo, and others would be left untreated. The results, announced on April 12, 1955, electrified the country; 200,000 American children had been vaccinated against poliomyelitis with no ill effects. The federal government's National Institutes of Health quickly licensed the Salk vaccine for general use. Within weeks *four million* Americans received the vaccine.

The triumph was not unalloyed, however. In the summer of 1955 a disturbing, if small, epidemic pattern of poliomyelitis appeared among some of those who had been vaccinated. It developed that over 200 cases of the disease could be traced to vaccines prepared by a single California laboratory. Three-fourths of the cases resulted in paralysis, and eleven died. This "Cutter incident," the result of production errors in the Cutter Laboratory, led to doubts about the speed with which the vaccine had been tested and approved. Did the foundation press its agenda too aggressively? Did the federal authorities license the vaccine too quickly?

Meanwhile other lines of research on vaccines were being pursued, especially those involving attenuated (as opposed to killed) viruses. Albert Sabin of the University of Cincinnati prepared such a vaccine and first tested it on himself, his family, and 200 inmates of a federal penitentiary. With the support of the World Health Organization (and the Kenny organization, still at odds with the National Foundation for Infantile Paralysis), the Sabin vaccine was widely tested in Mexico, Belgian African colonies, and the Soviet Union in 1957. Its results were also spectacularly successful. Sabin's vaccine had two advantages: it promised to confer lifetime immunity (the Salk vaccine needed repeated applications), and it could be administered orally rather than by injection. Although American government and philanthropy had originally backed the Salk vaccine, by the early 1960s the attenuated vaccine had become the world's choice.

The responses of American governments to the 1945–1955 epidemic reflected changing perceptions of the disease. In 1916 (see volume 2, chapter 37) U.S. city governments reacted with aggressive public health measures; John Paul, a leading poliomyelitis authority, later called 1916 "the high-water mark in attempts at enforcement of isolation and quarantine measures" (Paul 1971, 148). Those measures reflected a belief that germs spread disease and that public health could contain their spread. In subsequent years, the virus had proved more elusive than had been hoped, for its paths of infection remained debatable. Perhaps for that reason, much of the response to the 1945–1955 epidemic came from private agencies, not government ones. Private foundations supported the provision of therapeutic facilities and their instruments; a private foundation organized the sweeping field trials of a vaccine. Only after those trials were complete did the federal government agency license the results; government thus *permitted* action and did not *initiate* it.

UNRESOLVED HISTORICAL ISSUES

The application of vaccines that ended the poliomyelitis epidemic in the years after 1955 was an undoubted, and huge, success. Their development and application, however, raised important questions about the roles of biomedical science in modern society, and those questions remain matters of debate.

At some point in the development of such vaccines, they must be tested on human subjects. Which humans are chosen and why? Do those chosen give their consent freely for an experiment that may be perilous? How many people must be tested before results are conclusive? The Cutter incident illustrated other questions: How many safety checks are needed to guarantee a harmless product? Is such a guarantee possible?

Whenever a new cure or preventive measure is developed, should it be rushed to the widest public as soon as possible? In effect, American authorities in 1955 balanced the desirable immunization of several million against the possible spread of the disease to hundreds or more, if more Cutter incidents had occurred. Should the National Institutes of Health have withheld licensure of the Salk vaccine for another year so that more tests could be performed, or that more controls could be placed on production facilities? Had it done so, how many of the millions of those immunized in 1955 would have succumbed to poliomyelitis?

To what extent did the nearly hysterical pressure of aroused public opinion influence such decisions? How much was that public opinion manipulated by a philanthropic organization seeking to justify or aggrandize itself? Is the allocation of research resources, or of therapy, dependent on successful public relations? Such questions remain alive in the early twenty-first century.

As poliomyelitis has persisted in the world into the twenty-first century, these questions have persisted with it, and other uncertainties have joined them as well. For while mass vaccination halted the poliomyelitis epidemic in mid-twentieth-century America and elsewhere in the Western world, its eradication elsewhere has been more difficult. Those eradication efforts have included systematic vaccination of the population together with identification and isolation of active cases of the disease. Identifying active cases of a disease that may manifest itself as only a minor childhood ailment (thus differing from smallpox infections) poses a problem, in the absence of laboratory tests; the virus may have reached a victim either through the air or through food and water, so that its presence in the environment may be complex. The necessary public health infrastructure of a society may be crippled—or entirely incapacitated—by poverty, while geographic isolation may frustrate well-meaning attempts to reach it from without. Warfare as well as other civic turmoils certainly add further difficulties.

Active social or political resistance to eradication has also arisen. Vaccination may be opposed on religious or other ideological grounds, sometimes fanatically, by a society or some of its members. Recurring disputes about different vaccines and their efficacy, added to long-standing rivalries that persist among different nongovernmental agencies, also contribute to uncertainties in eradication campaigns. And overhanging all such efforts are very difficult questions about the allocation of resources. Can an all-out eradication effort on a disease, which however dramatic affects relatively few, be justified when scarce resources might be better employed on more general health initiatives?

Such difficulties may be illustrated by reviewing several twenty-first century examples of persistent poliomyelitis, undertaken by international eradication efforts. Such efforts evolved in the 1970s and 1980s, initially in Latin America, with the involvement of a variety of supporting organizations such as the World Health Organization, UNICEF, and Rotary International. In the early twenty-first century, those efforts were consolidated in the Global Polio Eradication Initiative (GPEI) as an arm of the WHO, and that organization has struggled since its founding with polio's apparent intractability. Those struggles were evident in a report issued by the GPEI in May 2014 that identified 10 countries in Africa thought to be at risk of a polio outbreak, which joined 7 other states already infected; critics argued that the report showed that the GPEI had been ineffective. Specific illustrative examples:

1. *Syria.* Resistance to the government of Bashar al-Assad became an outright civil war by 2011, which created a massive refugee crisis as what became millions of Syrians fled the zones of fighting. On the move they found themselves in squalid tent cities with minimal sanitation or sewage, in which epidemic diseases flourished—including polio, which appeared in Syria in 2011 after having apparently been eradicated 15 years earlier. Massive international efforts at vaccination followed, hampered by political tensions; for example, the Assad regime refused to allow vaccines brought from its international "enemies," such as Turkey.
2. *Nigeria.* The most populous country in Africa had been considered one of the last strongholds of endemic polio, but the disease had seemingly been eradicated by 2014. When cases were reported in August 2016, a huge response by GPEI followed, only to have another renewal of disease in June 2018, perhaps now originating with a mutant version of polio that had survived in the orally administered ("Sabin") vaccine. Nigeria's huge population, beset by ethnic and religious tensions and poverty, has made systematic vaccination a challenge, especially given the activities of the radical Islamic sect Boko Haram that is murderously opposed to vaccination.

3. *Democratic Republic of the Congo.* Another country with a large population, poverty, and serious levels of internal turmoil, Congo also has harbored the frightening Ebola virus (see volume 2, chapter 48), and recurrent polio outbreaks have furthered complicated public health. Here, as in Nigeria, a 2018 outbreak arose from a virus that had mutated from "Sabin" orally administered vaccine; such vaccines (see the "Responses" section) employ a live virus in their preparation. Poverty, combined with geographic isolation, have meant that many Congolese children remain entirely unvaccinated.
4. *Pakistan.* Pakistan had long been considered the strongest redoubt of persistent polio, but eradicators had made headway by 2012. Then in 2016 the number of cases suddenly reached 306, representing 85% of the world's total. The GPEI, through one of its arms, strongly criticized the Pakistan government for the failure. An important problem was the long-standing struggle between the government and the Taliban, the radical Islamic movement that effectively controlled swatches of the country; the Taliban opposed vaccination on religious grounds, killing vaccinators, especially women. Larger geopolitical issues entered as well. Beginning with the "9/11" attacks in the United States, what came to seen by some as a Western (and particularly American) war on Islam began: the invasion of Iraq, the bombing of Afghanistan, the capture of Osama bin Laden in Pakistan, and the use of drones in warfare. Was vaccination a Western plot, perhaps even an attempt to poison people?

REFERENCE

Paul, John R. *A History of Poliomyelitis.* New Haven, CT: Yale University Press, 1971.

SUGGESTED ADDITIONAL READING

Abraham, Thomas. *Polio: The Odyssey of Eradication.* London: Hurst and Company, 2018.

Closser, Svea. *Chasing Polio in Pakistan: Why the World's Largest Public Health Initiative Might Fail.* Nashville, TN: Vanderbilt University Press, 2010.

Gould, Tony. *A Summer Plague: Polio and Its Survivors.* New Haven, CT: Yale University Press, 1995.

Oshinski, David M. *Polio: An American Story.* Oxford: Oxford University Press, 2005.

Rogers, Naomi. *Dirt and Disease: Polio before FDR.* New Brunswick, NJ: Rutgers University Press, 1990.

Smallman-Raynor, Matthew R., and A. D. Cliff. *Poliomyelitis: A World Geography.* Oxford: Oxford University Press, 2006.

Smith, Jane S. *Patenting the Sun: Polio and the Salk Vaccine.* New York: William Morrow, 1990.

Wilson, Daniel J. *Living with Polio: The Epidemic and Its Survivors.* Chicago: University of Chicago Press, 2005.

40

Seventh Cholera Pandemic, 1961–

WHEN AND WHERE

The modern era's seventh widespread cholera pandemic began in Southeast Asia in 1961. The pandemic then advanced in two further phases, the first between 1970 and the early 1980s, and the next beginning in 1991. Each of those subsequent phases saw the spread of cholera into different areas of the world. Since 1991, cholera has continued to be endemic and at times epidemic, especially but not exclusively in Africa, and has surged in periods of social or ecological breakdown.

In 1961 cholera broke out on the island of Sulawesi (Indonesia), quickly reaching populous Java, and from there spread rapidly through Southeast Asia (including Sarawak, the Philippines, and Hong Kong) in the same year. In 1962 cases were reported in Borneo and New Guinea in Indonesia, and in Taiwan; by 1963 the disease reached into East Asia (Korea) and South Asia (Burma, Bangladesh). In 1964 and 1965 the wave of cholera moved westward, reaching first India and then Iran, Iraq, and Bahrain. The pandemic then apparently stalled, with no further advance in the late 1960s.

Then in the autumn of 1970, cholera began a new and dramatic expansion that rapidly carried it into both Africa and Europe. Three nearly simultaneous paths of infection occurred. The first followed an old cholera route from western Asia into the then-Soviet Union, reaching Astrakhan on the Caspian Sea and Odessa on the Black Sea. The second was also familiar from earlier cholera pandemics: from the Arabian Peninsula to both other places in the Near East and East Africa. The third path illustrated the new diffusing powers of modern transportation, for cholera suddenly appeared in the West African state of Guinea. It almost certainly arrived by air, brought by a passenger (or passengers) on an airplane. In the early stages of the pandemic in West Africa, about 50% of those infected by cholera died; 11 West African countries reported cholera cases by the end of 1970.

In 1971 cholera spread across East Central Africa (Kenya, Uganda), into southwestern Africa (Angola), and into Spain and Portugal in Europe. In that year the number of reported cases worldwide was 155,000. Particular attention in the West in 1972 focused on another example of aircraft transmission: cholera infected a flight carrying 393 people from London to Sydney, probably coming on the plane with food prepared in Bahrain, a stopover. Forty-three cases of cholera were subsequently reported in Australia and New Zealand. That frightened Westerners, but in the same year over 44,000 cases were reported in Indonesia alone.

Europe's principal cholera scare occurred in 1973, when the disease struck Naples, Bari, and Cagliari in Italy. Cases were relatively few, but Naples particularly had a tragic history of cholera and now, as had happened in 1910–1911, the Italian tourist trade was hurt by fears of an epidemic. In 1974 another historic reprise threatened, when Muslim pilgrims carried cholera from Mecca back to their homeland, in this case Nigeria, where 90 new cases were reported after a flight from Arabia arrived.

By the late 1970s a pattern of "widespread endemicity" had emerged, in which (by 1984) 93 countries in Asia, Europe, and Africa had reported cases of cholera. This pattern could be broken by "occasional recrudescences to serious epidemic proportions" (Barua 1992, 22). An example of such an epidemic occurred in the Maldives in 1978, when 11,000 people (in a total population of about 200,000) fell ill with cholera.

The third stage of this pandemic began abruptly in January 1991, when cholera reached the Americas. A sudden epidemic spread along the coast of Peru in that month, probably brought on by climatic changes that warmed Peru's coastal waters. In the following year, cholera spread through Latin America, and by the end of the year Latin America reported 391,000 cases of cholera, about two-thirds of the worldwide total. By February 1992, 18 American countries had been infected. A number of different human migrations may have carried cholera with them: for example, migrant shrimp workers moving from Peru to Ecuador, itinerant preachers within Central America, and drug smugglers, all the way from the Amazon basin to Mexico.

After 1991 cholera has become endemic in parts of the world, and reached epidemic proportions in some times and places as well. By the late 1990s, Africa had emerged as its prime locus; in 2009 that continent had 217,000 cases, representing 98% of the world total. Mortality rates have generally been much lower than those experienced in earlier pandemics; the 50% mortality found in west Africa in 1970 was exceptional, for it soon fell, both in Africa and elsewhere. In 1991 the African mortality rate was 9%, and by 2009 it had dropped to slightly over 2%. That 2% represented 4,900 African deaths. (Reasons for these declines will be discussed shortly.)

In the twenty-first century, however, major environmental and ecological changes have combined with social and political conflicts (including wars and failing states) to create zones where cholera flourishes. As will be seen below, a variety of countries in the world have suffered—and continue to suffer—the ravages of cholera.

SIGNIFICANCE

The seventh pandemic demonstrated that cholera was still a menace, even though both its cause and the effective means of prevention were apparently well understood in the late twentieth century. And despite that understanding, cholera still had the power to frighten, as the shock to the Italian tourist industry in 1973 and the more general damage to the Peruvian economy in 1991 (see the "Unresolved Issues" section) illustrate.

Public health and biomedical responses to the pandemic were in many ways effective, but events during the pandemic (especially since the 1990s) illustrate that their effectiveness depends on the preservation of a peaceful and prosperous civil society. As will be shown later, the dramatic cholera outbreaks in, for example, Congo (1994), Haiti (2010), Yemen (2017–), and Zimbabwe (2008–), demonstrate the consequences of the failure of such societies.

BACKGROUND

In the decades before the seventh pandemic, a mild form of cholera persisted as an endemic disease in Indonesia, with occasional outbreaks elsewhere in Southeast Asia. The spread of the pandemic after 1961 may have marked the first widespread appearance of a different variety of the causative organism *Vibrio cholerae* 01 El Tor. It differed from the previously dominant biotype in two ways: its immediate effect on its victim was less drastic, and it could thus remain with its still living human for a longer period. Those victims could therefore travel and excrete the organism into the environment without attracting attention. Cholera infections might thus be more likely to move distances and the continuing diffusion has thus continued.

Modern air transportation and international migration have played important roles in the pandemic. Perhaps even more important have been a panoply of environmental changes. In the largest sense global warming has cooperated with rising sea levels to create favorable conditions for *Vibrio cholerae*, especially in those coastal waters where sewage accumulates and where fertilizers have entered the mix.

HOW IT WAS UNDERSTOOD AT THE TIME

Medical opinion in general had accepted the ideas that a microorganism (*Vibrio cholerae*) was responsible for the disease, that it entered the body from infected food or water, and that epidemics most often spread when the infected individuals excreted the organism into water supplies. Understanding that different varieties of the microorganism exist has been increasingly realized during the seventh pandemic.

RESPONSES

At different times and in different places during the seventh pandemic, medicine responded to it with vaccinations, antibiotics, and therapies to replace body fluids. Of these the last emerged as the most successful; vaccines and antibiotics both had mixed records.

One approach, which combined mass vaccinations with the isolation of infected individuals and regions, was attempted in the early stages of the pandemic, for example, in Egypt in 1970. In general, such approaches seemed to have little effect on the spread of cholera. Thus in 1986 India chose not to insist on using the cholera vaccine to protect people on an internal pilgrimage; the Indian government chose instead to trust sanitation measures and careful surveillance to hold cholera at bay. And by the late 1970s, other countries placed growing faith in the curative power of antibiotics, especially tetracycline. But the over-prescription of tetracycline, especially in Africa, led to increasing the microorganism's powers of resistance to it, and a procession of new antibiotics attempted, with limited success, to keep pace with the organism's mutations. However, by 2013 greater reliance began to be placed on vaccination.

These approaches gave way to the highly successful fluid replacement therapy, the original idea for which went back to the nineteenth century. A cholera infection was so lethal because it led to a sudden and catastrophic loss of body fluids. Despite that fact, much nineteenth-century therapy was purgative, driven by the belief that humoral imbalance needed restoration. Initially, a small minority of healers disagreed and argued that fluids should be replaced, not purged. By the time of the sixth pandemic, early in the twentieth century, Leonard Rogers (a British scientist working in India) had developed a successful method of fluid replacement. During the seventh pandemic, the technique of fluid replacement administered orally supplanted the previous intravenous infusion, and that became the favored therapy. The much lower mortality from cholera in the seventh pandemic has been largely due to the use of fluid replacement therapy.

UNRESOLVED ISSUES

Conflicts between perceived national interests and responsibilities to world health have long characterized responses to cholera pandemics. The seventh pandemic was no exception. In 1980 Bangladesh stopped reporting cholera cases, and in 1982 the Philippines followed. They were reacting to "excessive trade restrictions applied by a few countries" (Barua 1992, 22); fear of cholera could quickly lead to trade embargoes and a decline in tourist business. The 1991 epidemic in Peru led to a 20% decline in the country's exports, so the tensions between national prosperity and international health remain.

Sanitation problems, especially the inadequate disposal of sewage and provision of clean water, account for much of the persistence of cholera. World poverty therefore remains an important and unresolved issue, and social breakdowns, states failing, and warfare continue to create conditions favorable for cholera epidemics; it may therefore be that possible eradication of cholera is an "unresolved question," as the following examples illustrate.

1. The Democratic Republic of the Congo (DRC), where in July 1994 a cholera epidemic commenced in which in a three-week period as many as up to 3,000 deaths occurred on some days, and by mid-August the toll had reached 13,000. The epicenter of this disaster was the city of Goma, which adjoins the border with Rwanda; in July 1994, it was overwhelmed by perhaps one million

refugees fleeing the genocidal slaughter that involved the rival Rwandan ethnic groups of Hutus and Tutsis. In that situation, water and sewage facilities in even the most advanced societies would have collapsed; the DRC—a large, populous country long struggling with poverty, its own tense ethnic mixtures, the legacies of former imperial rule, and government corruption—already had had dangerously endemic cholera outbreaks before 1994. So, while the 1994 refugee crisis illustrates an exceptionally fraught circumstance, it came to a country where a pattern of cholera had been set. By 2009 the DRC had suffered over 300,000 cases of cholera since 1991 (Echenberg 2011, 134).

2. Zimbabwe has become an example of a failed state in which cholera has found a home. Long under the increasingly despotic rule of Robert Mugabe (between 1980 and 2017), the country gradually slid into dire poverty, with rising mortality rates, rampant inflation, and homelessness. By 2004 the country—once a significant grain exporter—had become dependent on food imports. Since the 1980s, Zimbabwe had also been ravaged by HIV/AIDS (see volume 2, chapter 41), and cholera had joined in by 1992, appearing in strength annually. Then in August 2008 what became one of the worst cholera epidemics in African history began, not to wane until June 2009, by which time there had been 128,000 cases of cholera and 5,600 deaths. In its face, Mugabe's government only proclaimed an emergency in December 2008, while it also resisted international assistance. (Such aid, while sometimes ill-informed about local conditions, had been important in bringing the 1994 crisis in the DRC under control.) As late as September 2018, after Mugabe's ouster, sewers in Harare (the capital city) remained a "big problem" that had been blocked and "never repaired for at least two months" (Moyo and Perez-Pena 2018).

3. Haiti has suffered a series of natural disasters in the twenty-first century, including (but not limited to) hurricane-related floods in 2004 and 2008. Then in January 2010 a massive earthquake left 220,000 dead, over 300,000 injured, and a seriously damaged infrastructure that left a door open for cholera. As a result, 730,000 Haitians were sickened, and 9,300 deaths followed, but *Vibrio cholerae* had actually been inadvertently introduced in a way that illustrated the rapid movement of disease through international political and relief-related traffic. All the foregoing natural disasters had both contributed to and coincided with a long period of political turmoil and violence in Haiti that in turn fed a long-standing history of international intervention; in 2010 a team of United Nations peacekeeping troops had been dispatched to Haiti from distant Nepal, and they unwittingly were accompanied by the cholera organism. Genome evidence showed that "the Haiti strain is virtually identical to one circulating in Nepal at the time," and the United Nations offered a belated apology to Haitians in 2016 ("U.N. Makes U-Turn on Cholera" 2016).

4. Yemen became the site of one of the world's most serious cholera epidemics in 2017 (Volume 2, chapter 51, "Cholera Epidemic, Yemen, 2017–?"), an outbreak that occurred during a civil war—complicated by international rivalries—that resulted in massive destruction of cities and collapse of infrastructures. The country has been wracked by tensions and violence between factions for decades, and the most recent of those has pitted the reigning Sunni

> regime, backed by Saudi Arabia (with U.S. military assistance) against the breakaway Shiite, Houthi, population that is supported by Iran. The latter group has controlled the capital city, Sanaa, and the northern area of Yemen, and the capital (a city with perhaps three million people) has been relentlessly bombed by the Sunni government and its allies. Cholera began spiking there in April 2017; by June, the WHO estimated that 14.5 million people had lost access to safe water supplies, perhaps 5,000 new cases of cholera occurred daily, and the death toll stood at 7,300. It did not stand there long. In July, the number infected reached 320,000, and by February 2018 the total of the infected topped one million. Since 2013, determined international efforts have increased the manufacture of cholera vaccines; but in "conflict-torn places such as Yemen, vaccines don't help if vaccinators can't reach those who need them" (Kupferschmidt 2018).

Meanwhile, conflicted opinions about cholera's history and significance continue. Some of the issues raised in and about earlier cholera pandemics still draw historians to different conclusions; among those are the views of such epidemics as windows through which to assess class, ethnic, or cultural fault lines, now with an increasing emphasis on Asia and Africa; the use of cholera policies as an example of a "tool of empire," whether empire is politically official or unofficial; and the persistence of "us" versus "them" mentalities and policies. In addition to those continuing sources of controversy, the understanding of the multiplying varieties of *Vibrio cholerae* has reopened old questions about the relation between epidemics and their environments. Is it enough to say that cholera is "caused" by the actions of a bacterium, when changing climates or land-and-water configurations, for example, determine an epidemic's course or even origin? Do such environmental changes themselves contribute or cause the varieties of *Vibrio cholerae* to arise in the first place?(See also the earlier chapters 19, 21, 22, 25, 28, and 32 in this volume, in which continuing questions appear.)

REFERENCES

Kupferschmidt, Kai. "Use of Cholera Vaccines Expands, Raising Hopes." *Science* 359 no. 6376 (February 9, 2018): 620–621.

Moyo, Geffrey, and Richard Perez-Pena. "Zimbabwe Tries to Stem an Outbreak of Cholera." *New York Times*, September 12, 2018, A4.

"U.N. Makes U-Turn on Cholera." *Science* 353 no. 6302 (August 26, 2016): 850.

SUGGESTED ADDITIONAL READING

Barua, Dhiman, and William B. Greenough III, eds. *Cholera.* New York: Plenum, 1992.

Echenberg, Myron. *Africa in the Time of Cholera: A History of Pandemics from 1817 to the Present.* Cambridge: Cambridge University Press, 2011.

Hamlin, Christopher. *Cholera: The Biography.* Oxford: Oxford University Press, 2009.

Mukharji, Projit Bihari. "The 'Cholera Cloud' in the Nineteenth-Century 'British World': History of an Object-Without-an-Essence." *Bulletin of the History of Medicine* 86 (2012): 303–332.

41

Contemporary HIV/AIDS Pandemic, 1980–

WHEN AND WHERE

The syndrome later called AIDS first came to public attention in the United States. In the next several years, it seemed concentrated in that country, but by the end of the decade its worldwide spread began to be realized. Since then, AIDS and the HIV infection that leads to it have become a true pandemic. Its effects have especially ravaged sub-Saharan Africa. But, if anything, AIDS in the early twenty-first century has blanketed more of the world than ever.

While early medical attention focused on the United States, the worldwide HIV-AIDS pandemic had its origins in Africa in the early twentieth century. In about 1920, chimpanzees infected with a "simian immunodeficiency virus" (SIV) closely related to a "human immunodeficiency virus" (HIV-1) came in contact with people (perhaps hunters) in Cameroon, where infection spread from the apes to people. They, in turn, rapidly moved by river routes into the then-Belgian Congo (now the DRC) and from there diffused through both river and railway lines in the DRC. It is uncertain when the earliest cases of AIDS can be identified, but by the 1950s, they had appeared in Kinshasa (then Leopoldville); by the 1970s, an HIV epidemic existed in that city at least. The epidemic had remained "hidden" for two reasons: first, its long and uncertain incubation period (between the infection and the onset of symptoms) made the dating of its "appearance" impossible; and second, those "symptoms," when they appeared, were those of other infections, clearly identified with other ailments. Thus, in the 1970s and early 1980s, HIV-AIDS spread largely unrecognized through sub-Saharan Africa.

In June and July 1981, accounts of mysterious ailments appeared in the *Morbidity and Mortality Weekly Reports*, a publication of the U.S. government's Centers for Disease Control (as it was then called). The reports told of outbreaks of unusual infections and forms of pneumonia and cancer among previously healthy men in New York and California. In all the cases, the immune systems of the victims had collapsed, for then-unknown reasons. By the end of 1981, 189 such cases had been reported in the United States, and in the next few years the number escalated rapidly: 650 in 1982, over 2,100 in 1983, over 4,500 in 1984. Many of the cases proved to be fatal, as the victims could not resist their infections.

These cases of failed immune systems and subsequent infections seemed (at this stage) to concentrate in certain populations, above all among male homosexuals. As the search for the cause of the immune problem proceeded, for a time in 1981 and 1982 the syndrome was called Gay-Related Immune Deficiency (GRID), and research centered on the practices of, and substances used by, male homosexuals. Other populations seemed affected too, however, especially intravenous drug users such as heroin addicts, hemophiliacs, natives of Haiti, and people who had traveled to or lived in Africa. The fact that homosexuals were not the only victims made the term "GRID" seem inaccurate, and in the course of 1982 a new name for the syndrome came into use: AIDS, or Acquired Immune Deficiency Syndrome.

Between February and May 1983, two different research teams (one at the Pasteur Institute in Paris, the other at the National Institutes of Health in Maryland) independently identified likely culprits, examples of a curious class of viruses called retroviruses. After some dispute about priority, the two teams came to agree on the retrovirus responsible for the devastating attacks on human immune systems, and by 1986 international agreement had been reached on the name *human immunodeficiency virus*, or HIV. HIV, then, was identified as the cause of the syndrome called AIDS. And while some uncertainty about how HIV was transmitted persisted, expert opinion increasingly agreed that it passed from one person to another only through the exchange of body fluids, especially blood or semen. Transmission therefore might occur as a result of anal or vaginal sex, blood transfusion, or intravenous injection by a needle used by more than one person.

Meanwhile, the United States seemed in the grip of a new Black Death, a relentless disease that meant death for its victims and spread by uncertain means. By 1985 over 15,000 cases had been diagnosed in the country, and about half of them had already died. In that year, the celebrated film actor Rock Hudson was one of the victims of AIDS, and his death increased popular attention to the epidemic.

The discovery of the apparent causative agent did at least make possible tests to diagnose the presence of the virus, although not everyone wanted to learn that they carried the seeds of an incurable disease. But the tests that were made suggested that the virus had infected perhaps one million Americans; if so, a calamitous epidemic loomed. Some hope came in 1987, with the approval for use of a drug called Azidothymidine (AZT) that retarded the development of active AIDS in the HIV-infected.

By the end of the decade from 1981 to 1990, the number of diagnosed cases of AIDS in the United States had reached a total of over 160,000. That number continued to grow into the 1990s, but in 1995 the annual death toll reached a peak of about 50,000. In 1996 the number of deaths from AIDS fell to about 37,000, and the number continued to decline in subsequent years. More people continued to contract AIDS, but they lived longer. And by 1990 (if not earlier), the general conceptions of the epidemic were changing (see the "How It Was Understood at the Time" section). (For factors behind the declining mortality from AIDS, see the "Responses" section.)

The 1980s AIDS epidemic in the United States initially had a very disproportionate effect on male homosexuals (many white), but by the end of the decade the target population had changed significantly. One example illustrates the change: in New York City in 1981, 90% of the victims were male, and 50% of them were white. By 1999 males still made up 79% of the victims, but only 14% of them were white. After the initial 1980s epidemic, AIDS became increasingly a disease of men and women of color; homosexual contacts were increasingly joined by intravenous drug use and heterosexual contacts as the modes of transmission of the virus. And those characteristics of the AIDS epidemic were also true, on a frighteningly larger scale, in the African AIDS epidemic that continues to grow.

In 1982 about 1,500 cases of AIDS had been diagnosed in the world, the majority of them in the United States. By 1991 that number had risen to 800,000, and the United States was no longer the center of the epidemic. More startling still were the numbers of people in the world infected by HIV, which reached 6.5 million in 1992. Since that year the base number of those infected has soared: 23 million in 1999, over 25 million in 2000; in 2018 the estimated total was between 36 and 37 million.

Worldwide deaths from AIDS-related infections began exceeding two million by 2000. The peak year thus far seems to have been 2005, when UNAIDS estimates of deaths ranged between 2.3 and 2.7 million. After that, a combination of responses intermittently and regionally began reducing the toll, which was set at about one million in 2018. The final toll of the pandemic remains to be known.

Sub-Saharan Africa, where HIV-AIDS gained a huge head start on the population "before anyone knew the disease existed" (Iliffe 2006, 1) has borne the brunt of this pandemic.

By the 1990s, it was realized that about 80% of the world's AIDS deaths were occurring in Africa. Some examples illustrate the extent of the disaster: in 1997 between 25% and 30% of the adult population of Botswana was thought to be HIV-positive; in the same year, the number of AIDS cases per 100,000 population exceeded 500 in Zimbabwe, Zambia, and Malawi; in 2000 perhaps 4.2 million South Africans may have been HIV-positive, and that number rose to 6.6 million by 2010. South Africa's population was then about 54 million; about one-eighth, therefore, of the population of sub-Saharan Africa's most economically advanced society, the one with the highest per capita income, had been infected by HIV. The successes of some places could alternate with failure; thus, Uganda saw gradual reductions in new HIV infections between 1990 and 1998, but from that time until 2010 new infection numbers rose again, from perhaps 80,000 to 150,000.

Although Africa remains much the most-affected continent, since 2001 Asia (and especially Vietnam and Indonesia) has been claiming a larger share. In 2003 one-fourth of the new infections—1.2 million of the total of 4.8 million—were Asian. In 2005 HIV-AIDS related deaths in sub-Saharan Africa amounted to roughly 78% of the world total; by 2010 that proportion had dropped to about 74%, reflecting some comparative success for the world's most beleaguered region. South and Southeast Asia's share has remained at about 13%. The broadly defined area called "eastern Europe and central Asia" accounted for 3% in 2005, and over 4% in 2010, evidence of increasing concern about that part of the world.

SIGNIFICANCE

The U.S. AIDS epidemic in the 1980s marked a dramatic end to an era. In the years after World War II, Americans had become convinced that violent and uncontrollable epidemics were things of the past. That conviction stemmed in part from the remarkable application of antibiotics that apparently stamped out such diseases as tuberculosis and syphilis, and in part from the development of successful preventive vaccines. The most dramatic vaccine story was that of poliomyelitis in the 1950s; the most sweeping success, the eradication of smallpox from the human population by 1977. Biomedical science seemed to have conquered the world of epidemic disease. AIDS challenged, and in many ways overthrew, that optimism.

The AIDS epidemic also affected sexual practices, coming as it did after a period of two decades when sex seemed to have no unfortunate consequences. The contraceptive pill, introduced in the early 1960s and widely available by 1965, reduced the likelihood of unwanted pregnancy; antibiotics, especially penicillin, seemed to banish the danger of venereal infections such as syphilis. The 1960s and 1970s were therefore generally seen as an era of sexual liberation. That was true—perhaps especially so—for American homosexuals, for many of whom sexual liberation became part of a larger assertion of individual and civil rights as well as self-affirmation. AIDS led to increasing emphasis on safe-sex practices, both among homosexuals and the general population.

The AIDS epidemic also gave rise to a period of renewed stigmatization of homosexuals and a countervailing self-assertion and political activism among them (see the "Responses" section). That activism included movements to empower victims of the disease and to pressure political leaders for increased public commitment to research and assistance. In turn, other patient awareness movements sprang up, stimulated by the AIDS example. The victims came from groups suffering from such other ailments as breast cancer that had been (for whatever reasons) marginalized in the society.

AIDS also fueled new concerns about germs and their menace, especially in the period of the early and middle 1980s when the mechanism of transmission was not popularly understood. The adoption of electric-sensor bath and toilet fixtures in public restrooms began in that period, as people sought to avoid hand contacts with germs.

And, of perhaps the greatest significance, the American AIDS epidemic of the 1980s was a part of the much larger (and continuing) story of the worldwide spread of the disease, on a scale that dwarfs the American experience.

Very few epidemics or pandemics in history have had important and lasting demographic effects; that is, population levels have almost always rebounded fairly quickly after an epidemic. That rapid recovery may not have happened in the wake of the early stages of the second plague pandemic (the Black Death), but even that case remains historically controversial. The present AIDS pandemic, especially in Africa, may prove another exception to the rule. If so, the pandemic will stand as one of the most significant demographic events in history.

Under the pressure of AIDS, life expectancy in many of the countries of sub-Saharan Africa fell sharply by the early twenty-first century. Life expectancies for children born between 2000 and 2005 in a number of African states dropped below age 40. In some of those countries, life expectancy had earlier been over age 50. Thus, in Swaziland, where life expectancy at birth was about 55 in the early 1990s, life expectancy at birth fell to 34 by 2004. In at least eight other African states, life expectancies fell under age 40: Botswana, the Central African Republic, Lesotho, Malawi, Mozambique, Rwanda, Zambia, and Zimbabwe. Most of those countries have since crawled back from that precipice, and their life expectancies have risen above age 50, but the possibility of long-term demographic decline as a result of epidemic disease remains.

The pandemic has had those demographic effects in part because the disease has particularly struck the age groups of the population (between 15 and 45) responsible for both birth rates and childcare. The number of orphaned children (themselves at significantly greater risk of death from a variety of causes) has grown rapidly in sub-Saharan Africa.

The same age structure of the victims has also had important economic effects because young adults are generally the most economically productive group of the population. The consequences of the loss of young adult labor may be very great. For example, many African countries have become increasingly dependent on lucrative crops raised for export; those crops are often labor-intensive, and if so the scarcity of labor may imperil a country's already shaky economic well-being. Individual enterprises may be crippled as well.

And, as the "Responses" section will make clear, the costs of responding to the disease may seriously strain the budgets of both poor countries and poor individuals. Will the costs of therapy create a new "apartheid" (McGreal 2000, 5) in South Africa, one in which the wealthy receive drugs and the poor are left to die?

As is true of any contemporary phenomenon, these (and any other) points about historical significance must be understood as very tentative and subject to revision, addition, and subtraction.

BACKGROUND

AIDS originated in Africa, but its appearance and spread in the world were facilitated by a number of factors. Rapid international transportation and frequent migration between countries and continents had become a feature of the world by the 1970s. Another worldwide phenomenon was the international trade in blood for transfusions; effective blood transfusions had become possible in the early twentieth century, and in World War II the techniques of transfusion spread widely. Blood infected by viruses could thus fly around the world quickly. Syringes, both glass and later plastic, were used for medical procedures (including inoculations and administration of antibiotics) and injecting narcotics. Reusing syringes could move an infection from one person to another.

Particularly in the Western world, the decades after World War II saw the rapid disruption of many traditional mores, especially sexual ones. Antibiotics freed people of the fear of venereal disease; contraceptive pills freed them from unwanted pregnancies. At least in public discourse (and perhaps in private practice as well), a whole new air of sexual freedom and casual sexual encounters resulted. In some United States cities—notably San Francisco and New York—this sexual freedom was promoted among homosexuals as an aspect of their personal and civil rights.

As the American epidemic proceeded, it came to coincide (unfortunately) with trends in criminal law. The war on drugs declared by a series of U.S. administrations imposed lengthy prison sentences on drug users. Largely (but not entirely) for that reason, the U.S. prison population soared, a population that included a disproportionate number of drug users, some already infected with HIV. Prisons thus became a further locus for the spread of AIDS infections.

American political reaction to the AIDS epidemic may also have been conditioned by an earlier disease scare, the swine flu episode of the 1970s. A huge government program had been developed to resist the threatened outbreak, only to have the epidemic fizzle out. Many people (and political leaders) were therefore leery of sweeping (and expensive) government programs. Would AIDS also prove a false alarm?

A further background point of interest: AIDS appeared in a sort of disease vacuum, not just in the United States but in the world. Tuberculosis seemed to be in retreat; smallpox, as of 1977, no longer existed in human populations. Was AIDS therefore more visible? Did AIDS find victims who might earlier have fallen to those other diseases? Certainly AIDS and tuberculosis now work in concert, all around the world.

Other factors complicated the African situation. Some were political; until the 1950s and early 1960s almost all of sub-Saharan Africa had been controlled by European empires. Those European rulers, in place since the nineteenth century, had seriously disrupted traditional African social and political systems; the independent states that succeeded imperial rule often occupied territories—defined by the European powers—that lacked ethnic or tribal cohesion. Independence might therefore be succeeded by prolonged periods of ethnic conflict or civil war.

Colonial rule had also involved economic exploitation, as European powers (and international businesses) sought to extract resources and profits. Labor was concentrated in both agricultural plantations and mines; economies were brought forcibly into larger metropolitan markets. Those changes meant increasing commercialization and movement of goods, which continued after independence; an important factor in the diffusion of HIV infections was the sexual activity of long-distance truck drivers.

The growth of cities in sub-Saharan Africa in the second half of the twentieth century was very dramatic. What had been sleepy colonial administrative centers rapidly amassed populations over one million. The cities grew in large part as a result of in-migration—people poured into them from the countryside. Economic necessity made many of the migrants leave their spouses behind; most of them, in coming to the cities, also left behind a world of traditional social customs and sanctions. Economic necessity drove others to prostitution. In these circumstances, restraints on sexual behavior weakened, and the opportunities for venereal disease—including AIDS—magnified. From the start, AIDS in Africa was associated much more thoroughly with heterosexual contacts than with homosexual ones.

Human blood transfusions may have also played a role in diffusing AIDS in Africa. Between 1950 and 1985, the total number of transfusions in sub-Saharan Africa increased from about 600,000 per year to 6.8 million per year; by 1970 the rate of transfusions in sub-Saharan Africa approached that of the developed cities of North America and Western Europe. As two modern scholars put it: "All known epidemic strains of HIV emerged in [sub-Saharan Africa] between 1959 and 1965, and over 50% of all transfusions in sub-Saharan Africa's history occurred before 1985—when HIV tests for blood first became available. It is likely that transfusions in Africa contributed significantly to the growth of AIDS in this region" (Schneider and Drucker 2004).

Also contributing was the widespread use of hypodermic needles in health care procedures and among drug users. The needle was the symbol of modern Western biomedicine, used for both preventive vaccines and therapeutic antibiotics. The poverty of African societies made the frequent reuse of needles more likely.

HOW IT IS UNDERSTOOD AT PRESENT

When what is now called AIDS surfaced in 1981, it seemed to be concentrated in particular populations, and so first thoughts about the disease (or syndrome) focused on those groups, their lifestyles, and the products they used. Researchers (and the American public at large) especially considered homosexuals, their sexual practices, and the products some of them used as recreational drugs (such as amyl nitrites, or "poppers") as the potential sources of the ailment and/or as the means of its transmission.

But other groups attracted attention as well, notably Haitians both in Haiti and in North American cities such as New York and Montreal. As late as 1986, an article in the *Journal of the American Medical Association* considered this question: "Do necromantic zombiists transmit [HIV] during voodooistic rituals?" in an article entitled "Night of the Living Dead II" (Greenfield 1986).

From the start, the biomedical community assumed that a causative agent—a microorganism of some sort—*could* be found. Researchers in France discovered the causative agent, the retrovirus called at first lymphadenopathy associated virus (LAV) in the spring of 1983; U.S. researchers simultaneously discovered human T-cell leukemia virus-I (HTLV-I), and then in 1984 the same U.S. team put forward human T-cell virus-III (HTLV-III), which proved to be identical to LAV. By 1986 the name "human immunodeficiency virus," or HIV, was agreed on. And in the late 1980s, it was realized that two varieties (HIV-1 and HIV-2) existed.

The discovery of the virus led biomedical thinking away from groups of the population and toward specific actions or behaviors that might facilitate its spread, although the line between a general fear of all gays as risky and only certain gay practices as risky was not always clear, especially in the popular mind (see the "Responses" section for some examples of such fears). Before the end of the decade, however, the fact that the virus only spread through the exchange of human body fluids, especially blood or semen, was widely accepted.

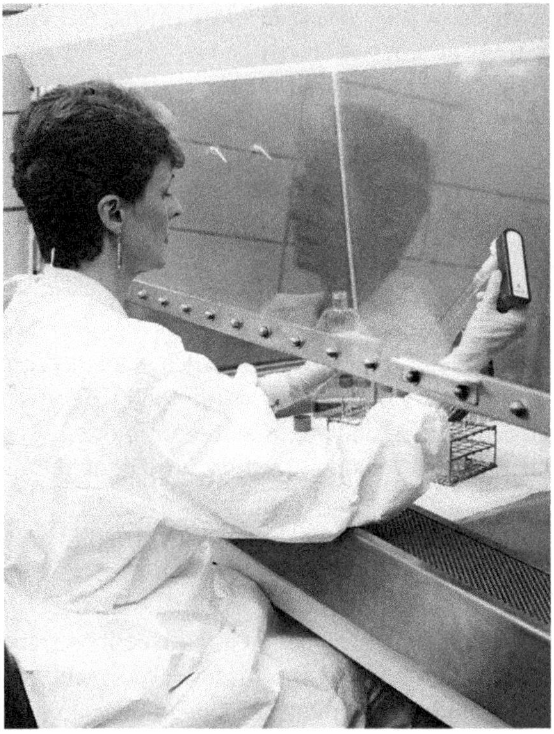
An AIDS researcher at the Centers for Disease Control and Prevention (CDC). Since the beginning of the AIDS epidemic, the CDC has been at the forefront of HIV investigation and laboratory research. (Centers for Disease Control and Prevention)

The discovery of the virus also made possible blood testing to discover infection and that in turn led to a realization that not everyone infected by HIV had developed the symptoms of AIDS. That is, infection with HIV and a case of AIDS were not synonymous. That contributed to the shift from thinking about AIDS as a sudden and terrifying plague, a new Black Death, to considering it as a chronic or even latent condition. Its true historical analogy was not with plague, smallpox, or cholera, but with tuberculosis, leprosy, or syphilis. Could it be *managed?*

As the AIDS epidemic became worldwide, it was generally understood that HIV passed from one person to another when body fluids (blood, semen) were exchanged, and that those exchanges might accompany sexual contact, injections from reused needles, or blood transfusions. Many social, political, and economic issues interfered with action on that understanding, however (see the "Responses" section).

By the late 1980s, researchers realized that HIV had at least two variants. The variant that was responsible for the devastating epidemic became known as HIV-1; another, and apparently milder, variant, found especially in West Africa, was called HIV-2. The existence of variations of the virus in Africa reinforced the growing conviction that HIV had originally evolved on that continent, and that its earliest human victims had perhaps been found there. Related viruses were shown to affect apes, and one in fact received the name simian immunodeficiency virus (SIV); its relation to HIV-2 is very close. That discovery therefore led to the theory that AIDS began as a disease of apes and crossed over into human populations that had contact with apes.

RESPONSES

Responses to the AIDS pandemic have reflected the general understanding of the cause and epidemiology of the disease, at least in theory. Involved have been a variety of preventive measures, including both attempts to modify behavior and to find an effective vaccine, and the development (and provision) of therapeutic drugs for those already infected. Political, social, and economic controversies have arisen over both the preventive and the therapeutic approaches.

Many early responses, both of the public and of medical professionals, illustrated the fears that accompanied the epidemic. Fear of Haitians led to a dramatic fall in the number of American tourists traveling to Haiti: from 75,000 in the winter of 1981–1982 to 10,000 in the winter of 1982–1983. Fear of homosexuals was particularly widespread. Thus, the city of Tulsa ordered a public swimming pool drained and disinfected after a gay group used it; the political commentator Patrick Buchanan urged (in 1983) that gays be barred from jobs involving food handling or childcare. Some religious and/or political conservatives saw the AIDS epidemic as a judgment of God on the sins of homosexuals and drug addicts.

Fears surrounded a variety of intimate human situations. In 1985 the Screen Actors Guild ruled that its members could refuse to take part in scenes involving heavy kissing, while the Washington National Cathedral (Episcopal) began offering alternatives to common cups in its communion services. Delta Airlines proposed (and later withdrew the idea) that sufferers with AIDS be forbidden on its flights. And even the most mundane action might be a fearful one; as late as 1995 a letter carrier in Charleston, West Virginia, refused to deliver mail to the residence of an AIDS sufferer.

The medical and health care professions expressed fears as well. In some cases, hospitals refused to treat AIDS patients or their staffs refused to work with them; in at least one instance a pathologist refused to examine a deceased AIDS victim. In an effort to overcome these fears, the New York state government in 1983 began distributing more public money to hospitals if they agreed to join an AIDS treatment network.

Drastic public health remedies, notably ideas about quarantine, seemed to have little point, owing to the rapidly increasing size of the affected population and the early uncertainty surrounding the disease's transmission. But the discovery of the virus opened the possibility of testing the population and that in turn raised important doubts about the freedom of the individual from state interference. Gay activists (and others) objected that a mandatory blood test could result in people losing their jobs or being denied health insurance. A Chicago court case in 1986 considered whether a divorced gay father, seeking overnight visitation rights with his children, could be compelled to undergo a blood test (Tybor 1986).

Medical attention fairly quickly moved from concerns about whole populations at risk (homosexuals, for instance) to an emphasis on individual behavior. In a way, the discovery of HIV led to more focus on individual responsibility; if you got AIDS, it was your fault, although it was difficult to make that argument about people who innocently became infected through blood transfusions or about infants who were infected by their mothers before their births. But clearly one response, therefore, was moral: reform your habits, especially your sexual habits and/or your use of intravenous drugs. The adoption of safe-sex practices divided the gay community, with some of its members urging that life itself depended on doing so, while others objected that their identity would thus be compromised.

Still another moral response generated more general controversy. Should drug addicts be supplied with clean needles, at public expense and with the urging of government? New York City undertook a needle exchange program in 1988 that generated formidable opposition. Addicts feared identifying themselves to authorities; opponents of the program accused the health department of licensing, and even facilitating, drug abuse. What was more important: bringing the AIDS epidemic under control or stamping out heroin addiction? Something of the same question arose about the distribution of condoms in schools. Did doing so halt the spread of venereal diseases (among which AIDS might be numbered) or encourage youth sex? Which goal was the more important?

Until 1987 responses to the AIDS epidemic were limited to prevention, but in that year the first drug for the treatment of the disease, AZT, was licensed for use in the United States. It did not cure the syndrome, but it did apparently delay the progression of an HIV infection to an active case of AIDS. One result of the drug's appearance was to give people more reason to have a blood test; they might no longer fear simply learning about a death sentence but about a disease that might be managed.

The introduction of AZT also contributed to the changing conception of the disease, away from the fearsome sudden plague and toward a chronic disease with which people might live for years. Further drug therapies in the 1990s made such an outcome ever more likely. An AIDS "cocktail" came to include more than one drug and also to include a protease inhibitor (another development of the 1990s) that had the effect of stopping HIV replication in the body.

But these therapies were not universally applied, in part because their costs remained very high and in part because some of the most vulnerable and affected people remained reluctant to accept treatment by modern biomedicine. That seemed especially true of African American women, who were more likely to consult holistic and alternative healers. And by 2001, the disproportionate toll of AIDS on the African American population had become severe. Among white women in the United States between the ages of 25 and 44, 1.9 per 100,000 population died of AIDS; among black women the number was 26 per 100,000. (For men in the same age group, the rate for whites was 8.3; for blacks, 53.5.)

Still another category of response was the effort to develop a preventive vaccine. Several dozen such vaccines were tried in the years after 1987, none with much success. Serious ethical questions surrounded trials of such vaccines, for the nature of the retrovirus posed different problems from those of other viral diseases for which vaccines had been produced and applied. Such earlier vaccines remain some of the great triumphs of humanity over disease: the eradication of smallpox from the human population by 1977; the rapid development of vaccines against poliomyelitis in the 1950s. But each of those diseases (and others such as measles) shared the characteristic that one case of the disease conferred on the individual immunity from further attacks. A vaccine could therefore work because it gave the recipient a mild case of the disease, strengthening the immune system. But AIDS itself caused *destruction* of the immune system; how to mimic it without bringing on that disaster?

The World Health Organization (WHO) began proposing world strategies to combat AIDS in 1986. In the following years, with the WHO's encouragement, many African countries organized national control programs for AIDS, but resources lagged well behind intentions. Some African political leaders thought that taking action against AIDS would tell the world that their countries were infected. Because they feared that international stigma would follow, they delayed action or even denied the existence of the epidemic altogether. Such attitudes discouraged donors from making contributions. Annual global resources for AIDS had grown from $44 million in 1986 to $165 million in 1990, but that growth then slowed and stagnated by the mid-1990s.

Worries grew that the international response to the epidemic had failed, and those fears led to the formation in 1996 of UNAIDS, a program that combined the activities of a number of UN agencies in the hope that the different specialties of those agencies could be coordinated in a campaign against AIDS. At the least, this program did produce more reliable statistics about the spread of the disease, and the wide publication of those statistics created a sense of urgency among agencies, foundations, and some governments. Funding increased dramatically, but whether it has been enough remains uncertain. The WHO proposed to spend $5.5 billion to provide anti-AIDS drugs to 3 million Africans by 2005. But by early 2004, it had raised only $2.3 billion, and the United States was withholding contributions because its officials remained unconvinced of the safety of the drugs to be used.

Prevention programs aimed at changing some sex habits, especially focusing (first) on sex education for the young and advocating the use of condoms, and (second) on the reformation of drug habits by offering treatment programs for addicts (perhaps to wean them from their dependency) and needle exchanges, ensuring that needles are not reused. Another preventive strategy has been to urge (and make available) blood testing for the general population. If people know that they are HIV-positive, they may modify their behavior to protect others.

Accompanying these prevention programs are parallel attacks on other venereal diseases and on tuberculosis. The lesions of other venereal diseases may be another entry point for HIV-infected blood or semen, and tuberculosis is just the sort of infection that the HIV-positive person may be unable to resist.

In some countries, these programs seemed to have worked well. In 1997 Uganda was a bright spot, where sex education and condom distribution had an effect on disease rates. Thailand had even greater success with such measures. But in too many places in Africa (and elsewhere) real barriers remained. Some donors and governments remained opposed to the distribution of condoms and needle exchanges, for fear that such programs simply encouraged the behaviors (sex, drugs) that furthered the epidemic. Would it not be better to preach abstinence? (The short historical answer to that question is that abstinence programs have not worked.) Resistance to the use of condoms remains widespread throughout Africa; their use is often taken to imply a lack of trust in one's partner. Similarly, blood testing is widely feared; many people do not want to know that they are HIV-positive, if only because their communities (including their lovers) may shun them. Social restraints (and lack of resources) thus hamper many preventive efforts.

Political pressures and the demands of commerce have complicated the use of therapeutic drugs. The first therapeutic drug for AIDS, AZT, became available in 1987.

It has since been joined by a variety of other drugs, many of which are now supposed to be used together in what has been dubbed a "cocktail." A variety of drugs may lessen the chance that HIV can develop resistance to any one in particular and the addition of protease inhibitors to the cocktail may slow or stop the replication of HIV in the body. And while these drugs have not promised to cure AIDS, they may make it manageable, prolonging the lives of those infected.

But their use in sub-Saharan Africa has met many obstacles, beginning with their costs. In 2000 a triple cocktail in South Africa cost about $600 (U.S.) per month, and one source estimated that only about 10,000 of South Africa's 4 million-plus HIV-positive people could even remotely afford that. Making drugs available more cheaply has been a very contested issue. The manufacturers—mostly European or American—have argued that their research and development costs have to be recouped. Some African governments—most notably South Africa's, as late as 2000—refused to negotiate with the manufacturers because their political leaders did not want to admit that AIDS was a problem.

A few examples from a period of months, in 2000 and 2001, illustrate the cross-currents of commerce and politics. In late 2000 a pharmaceutical company announced it would take legal action to block the sale of a generic version of one of its AIDS drugs in Ghana; the company cited the need to cover research and development costs. Nongovernmental AIDS organizations, such as Doctors Without Borders, argued that the drugs concerned had been developed back in the 1980s and that American government funds had assisted in that development. It was left up to individual African governments to negotiate with pharmaceutical companies, and the Ghanaian government chose not to offend the powerful pharmaceutical company. At the same time that Ghana's attempt to obtain generic copies was being contested, another company agreed to provide a certain AIDS drug to South Africa free, rather than face the importation of a generic copy.

In the early months of 2001, a legal case was contested in Pretoria, South Africa. At issue was another attempt by pharmaceutical companies to block the importation of cheap, generic, anti-AIDS drugs. In April the companies abruptly abandoned the case. But the political position of the South African government complicated the situation. That government had, for several years, been at best ambivalent about the AIDS epidemic within its borders. The president, Thabo Mbeki, had doubted the connection between HIV infection and the disease AIDS, and had also lashed out at Western perceptions of Africans as people whose habits spread the epidemic. His government, therefore, had at times downplayed the importance or the extent of AIDS and had refused to use public money to provide anti-AIDS drugs. Its reaction to the April 2001 Pretoria case in a sense persisted in denial: the case, it claimed, was not about the importation of anti-AIDS drugs, but about many different medicines used for many different ailments. Would the government now spend public money on anti-AIDS drugs? Or would it rely on the private sector to provide them?

In the succeeding years, a variety of international and nongovernmental agencies have attacked the worldwide pandemic both in the crucial lands of sub-Saharan Africa and elsewhere. The "Joint United Nations Programme on HIV-AIDS," or UNAIDS, organized in 1995, has been especially influential. In

2015 it set a goal of ending AIDS as a global health menace by 2030 and established statistical standards that would track progress toward that goal: 90% of the world's living HIV-infected should know of their infection, the same percentage should have begun treatment, and the same percentage should continue treatment. Achieving those targets has been difficult and has proceeded erratically in different regions and countries, for political, economic, and social enabling (or disabling) factors have persisted. Treatments—antiretroviral drugs or still-uncertain vaccines—remain expensive for poor countries or populations; social stigmas may lead those infected to deny their condition or resist treatment; active political opposition may resist perceived international interference with local autonomy.

Responses have also been complicated by the realization that AIDS and some other diseases work in tandem. Tuberculosis especially feeds on the HIV-positive. Venereal diseases such as syphilis provide more opportunities for HIV infection. Campaigns against AIDS have thus had to be linked with responses to those diseases as well (see volume 2, chapter 44).

UNRESOLVED ISSUES

As suggested in the "Responses" section, many political issues surrounding the pandemic remain unresolved. Individuals and governments remain (often for understandable causes) in denial about the seriousness or even existence of the disease. The costs of therapy remain daunting, and the demands of philanthropy and humanity face the countervailing pressure for profit. The AIDS pandemic provides an especially clear example of the tension between beliefs that health is a universal human right and that unfettered markets must be permitted to supply goods.

Other political questions remain as well. Are the responses to AIDS of poor sub-Saharan governments limited by austerity programs imposed on their spending by the International Monetary Fund or the World Bank? Has the extent of the pandemic been exaggerated or downplayed for political reasons? Has the relative success in slowing the spread of AIDS in developed countries and the successful application of anti-AIDS drugs there lessened Western interest in the problems of Africa and now Asia—or even in marginalized Western populations?

Another possible unresolved issue is the potential epidemic role of retroviruses related to, but distinct from, the HIV-1 that has ravaged the globe.

REFERENCES

Greenfield, William R. "Night of the Living Dead II." *JAMA* 256 (1986): 2199–2200.

Iliffe, John. *The African AIDS Epidemic: A History.* Athens: Ohio University Press, 2006.

McGreal, Chris. "AIDS: South Africa's New Apartheid." *Manchester Guardian Weekly*, December 28, 2000, 5.

Schneider, William H., and Ernest Drucker. "The History of Blood Transfusion in Sub-Saharan Africa: Implications for the Emergence and Course of the AIDS Epidemic." May 1, 2004. Paper read at American Association for the History of Medicine meeting, Madison, Wisconsin.

Tybor, Joseph R. "Fear of AIDS Shadows Visitation Fight." *Chicago Tribune*, April 28, 1986, 1.

SUGGESTED ADDITIONAL READING

Good sources of information on the AIDS pandemic are the annual World Health Reports, *issued by the WHO. Also helpful is the WHO's website:* http://www.who.int.en.

Alcamo, I. Edward. *AIDS in the Modern World.* Malden, MA: Blackwell Science, 2002.

Altman, Dennis. *AIDS in the Mind of America.* Garden City, NY: Anchor/Doubleday, 1986.

Berridge, Virginia, and Philip Strong, eds. *AIDS and Contemporary History.* Cambridge: Cambridge University Press, 1993.

Epstein, Helen. *The Invisible Cure: Africa, the West, and the Fight against AIDS.* London: Viking/Penguin, 2007.

Essex, Max, Souleymane Mboup, Phyllis J. Kanki, Richard G. Marlink, and Sheila D. Tlou, eds. *AIDS in Africa.* 2nd ed. New York: Kluwer Academic/Plenum, 2002.

Farmer, Paul. *AIDS and Accusation: Haiti and the Geography of Blame.* Berkeley: University of California Press, 1992.

Fee, Elizabeth, and Daniel M. Fox, eds. *AIDS: The Burdens of History.* Berkeley: University of California Press, 1988.

Fee, Elizabeth, and Daniel M. Fox, eds. *AIDS: The Making of a Chronic Disease.* Berkeley: University of California Press, 1992.

Gostin, Lawrence O. *The AIDS Pandemic: Complacency, Injustice, and Unfulfilled Expectations.* Chapel Hill: University of North Carolina Press, 2004.

Goudsmit, Jaap. *Viral Sex: The Nature of AIDS.* New York: Oxford University Press, 1997.

Grmek, Mirko D. *History of AIDS: Emergence and Origin of a Modern Pandemic.* Princeton, NJ: Princeton University Press, 1990.

Piot, Peter. *AIDS between Science and Politics.* New York: Columbia University Press, 2015.

Schneider, William H., and Ernest Drucker. "Blood Transfusions in the Early Years of AIDS in Sub-Saharan Africa." *American Journal of Public Health* 96 (2006): 984–994.

42

The Mad Cow Crisis and Transmissible Spongiform Encephalopathies, 1985–

WHEN AND WHERE

Beginning in early 1985, a mysterious ailment began to be noticed among cattle in Great Britain. The number of animals affected multiplied rapidly in the next several years, and the name "mad cow disease" came into popular use to describe the problem. The British cattle population was reduced as a result of both the disease and the subsequent systematic slaughter of animals believed infected. That slaughter was undertaken as mad cow disease came to be linked with a fatal (and previously rare) neurological disease in humans, Creutzfeldt-Jacob disease.

The first observations of mad cow disease came from southern England in April 1985. A veterinarian was called to examine a cow that "had become hypersensitive to noise, apprehensive, unpredictable, and aggressive, and was having difficulty walking" (Ridley and Baker 1998, 150). The cow was euthanized and its brain sent to a laboratory. In the following months, some other similar cases appeared, but it was not until 1987 that a report analyzing the pathology of the cases appeared. The pathology reports suggested that the cows suffered from a disease akin to one long familiar among sheep and called *scrapie* (see the "Background" section) but apparently new to cattle. The new disease was formally called bovine spongiform encephalopathy or BSE in October 1987.

In 1988 evidence accumulated that the disease had spread as a result of cattle being fed meat and bone meal that included scrapie-infected sheep remains. The question was then posed: If an encephalopathy could cross from one species to another (sheep to cattle), could it cross to humans? Were people who consumed beef (or lamb) at risk? Some human diseases were caused by agents of the same type (prions; see the "How It Is Understood at Present" section) as those responsible for scrapie and BSE.

Of these, the most notable was Creutzfeldt-Jacob disease (CJD). Could eating beef bring on CJD? CJD was invariably fatal; it manifested itself in a variety of increasingly severe neurological problems, difficulty in walking, falling, tremors, dementia, and eventual paralysis and death. Could it have causes other than genetic?

Meanwhile the number of infected cattle rose steadily. A few hundred cases per month were diagnosed in Britain in 1988; in that year the British government began the compulsory slaughter of all animals suspected of the disease, and it also banned the addition of animal protein matter derived from ruminants (such as sheep or cattle) from animal feed. But despite these measures, by 1992 the number of cattle infected with BSE had risen to about 3,000 per month.

From that point, the number of infected cattle began to decline, but in March and April 1996 came the next great shock. A study analyzed 10 recent cases of a new variant of CJD and suggested that the cases *were* linked to the consumption of BSE-infected beef. Beef prices in Britain plummeted, and British beef faced embargoes first from France and then from the entire European Community. In 2000 a study forecast that somewhere between 100 people (bad enough) and 136,000 people (appalling) in Britain would fall victim to the new-variant CJD as a result of the infection of the British beef supply. Such estimates were admittedly difficult, both because how many people had consumed infected beef could not really be known (when, for instance, did the BSE epidemic really begin?) and because the incubation period of the disease was of an unknown length.

By the early years of the twenty-first century, the BSE outbreak had greatly eased, but the projections of eventual CJD cases remained uncertain. The total number of British cattle that had fallen victim to BSE was between 180,000 and 200,000 as of 2001; some new infections continued to appear (about 500 total in 2003), but the incidence had declined sharply. (And a far larger number of British cattle had been slaughtered to halt the outbreak since 1988.) Some cases of BSE, numbering in the hundreds, had also been found in France, Switzerland, Ireland, and Portugal. The first U.S. case appeared in the state of Washington in December 2003.

Since 1995 the number of British deaths from the new variant CJD has reached about 260 (as of May 2019). Some of those people had donated blood, and some recipients of that blood have been identified. The frightening forecast of 100,000 or more future deaths has therefore not materialized, although the future of the "epidemic" remains in doubt.

(Meanwhile other cases of CJD had arisen from another source. Between 1959 and 1985, thousands of children had been treated with human growth hormone, derived from human pituitary glands. Some of the hormone was infected with CJD. See the "Background" section.)

SIGNIFICANCE

The linkage of BSE and the new variant CJD generated a major international panic. An unknown and potentially enormous human mortality seemed possible, given the gigantic consumption of beef in some countries in the world. Beef eaters were threatened by an inexorable and incurable disease. And that disease was caused by an agent against which it was difficult to imagine a remedy (see the "How It Is Understood at Present" section).

The fear of beef (as a bearer of a fatal disease) therefore led to a major disruption of dietary habits, especially in Britain. In British culture, beef has long occupied a central place; the "roast beef of Olde England" is a familiar cliché and thinking about giving it up was particularly wrenching for many of the British. And a similar disruption would have been very difficult elsewhere as well; in the United States, the beef hamburger had become one of the chief national dishes. The episode also led to what the European Commissioner for Agriculture called "the biggest crisis the European Union had ever had," as the Union debated internal embargoes against one of its largest and most influential members (Ratzen 1998, 95). BSE (and CJD) therefore disturbed international relations, as well as crippling export businesses.

(The massive culling of cattle in Britain repeated an earlier twentieth-century slaughter. That campaign had been undertaken to eradicate bovine tuberculosis (*Mycobacterium bovis*), stimulated by fears that tuberculosis could reach humans through consumption of cow's milk; see volume 2, chapter 44.)

The epidemics also illustrate the apparently seamless web of infections between humans and other species. In that way, it was analogous to other contemporary disease concerns, such as avian influenza.

BACKGROUND

Both BSE and CJD are examples of a general class of diseases called transmissible spongiform encephalopathies, and some background about three of such diseases will clarify the history of this particular set of epidemics.

Scrapie, a disease of sheep, was first described in the eighteenth century. Sheep acted in a wild manner, rubbed themselves against posts, became dizzy, and then sank into lethargy, dying within two to six months. Nineteenth-century thinkers speculated about its cause, without coming to agreement. They also argued about what to do about it, with some advocating the isolation and/or slaughter of the ailing animals. In 1898 lesions were discovered on the nerve cells of the victims, and those lesions became the identifying mark of the disease. By 1960 a great deal had been learned about scrapie: it was contagious; material from nervous tissue in scrapie cases could be inoculated into other sheep and scrapie would result, so the nervous tissue must contain some virus; the disease could be transmitted from sheep to goats, and then (in 1961) to mice. (The last point made possible faster and cheaper experiments on animals.) By the late twentieth century, scrapie was found in many sheep herds in many countries.

Creutzfeldt-Jacob disease, a fatal human neurological disease, was first described in the early 1920s. An apparently rare genetic phenomenon, it attracted little attention for some time. In the 1970s, several circumstances occurred. Two cases were traced to infection in medical-surgical procedures, which suggested that CJD was not simply genetic. A high incidence of CJD among a population of Libyan Jews was tied to their consumption of sheep parts; could CJD be a product of what you ate? The first worldwide epidemiological study of it, completed in 1979, confirmed its rarity: one case per one million people per year.

Kuru was a disease found among the members of an isolated people, the Fore, on the island of New Guinea. In 1955 an American researcher Vincent Zigas discovered it there and described its symptoms: spasmodic trembling and eventual death, blamed by the Fore on sorcery. In the next several years, Zigas and Carleton Gajdusek studied it more thoroughly and suggested that it had been responsible for several thousand deaths in the limited area of New Guinea inhabited by the Fore.

Beginning in the late 1950s, some researchers began to connect these three diseases. William Hadlow (in 1959) suggested a link between scrapie and Kuru (Schwartz 2003). Then Gajdusek succeeded in transmitting Kuru to chimpanzees, with symptoms that resembled scrapie; he then linked them to CJD as well. In the years after 1966, Michael Alpers successfully traced Kuru among the Fore to cannibalism; when cannibalism declined among those people, Kuru declined as well. Kuru was apparently transmitted by the consumption of animal parts, of a particularly unusual sort. By the late 1960s, Kuru, scrapie, and CJD had been collectively called transmissible spongiform encephalopathies. But no agreement had been reached on the cause or agent, of any of the diseases. They all seemed transmissible, but what drew them together was not a known causative agent or virus, but their similar cellular pathologies—results, not causes.

Meanwhile human growth hormone began to be used in 1959 to treat dwarfism. The therapy seemed very successful and demand for the hormone soared. Human pituitary glands supplied the hormone. Between 1959 and 1985, about 25,000 children, worldwide, were so treated. By the end of 2000, 139 of them had contracted CJD.

HOW IT IS UNDERSTOOD AT PRESENT

When the mad cow crisis began in 1985, some understanding had been reached about the causes of transmissible spongiform encephalopathies, of which BSE proved to be one. In the late 1970s and early 1980s, Stanley Prusiner, an American biochemist, had shown that the causative agent of scrapie was a curious protein called a prion. Many prions exist in the protein world, most of them harmlessly; some abnormal prions, however, are infectious, and once in the body, accumulate and ultimately result in lesions in the nervous system. Kuru, CJD, scrapie, and BSE were soon all shown to be prion diseases.

All these diseases were therefore infectious, in the sense that the offending prions could be inserted into the body. But a number of CJD cases seemed instead to be genetic, or caused by the mutation of a gene. CJD might be infectious, or genetic, or spontaneous.

From 1988 on, BSE and CJD were linked in people's minds by the possibility that the former could spread to humans and thus cause the latter. Was there an adequate "species barrier" that would prevent that? Was each prion specific to one species? In May 1990 a British domestic cat was infected by BSE, which suggested that the disease could cross a species barrier (as had been known to be true of scrapie since the 1950s).

The idea of a linkage between BSE and CJD got much stronger in April 1996, when a group of British patients were diagnosed with what proved to be a variation of CJD. This *new variant* Creutzfeldt-Jacob disease (or nvCJD)—unlike other cases of CJD—shared a pathological resemblance to scrapie. Since BSE had emerged as a largely British problem, infecting the British meat supply, thinkers inferred that BSE likely was linked to the new form of CJD, which appeared in Britain as well. Subsequent experiments supported that conclusion, although the exact links remain in question.

RESPONSES

The practice of isolating and slaughtering infected animals had a long history, not just with scrapie but with other diseases as well. In the summer of 1988, the British government responded to the BSE crisis by ordering the compulsory slaughter of all animals suspected of infection. It also banned the use of animal feed that contained animal proteins derived from ruminants.

It proved difficult to implement these orders thoroughly. Animal feed containing meat and bone continued to be used. In 1988 the government originally offered 50% of the value of the slaughtered cattle as compensation for the farmers. Did that provide adequate incentive to comply? Perhaps not, and the government agreed to increase compensation to 100% in 1990. By that time, the crisis had become a political issue, as the Labour Party (then in opposition to the ruling Conservatives) accused the government of concealing the true number of infected animals.

Meanwhile, other segments of British opinion reacted angrily to French (and other European) embargoes on British beef; newspapers resounded with anti-French statements. European states lifted their bans on British beef in June 1990, after the British government agreed that only British beef from herds certified as free of BSE for two years would be exported. (In the previous year, another British policy had decreed that no cattle over 30 months old could be used for food. This policy reflected the belief that halting the use of meat and bone meal in cattle feed in 1988 would end the epidemic.)

But the intensified crisis of the spring of 1996 brought new and more stringent embargoes on the import of British beef into Europe. By 1999 the embargoes had eased.

By the end of 2003, it was estimated that Britain had destroyed about 4.5 million cattle in response to the BSE crisis, at a point when the total cattle population of the country was perhaps 10 million. And also, by the end of 2003, BSE had reached the United States. The discovery of an infected animal in Washington state led the U.S. government to recall meat products from eight states. A second American case of BSE was reported by the U.S. Department of Agriculture in June 2005.

The response to BSE, therefore, involved the slaughter of infected animals, increasingly strict limits on the sources of beef that could be sold, and attempts to ban the use of animal parts in animal feed. Some of these responses, especially after 1996, also grew out of fear of CJD. Much concern gathered around cattle products; what should be avoided? Cow's milk seemed safe; so too did muscle-tissue meat. The safety of meat from other organs of cattle remained more problematic.

Direct responses to the possibility of CJD took several forms. In the international blood trade, transfusions using blood from Britain, or from people who had been to Britain, began to be limited or stopped. After 1988 human growth hormone was no longer derived from pituitary glands, but from recombinant genetics. Those steps closed some of the doors through which CJD might pass. A more general closure of the doors, through a preventive vaccine, has been called (by a modern authority) "difficult to conceive of" because of the peculiar properties of prions (Schwartz 2003, 183). The disease remains considered untreatable and inevitably fatal, and responses are limited to the relief of pain through drugs.

UNRESOLVED ISSUES

The most immediately important unresolved questions concern the future. How many people, especially but not exclusively in Great Britain, remain at risk of nvCJD? The numbers quoted earlier (in the "Where and When" section) remain tentative. Other unsolved issues relate to future mortality predictions. Are some people more susceptible to infectious prions than others? If so, why? When will the BSE epidemic end? And a parallel question persists about the number of people still at risk of CJD from human growth hormone treatments before 1985.

Some answers to those questions will depend on learning more about the mechanism of the spread of infectious prions, both within the body and between one species and another. How do prions find their way into the central nervous system? Are other animals that get animal-based feed—hogs, chicken, fish—at risk? Can nvCJD conceivably pass from mother to unborn child?

Research continues on the development of possible vaccines, diagnostic tests, and even therapies for what has thus far been an incurable disease. But for some, such research raises another issue: In the world of public health, how significant is the nvCJD epidemic? Even the highest estimates of possible mortality place it far below contemporary AIDS, malaria, and tuberculosis. If public resources are scarce, how should they be apportioned?

For the historian, the origins of the BSE epidemic remain unresolved. Why did it occur when and where it did? Why did BSE suddenly appear (apparently in 1981–1982, given its two- or three-year period of incubation) in Britain, and nowhere else? The use of animal-based feeds for livestock began in the nineteenth century and was common across the Western world. What contributed to the contamination of British animal feed in 1981? Anything? Or did the infectious prions of BSE simply appear?

REFERENCES

Ratzen, Scott C., ed. *The Mad Cow Crisis: Health and the Public Good.* New York: New York University Press, 1998.
Ridley, Rosalind M., and Harry F. Baker. *Fatal Protein: The Story of CJD, BSE, and Other Prion Diseases.* Oxford: Oxford University Press, 1998.
Schwartz, Maxime. *How the Cows Turned Mad.* Translated by Edward Schneider. Berkeley: University of California Press, 2003.

SUGGESTED ADDITIONAL READING

Prusiner, Stanley B. "The Prion Diseases." *Scientific American* (January 1995): 48–57.
Rhodes, Richard. *Deadly Feasts: Tracking the Secrets of a Terrifying New Plague.* New York: Simon and Schuster, 1997.
Zigas, Vincent. *Laughing Death: The Untold Story of Kuru.* Clifton, NJ: Humana, 1990.

43

Contemporary Malaria

WHEN AND WHERE

In 2001 malaria had resulted in 1,124,000 worldwide annual deaths, about 960,000 in Africa alone. Those frightening numbers had become typical of malaria's annual toll in the late twentieth century. Some other statistics were even more awesome: in 1998, for example, perhaps 300 million clinical cases of malaria occurred in the world, and as many as 550 million people were said to live at risk of the disease. Malaria was highly endemic in about three-fourths of the land of sub-Saharan Africa, where it accounted for about 20% of the childhood deaths there. As this chapter will discuss, some uncertain progress against malaria has occurred in the twenty-first century, but in 2017 the World Health Organization estimated 220 million cases worldwide, and 435,000 deaths—262,000 of them children under the age of five. Sub-Saharan Africa remained the epicenter of malaria, the scene of both remarkable individual, national, and international efforts, on the one hand, and recurring periods of ethnic violence that imperil the implementation of anti-malaria programs, on the other. For example, in Burundi, which had endured horrendous ethnic massacres in the mid-1990s, malaria sickened three million people in 2001 and 2002—nearly half the then population of the country.

Sub-Saharan Africa especially remains the main focus of the *Plasmodium falciparum* parasite, but it has been relatively spared the ravages of the *Plasmodium vivax* variant, owing to the fact that many of its people lack a blood protein (the "Duffy antigen") susceptible to *P. vivax.* Of the two different malarias, *P. falciparum* (causing "malignant tertian fever") has most often been fatal, while *P. vivax* (and its "benign tertian fever") is less often fatal but can also lie dormant in the body for up to two years and thus poses both the danger of persistent illness and the threat of continuing infection of others. A sub-Saharan exception to the general infection pattern has been Ethiopia, where *P. vivax* persists.

Many other places (chiefly in Asia and Latin America) remain prone to seasonal or annual outbreaks of the disease. In Southeast Asia, *P. vivax* continues to infect Indonesia, Vietnam, Cambodia, and the Philippines. Some successes have been reported; in 2016 Sri Lanka had been malaria-free for three years, but in 2017 a more drug-resistant *P. vivax* appeared in Vietnam, illustrating the fluctuating and complex history of the struggle with malaria. In Latin America, similar triumphs alternated with failures: in 2018 the World Health Organization reported that Paraguay had eliminated malaria completely, the first American country to do so in nearly 50 years, but several months earlier malaria had returned to Venezuela, which ironically had declared its eradication about 50 years ago (Baumgaertner 2018; Grillet et al. 2018).

SIGNIFICANCE

Malaria is one of the great contemporary infectious epidemic killers, along with tuberculosis and AIDS. Its effects on the societies and economies of sub-Saharan Africa remain especially severe. The cost of even relatively inexpensive treatments can strain the resources of a poor family, and relieving the large number of victims certainly strains the budgets of poor governments. As a chronic and weakening disease, malaria affects an individual's ability to work, and so stunts the whole society's economic productivity. In heavily endemic malaria areas, malaria especially concentrates on young, previously unexposed, children, and that fact weakens educational effectiveness in entire countries. Fears of malaria depress tourism, while businesses from the developed world hesitate to invest in malarial areas (or send their technical skills to them).

The earlier successful eradication of malaria from much of the developed world had made it invisible to some Western opinion, which may have assumed that malaria (rather like tuberculosis) was a disease of the past. But international organizations, nongovernmental bodies and philanthropies, and scientific communities have also been increasingly mobilized against the disease.

BACKGROUND

Malaria epidemics have an ancient history. Human settlements in tropical and sub-tropical lands throughout Eurasia from Western Europe to East and Southeast Asia experienced it. Thus, the disease was known to the people of classical Greece and Rome throughout their earliest history, and they clearly described it; the Roman Empire in particular suffered from repeated attacks of malaria. It continued to affect the medieval and Renaissance Mediterranean lands. Its presence in the tropics became an obstacle to European exploration and settlement of, for example, the West Indies and the interior of sub-Saharan Africa well into the nineteenth century.

The use of cinchona bark (adopted from the Indians of Peru) offered some relief as both a preventive measure and a cure; in the early nineteenth century, its active ingredient was isolated as quinine and became the chief remedy for the disease. Nevertheless, malaria was still a major world problem in the early twentieth century. In the years before 1945, the world death toll from malaria probably averaged two million annually.

Then a dramatic decline occurred in the decades following World War II. Some figures illustrate the change: in 1900 the annual mortality rate from malaria has been estimated at 194 deaths per 100,000 population; in 1930 the number was 174; by 1950 it had fallen to 48, and then in 1970 it was 16. That is, in a 40-year period (1930–1970), the death rate from malaria fell about 90%.

Three factors accounted for this remarkable improvement. The first was the application of new insecticides, above all DDT (developed in the United States during World War II), and their widespread use in malarial areas of Asia and Latin America. People in effect waged a successful war of eradication against the *Anopheles* mosquitoes that carried malaria parasites. Second was the use of more effective quinine-derived remedies, especially chloroquine, which greatly reduced malaria's severity. Such remedies were combined with the third factor, called active case surveillance, in which malaria cases were monitored and (if possible) isolated from mosquitoes that might continue a chain of infection. In some places the results of these approaches were extraordinary. In Ceylon (later Sri Lanka) malaria had infected perhaps one million people before World War II; by 1963 the number of malaria cases in the country totaled only *20.*

After the 1960s, however, the assault on malaria died down for a number of reasons. Fears about the environmental effects of DDT began in the 1950s, and *Silent Spring*, a 1962 book by the American biologist and writer Rachel Carson, called attention to the insecticide's lethal effect on bird populations. The historian J. R. McNeill later said of *Silent Spring* that it "might be the most important [book] ever written by an American" (McNeill 2000, 339). In the Western world, public opposition to the use of DDT grew, and by 1972 its use had been banned in the United States. Many other countries followed suit.

At the same time that DDT was being abandoned, the causative microorganism of the most dangerous type of malaria—*Plasmodium falciparum*—began to evolve strains that resisted the effects of chloroquine. Even in countries where the number of mosquitoes had been sharply reduced, death rates stabilized (or crept up again) as therapeutic drugs proved progressively less effective.

And sub-Saharan Africa had remained the exception in the period between 1945 and 1965. Malaria mortality rates illustrate the growing gap between it and the rest of the world. In 1900 the sub-Saharan rate was 223 per 100,000 (marginally higher than the world's 194); in 1930 it was 216 (the world's, 174); but in 1950, when the world rate had fallen to 48, Africa's remained 184, and by 1970 sub-Saharan Africa's malaria mortality rate was over six times as high as the world's (107 to 16). After 1970 the gap grew wider yet; in 1997 the rest of the world's malaria mortality rate (excluding sub-Saharan Africa) was one death per 100,000 population per year, while in Africa the rate had climbed back up to 165. Sub-Saharan Africans were therefore 165 times more likely to die of malaria as people in the rest of the world.

Malaria has been highly endemic in much of sub-Saharan Africa probably since prehistoric times. Some Africans (as well as some Mediterranean peoples) carry the genetic trait called sickle cell anemia, a recessive gene that carries some protection against malaria. (If they are heterozygous all is well, but if they are homozygous sickle cell anemia results in death.) Many do not possess the gene, however, and so remain vulnerable to the disease, especially as children (adults, even without the sickle cell trait, may develop some immunity from previous exposure).

In the 1890s both the identity of the causative organisms (*Plasmodia*) and the role of mosquitoes in their transmission were discovered, and attempts to eradicate mosquitoes began. American authorities triumphantly cleared mosquitoes out of Havana (Cuba) and central Panama (during the construction of the Panama Canal, 1905–1914), but the huge mosquito population of Africa discouraged attempts to duplicate those feats. European colonial governments in Africa opted instead for a limited attack, making a relatively small area of coastal cities (such as Dakar) safe for Europeans, and not attempting anything more ambitious. Uncertainty about the possibility of eradication persisted even after the introduction of DDT, and no continent-wide efforts occurred in the years after 1945.

Some reduction in malaria mortality rates did occur in Africa after 1945, probably owing more to the greater availability of cheaper chloroquine (see the "Responses" section) than to mosquito eradication. But by the 1980s African malaria mortality again rose, as strains of drug-resistant *Plasmodia* spread.

African colonial and postcolonial political and economic conditions aided malaria's spread. War and civil unrest deepened poverty, disrupted health systems, crippled sanitation and drainage, and caused massive population movements. Such tragic episodes as the Biafran secession struggle in Nigeria between 1967 and 1970, the 1979 uprising against Idi Amin in Uganda, civil war and factional turmoil in Liberia starting in the late 1980s, repeated coups in Sierra Leone after 1992, and the ethnic violence that tore Rwanda in 1994 and then spread its results into Congo, all created favorable conditions for disease.

Some worldwide conditions have affected the prospects of malaria in other places as well as Africa. Global warming may make cities and regions in presently temperate zones more akin to the subtropics, and so *Anopheles* mosquitoes might return to (for example) southern Europe and southern North America. And worldwide transportation links make possible the quick movement of infections and disease vectors. The airport malaria phenomenon illustrates that. In France 26 cases of malaria were reported between 1970 and 2000 "among people who had never visited a malarious country but who lived near or worked at airports"; in 1994, "epidemiologists counted six malaria cases in three weeks near Charles de Gaulle Airport outside Paris, and calculated that eight to 20 anopheles mosquitoes had been on each of 300 arriving flights" (McNeil 2000, 11).

Without treatment, malaria—especially the variety caused by *Plasmodium falciparum*, sometimes called malignant tertian fever—can be a very serious disease. Its victim suffers debilitating weakness and anemia, and the disease may progress to organ failure and (in perhaps 10% of cases) death.

HOW IT IS UNDERSTOOD AT PRESENT

Since the 1890s, the roles of both the causative agents (*Plasmodia*) and the insect vectors that carry them (*Anopheles* mosquitoes) have been generally understood. Several varieties of the microorganisms exist: *Plasmodium falciparum* (the most serious), *Plasmodium vivax* (less serious but able to persist for years), and *Plasmodium malariae. P. falciparum* requires temperatures above 19°C, but *P. vivax* can flourish with seasonal temperatures above 15°C and can lie dormant throughout colder periods only to reemerge. The number of *Anopheles* mosquito species is very large, and their preferred habitats vary; for example, some feed indoors while others are found in the open, a circumstance that complicates attempts to control or eradicate them. More recently attempts have been made to genetically interfere with mosquito breeding (Wade 2018) and—similarly—to genetically uncover "essential genes" of *P. falciparum* whose identification might aid the development of therapeutic remedies (Zhang et al. 2018).

RESPONSES

Vector eradication, meaning attacks on mosquitoes, remains an important response. It has involved both spraying with insecticides and managing water sources to discourage places and conditions where mosquitoes might breed. Window screens and bed nets protecting sleepers, perhaps treated with insecticides, have formed another line of defense. DDT, although widely distrusted as a symbol of environmental havoc, is still used in some countries; South Africa used DDT with great effect in its 2000–2001 malaria epidemic. The World Health Organization's recent anti-malaria programs (such as "Roll Back Malaria," declared in 1998) have not endorsed DDT, however.

Several therapeutic drugs have been employed against contemporary malaria. Chloroquine, the drug of choice until the 1980s, began to be replaced (first in Asia and Latin America, and then in Africa) as strains resistant to it developed. Pyrimethamine, perhaps together with a sulfa drug, was one option; other drugs (such as mefloquine) appeared as well, but resistant strains of *Plasmodium falciparum* persisted. And newer drugs often might cost 5 to 10 times as much as the older ones, further crippling the ability of poor African individuals and governments to resist malaria. In the 1990s, some rediscovered "natural" drugs that were extracted from plants came into use, especially artemisinin; that class of remedies has joined the quinine-related ones in the continuing evolutionary struggle between microbes and their foes.

An important aspect of therapy is early recognition and treatment, especially for children. Again, poverty, together with lack of available medical facilities, makes early treatment difficult in many African places. Inadequate resources often have posed painful dilemmas: On what basis are they employed? Can young children be saved with stop-gap measures until more help can arrive?

Preventive vaccines remain a possibility, and a number of them have been tried. As they appear, however, poverty raises its head. For example, in 2015 a new vaccine ("RTS,S") was approved by the European Medicines Agency and a large African field trial was held. Would its use confer enough benefit to outweigh its costs, or would resources be better used to widen the use of bed nets ("Malaria Vaccine Clears Hurdle" 2015)

UNRESOLVED ISSUES

The effectiveness of therapeutic drugs against malaria is unclear and will likely remain so. *Plasmodium falciparum* has proven very adaptable, and a continuous evolutionary struggle between it and pharmaceutical research looms. Vaccines that would immunize people against malaria remain unproven, especially amid limited resources.

More generally, political issues remain unresolved. Will the rich nations of the developed world commit adequate resources and aid so that the poor nations (those most stricken by malaria) can deploy the ever-more-expensive therapeutic drugs made necessary by evolving strains of malaria? Will research on malaria vaccines receive adequate funding? Can poor nations find the resources to (for example) provide screens for dwellings? Will the ability and willingness of private philanthropy and nongovernmental organizations to invest in campaigns against malaria continue?

The use of DDT remains another unresolved (and in many ways political) question. Some malaria experts urge that a "worldwide ban on DDT would be a mistake . . . DDT can be uniquely helpful" (Spielman and D'Antonio 2001, 204; see also Rosenberg 2004). But its use is strongly opposed by environmental organizations (for whom DDT remains a prime example of the evils of human environmental manipulation), and the United States has banned its use. The World Health Organization has not supported its application.

Global warming may extend mosquito ranges and bring malaria back within some territories from which it has been eradicated, especially in southern Europe. If and when that happens, how will world responses and resources be changed?

REFERENCES

Baumgaertner, Emily. "In a Rare Success, Paraguay Conquers Malaria." *New York Times*, July 10, 2018, D4.

Grillet, Maria Eugenia, Leopoldo Villegas, José Felix Oletta, Adriana Tami, Jan E Conn. "Malaria in Venezuela Requires Response." *Science* 359, no. 6375 (February 2, 2018): 528.

"Malaria Vaccine Clears Hurdle." *Science* 349, no. 6247 (July 31, 2015): 456.

McNeil, Donald G., Jr. "Mosquito-Borne Illness: The Right Bug and an Unlucky Series of Coincidences." *International Herald Tribune*, September 4, 2000, 11.

McNeill, J. R. *Something New under the Sun: An Environmental History of the Twentieth-Century World.* New York: W. W. Norton, 2000.

Rosenberg, Tina. "What the World Needs Now Is DDT." *New York Times Magazine*, April 11, 2004, 38–43.

Spielman, Andrew, and Michael D'Antonio. *Mosquito: A Natural History of Our Most Persistent and Deadly Foe.* New York: Hyperion, 2001.

Wade, Nicholas. "Nudging a Species to Self-Destruction." *New York Times*, September 25, 2018, D6.

Zhang, Min, Chengqi Wang, Thomas D. Otto, Jenna Oberstaller, Xiangyun Liao, Swamy R Adapa, Kenneth Udenze, et al. "Uncovering the Essential Genes of the Human Malaria Parasite *Plasmodium falciparum* by Saturation Mutagenesis." *Science* 360, no. 6368 (May 4, 2018): 506.

SUGGESTED ADDITIONAL READING

Good sources of information on contemporary malaria are the annual World Health Reports, *issued by the World Health Organization. See especially "Rolling Back Malaria," in the WHO's* World Health Report 1999, *49–63. Also helpful is the WHO's website:* http://www.who.int/en.

Background may be gained from the following:

Desowitz, Robert S. *The Malaria Capers: More Tales of Parasites and People, Research and Reality.* New York: W. W. Norton, 1991.

Humphreys, Margaret. *Malaria: Poverty, Race, and Public Health in the United States.* Baltimore, MD: Johns Hopkins University Press, 2001.

Packard, Randall M. *A History of Global Health: Interventions into the Lives of Other Peoples.* Baltimore, MD: Johns Hopkins University Press, 2016.

Packard, Randall M. *The Making of a Tropical Disease: A Short History of Malaria.* Baltimore, MD: Johns Hopkins University Press, 2007.

Webb, James L. A., Jr. *Humanity's Burden: A Global History of Malaria.* Cambridge: Cambridge University Press, 2009.

44

Contemporary Tuberculosis

WHEN AND WHERE

In the early twenty-first century, tuberculosis remains one of the most widespread and dangerous diseases in the world, with an annual death toll that far outstrips some epidemics that attract more popular attention. In 2017 about 10 million new cases of it occurred in the world. Since 1998 the number of annual world deaths has ranged between 1.5 million and 2 million; in 2017 the figure was 1.6 million, a toll that exceeded that of HIV-AIDS. Estimates of the total number of people infected with the bacillus have been staggeringly high, some exceeding one *billion,* but the uncertain ground between "infection" and "symptoms of tuberculosis" makes such figures problematic.

Although tuberculosis is a worldwide problem, its incidence varies widely across different areas. The highest rates of morbidity and mortality are in countries of sub-Saharan Africa and Southeast Asia: the Central African Republic, the Congo Republic, Lesotho, Liberia, Namibia, Sierra Leone, Zambia, and Zimbabwe, and Cambodia and Papua New Guinea. The largest numbers of cases are found in populous Asian nations; in 2017 two-thirds of the world's new cases occurred in India, China, Indonesia, the Philippines, Pakistan, Nigeria, Bangladesh, and South Africa, all but the last of those being among the largest world populations. In 30 countries in 2017 the rate of new tuberculosis cases varied between 150 and 400 per 100,000; in three of them—Mozambique, the Philippines, and South Africa—the rate exceeded 500. And in 2018 when the rate in North Korea reached 640 the World Health Organization's (WHO) Global Fund suspended grants to the country, hoping—diplomatically—that the "operating environment" would improve.

Although its incidence dramatically declined in the developed West in the twentieth century (see the "Background" section), tuberculosis persists there as well. In the developed world, the rate of new infections per year is generally less than 10 per 100,000 per year, but deaths from tuberculosis occur annually in Europe (many of them in Eastern Europe, including Russia and Ukraine). In 2017 about 9,100 new cases of tuberculosis were reported in the United

States—fewer than AIDS (38,000 in 2017) or whooping cough (48,000 in 2012), but far ahead of such historic horrors as the now-rare plague, cholera, and yellow fever.

SIGNIFICANCE

The sheer worldwide extent of the contemporary tuberculosis epidemic marks it as one of the most serious disease events in human history. Any epidemic that kills over a million people a year and has infected untold millions of others deserves attention.

The contemporary tuberculosis epidemic also stands as an important example of a disease whose mortality has persisted despite the apparent success of curative remedies. By about 1960, many observers (in the Western world at least) believed that tuberculosis was a disease of the past. Its continued power demonstrates the importance of the relation between poverty and epidemic disease, as well as the danger of false promise fed by apparent local success (see the "Background" section).

Contemporary tuberculosis also illustrates the continuing biological evolution of disease microorganisms in response to human measures against them (see the "Responses" section).

Tuberculosis and the contemporary AIDS epidemic have fed on each other, for tuberculosis is the leading infection to which the immune-weakened AIDS patient succumbs, and an HIV infection weakens resistance to tuberculosis (see also volume 2, chapter 41).

BACKGROUND

It is now believed (and has been since the late nineteenth century) that pulmonary tuberculosis results from an infection of the lungs by the microorganism called *Mycobacterium tuberculosis.* Many people are infected by that bacterium but do not develop disease symptoms. In such cases, the body's immune system successfully isolates the invading germs and no harm results, even though a blood test will give a positive reading for tuberculosis. The disease, therefore, involves an infection that is a *necessary* cause but evidently not a *sufficient* cause. Many different possible factors may account for a body's successful resistance, and those factors will be discussed shortly.

Mycobacterium tuberculosis was discovered in 1882 by Robert Koch, which made possible a new and more precise definition and diagnosis of the disease. Previously, its identification had depended on a judgment of clinical symptoms, but by the beginning of the twentieth century the presence of the bacterium defined the disease; if it was absent, the disease was not tuberculosis.

This discovery did not, however, play much role in the decline of tuberculosis mortality that began in the Western world at the end of the nineteenth century. That decline was sustained largely by improvements in standards of living. Better nutrition increased powers of resistance, and so too did declining birthrates that meant fewer pregnancies for women. More spacious living quarters (and better ventilation of homes and workplaces) reduced the chances of exposure to the bacterium, which was most often airborne. Death rates may have also receded from their high nineteenth-century levels in part through natural selection; if powers of resistance had a genetic component (still an uncertain point), then the survivors (and their descendants) may have been more resistant.

Human interventions against tuberculosis played a secondary role in the fading of the disease between 1900 and 1950. Sanatoriums (popular especially in Britain, Germany, and the United States) did isolate some sufferers from contact with others; a vaccine (called BCG) began to be used in the 1920s in some countries, but it was not universally accepted. Another human intervention grew out of the realization that tuberculosis could be found in other animals. Very old traditions had associated human and animal diseases, and in the 1860s tuberculosis had been inoculated from one species to another. Then in the 1890s, the American researcher Theobald Smith successfully isolated *Mycobacterium bovis* in cattle. Could humans be infected by bovine tuberculosis? Authorities differed, but (especially in the United States) pressure grew to err on the side of safety. The response proceeded on two fronts: cattle shown to be tubercular were to be slaughtered (at potentially huge costs), and the "pasteurization" of milk began, in which heat killed microorganisms in it. Between 1917 and 1922, the incidence of tuberculosis in American children had fallen to one-half the rate experienced by their British counterparts, a triumph credited to the "pasteurization" campaign, although many other environmental factors may have been involved.

Mortality from tuberculosis fell appreciably, for a combination of those reasons, into the 1950s. At that point antibiotics intervened to dramatic effect, especially streptomycin, first isolated in 1944. Streptomycin, and later antibiotics that also proved effective against tuberculosis, opened the possibility of a genuine cure that would kill the microorganisms and hence end the disease. By the 1960s—in the developed West at least—tuberculosis was rapidly forgotten, apparently a disease of the past.

Tuberculosis did not, however, disappear so rapidly from other parts of the world. The disease remained the single most important killer in China throughout the first half of the twentieth century (Yixia and Elvin 1998). Many places in the world did not share in the industrializing West's prosperity, and so the Western improvements in standards of living were not mirrored elsewhere.

And after the introduction of antibiotics, many places lacked the resources to provide such treatments to their populations. In addition to the provision of antibiotics themselves, their administration had to be monitored and patients reminded to complete the treatment. Administration of antibiotics required some widespread level of primary health care, and also some level of medicalization of the population as a whole. Some or all of those necessities remained absent in many poor or developing countries.

In some places, therefore, antibiotics were not available at all. In others, their administration was incomplete, with some people untreated and others only partially treated leaving their dosage unfinished. Such circumstances encouraged the spread of strains of *Mycobacterium tuberculosis* that were resistant to antibiotics. Survival of such strains would probably have happened anyway through natural selection, but the incomplete administration of dosages accelerated the process.

HOW IT IS UNDERSTOOD AT PRESENT

Since the late nineteenth century, tuberculosis has been linked with infection of the body by the microorganism *Mycobacterium tuberculosis.* Tuberculosis is often equated with a specific infection of the lungs, called pulmonary tuberculosis, but the microorganism can infect other parts of the body as well; for example, the disease sometimes called scrofula is a tuberculosis infection of the lymph glands.

Why some people infected by the microorganism develop the clinical symptoms of tuberculosis (of the lungs or elsewhere) remains a topic of discussion. In 2018 an authoritative journal reported that "our understanding of how 90 to 95% of infected individuals live with chronic TB is extremely limited" (Fogg 2018). Heredity, living standards (including diet), and stress may all play a role, as (obviously) does any weakening of the body's immune system, such as that resulting from an HIV infection.

RESPONSES

In the early stages of the contemporary epidemic, some health authorities hoped to immunize infant populations with the BCG vaccine. Some of those efforts have persisted, but attention has shifted to the effective administration of antibiotics to cure tuberculosis patients.

The first successful antituberculosis antibiotic, streptomycin, was soon joined by isoniazid, and their combination became the remedy of choice. Two other antibiotics were added to these, forming what is sometimes called a four-part antituberculosis "cocktail": rifampicin and ethambutol, and the development of still others continues. These antibiotics confront a microorganism whose powers of resistance evolve, which inhibits or nullifies the drug's efforts. In early 2019, the WHO reported that one-third of world TB deaths were inflicted by "Multi-Drug Resistant Tuberculosis" (MDR-TB), illustrating the difficulties facing curative remedies. Costs of drugs rise, and treatment regimens evolve; for example, in 2018 the WHO encouraged the use of "less harmful drugs in regimens lasting as little as 9 months" instead of one that lasted twenty months and had "serious side effects."

In the late 1980s, some countries evolved a strategy called DOTS (directly observed treatment, short course). The concept centered on the careful monitoring of each patient's consumption of antibiotic pills. An individual—perhaps a family member, a nurse, a local traditional healer—personally watched each pill being consumed by the patient for a full dosage of (usually six) months. Where it was introduced, this system achieved dramatic increases in the rate of cure, and it remains a widely accepted international standard, adopted by the WHO in 1993.

An interesting surge in tuberculosis in the United States between 1985 and 1992 illustrated that social and political factors remained important. After steady declines in tuberculosis rates (and cases) since World War II, the numbers of cases (and the rate) leveled out in 1984, and then rose irregularly until 1992. That increase followed a change in federal policy, which until those years had made available federal funds for tuberculosis control. The new approach offered block grants to states to use as they wished; federal authorities in effect said that if states chose to downplay antituberculosis efforts, doing so was up to them. Some did, and tuberculosis rates rose, especially among the populations of prisons and those infected with HIV, both groups stigmatized by elites. In 1993 direct federal funding for tuberculosis control resumed, and tuberculosis rates once again declined. Effective measures against the tuberculosis epidemic remain, therefore, subject to political whims.

Did the success of biomedical cure weaken interest in preventive measures? What has been called a "U-Shaped Curve of Concern," in which a fall in mortality and morbidity rates create a corresponding fall in public health funding and attention, may have been at work. In Germany in the 1980s city planning manuals and educational curricula no longer discussed issues of public health; had the problems been solved? (Rodenstein 1988; Reichman 1991).

For many people and authorities, especially in the developed West, tuberculosis remains a disease of the *past* and is therefore easily ignored. It does not generate the fears or stimulate the excitement of other newer ailments, even though its toll far exceeds theirs. Resources to combat tuberculosis therefore may have a lower priority than they should.

UNRESOLVED ISSUES

The prevalence of worldwide poverty, related to dramatic disparities in income, remains the most general underlying issue in the tuberculosis epidemic. As long as ill-nourished people live in congested quarters, the conditions favorable to tuberculosis will continue to exist. And although the possibility of cure for many (or even most) tuberculosis patients is real, making antibiotics available and organizing their effective administration has required political commitments that both governments and social elites have not always been willing to undertake. Historically, elites and governments have often been indifferent to diseases that affect the poor or the otherwise marginal members of society.

Historically tuberculosis flourished in crowded cities and housing conditions, and such conditions persist in much of the world. In some ways they are more widespread than ever, for a higher proportion of the world's population is now urban, and the cities of the developing countries of Asia and Africa have grown especially rapidly. The gulf between the rich nations of the developed world and some of the poor nations elsewhere remains very wide. Rapid means of transportation and massive worldwide labor migration, as well as flight from warfare or internal political turmoil, all contribute to the spread of disease, especially a disease such as tuberculosis, which may be carried by people who have not yet shown symptoms.

An important background complication of the contemporary tuberculosis epidemic is the enormous number of people infected with HIV, estimated in 2003 at between 34 and 42 million. Those many millions are therefore at greater risk from infections such as tuberculosis, which is in fact the greatest single killer of the HIV-infected.

REFERENCES

Reichman, L. B. "The U-Shaped Curve of Concern." *American Review of Respiratory Disease* 144 (1991): 741–742.

Rodenstein, M. *"Mehr Licht, Mehr Luft": Gesundheitskonzepte im Stadtebau seit 1750.* Frankfurt: Campus, 1988.

Fogg, Christiana N. "Mycobacteria and Metabolism." *Science* 360, no. 3690 (May 18, 2018): 748..

Yixia, Zhang, and Mark Elvin. "Environment and Tuberculosis in Modern China." In *Sediments of Time: Environment and Society in Chinese History*, edited by Mark Elvin and Lin Ts'ui-jung, 520–542. Cambridge: Cambridge University Press, 1998.

SUGGESTED ADDITIONAL READING

Good sources of information on the contemporary tuberculosis situation are the annual World Health Reports, *issued by the World Health Organization. The websites of the WHO and of the U.S. Centers for Disease Control and Prevention are also helpful.*

Bynum, Helen. *Spitting Blood: The History of Tuberculosis.* Oxford: Oxford University Press, 2012.

Condrau, Flurin, and Michael Worboys, eds. *Tuberculosis Then and Now: Perspectives on the History of an Infectious Disease.* Montreal: McGill-Queen's University Press, 2010.

Waddington, Keir. *The Bovine Scourge: Meat, Tuberculosis and Public Health, 1850–1914.* Woodbridge, UK: Boydell Press, 2006.

Zumla, Alimudden, and Matthew Gandy. *The Return of the White Plague: Global Poverty and the "New" Tuberculosis.* London: Verso, 2003.

45

SARS Epidemic, East Asia, 2002–2003

WHEN AND WHERE

The ailment eventually entitled SARS first appeared in Guangdong province of southern China, where its first known case apparently occurred on November 16, 2002. A mounting number of cases developed throughout the province in November and December, and by the end of the year provincial medical authorities in Guangzhou (formerly Canton) had become concerned. In January 2003 the first case surfaced in the nearby autonomous city-state of Hong Kong, and from there the disease rapidly diffused around the world; infections had developed in a Hong Kong hotel, and on February 21 guests of the hotel began returning to their homes. Between February 23 and 25, infected air travelers had reached Singapore, Hanoi, and (remarkably) Toronto. Cases of the disease also spread through China; Beijing reported cases on March 5.

By that time, international concern and responses had rapidly grown, and the epidemic was quickly contained. By late April, Vietnam was free of SARS; Singapore followed in May, Hong Kong and Beijing in June, and by July 5, when both Toronto and Taiwan had eliminated SARS, the World Health Organization declared that the worldwide epidemic had been contained.

The WHO enumerated the toll as of July 31, 2003: 8,098 worldwide cases of the disease, resulting in 774 deaths. Of these cases, 7,083 had occurred in China, which suffered 648 of the deaths. Taiwan, Canada, and Singapore had, respectively, 344, 251, and 238 cases, and 37, 43, and 33 deaths. Twenty-nine cases occurred in the United States, none of them fatal.

After some early confusion about naming the ailment, on March 15 the WHO decided on calling it "Severe Acute Respiratory Syndrome," or SARS.

SIGNIFICANCE

This epidemic was the "first new infectious disease to cause a global health scare since the emergence of AIDS" (Abraham 2005, 120). Its rapid worldwide diffusion illustrated the hazards posed by the freely employed means of distance travel for international business and professions, as well as the mass internal movement of labor demanded by economic modernization. And the almost equally rapid containment of SARS showed the power of international biomedical organizations to discover a disease's cause and institute appropriate responses.

BACKGROUND

The SARS epidemic occurred at a time of severe international tensions and conflicts. The 2001 "9/11" terrorist attack in the United States precipitated the U.S.-led invasion of Iraq, which got underway in March 2003—as the epidemic seemed to be spreading across the world. Reactions to the epidemic reflected the war atmosphere. They also reflected a long-standing Western belief that the "East" in general, and China in particular, was the source of world diseases. In 2003 "Chinese-owned businesses in some North America cities were boycotted as sites of possible infection, even though there had been no cases of disease there" (Peckham 2016, 8).

The location of the original epidemic also made relevant the ambiguous relationship of the Peoples' Republic of China and the semi-autonomous territory of Hong Kong that immediately adjoins Guangdong and is only 90 miles from Guangzhou. Responses to the disease differed between them, and the international position of Hong Kong gave it a prominent role. It had long been a center of international trade and travel, and so could serve as both a potential diffuser of an epidemic and a focus for international response to it. In 2017 an estimated 250,000 people passed to or from Guangdong and Hong Kong *daily*, illustrating the remarkable volume of traffic between them.

HOW IT IS UNDERSTOOD AT PRESENT

SARS first appeared as a respiratory illness that did not respond to attempted remedies; an early term for it was "atypical pneumonia." In 2002—and since 1997—widespread concerns about an "Asian flu," H5N1, hovered in the background, and so possible influenza theories arose. In March 2003 many researchers, both in China and Europe, argued that a "paramyxovirus" was responsible, but by the end of that month, the WHO, adopting an argument made by Malik Peiris of the University of Hong Kong, had agreed that the culprit was a previously unknown coronavirus.

The virus is droplet-borne from the respiratory organs of the victim and so does not travel far. That circumstance explains why caregivers—nurses, physicians, hospital staff—were especially at risk, as were others in close contact with the victim—including relatives and those in the crowded public rooms of hotels.

RESPONSES

Initial responses in Guangdong confronted the evident symptoms: respiratory distress, fever, coughing. Steroids were prescribed, with uncertain effects. Fear of

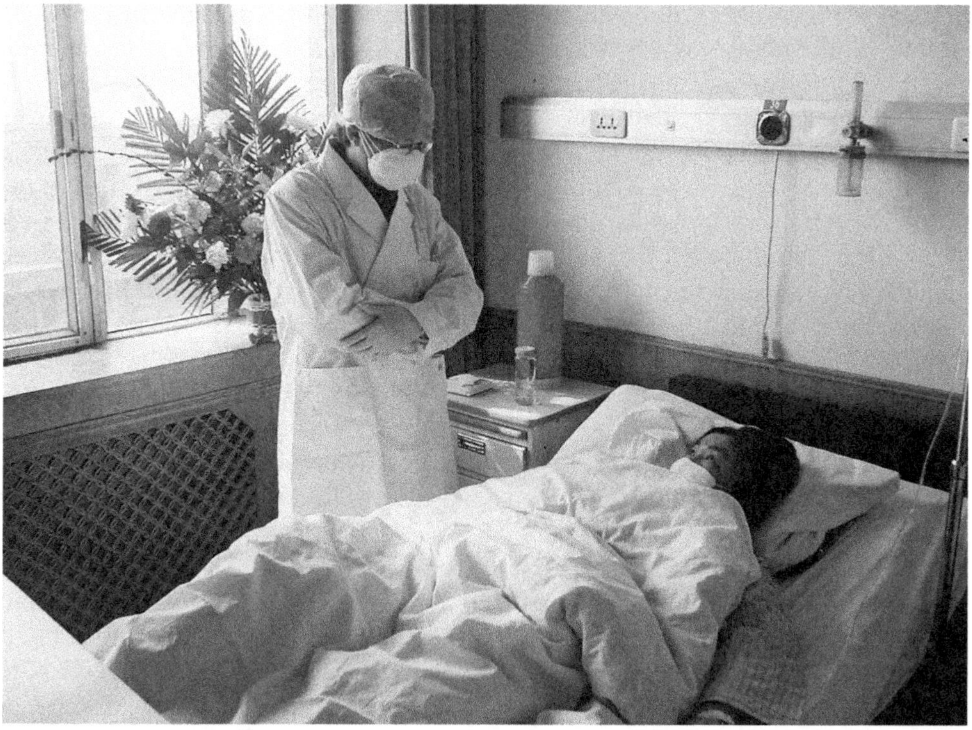

During a SARS outbreak in China in 2003, a doctor obtains information from a SARS patient. Both wear protective facemasks to minimize possible cross-contamination of the contagious SARS virus. The doctor also wears a gown, latex gloves, and a head covering as part of his personal protective equipment. (Centers for Disease Control and Prevention)

contagion quickly led to quarantines and isolation facilities, while caregivers girded themselves with gloves, masks, and protective gowns. In the belief that air conditioning systems might spread droplet-borne viruses, they were turned off—making the work of the caregivers, already heavily clad in gear, more difficult. The search for the causative organism proceeded, marked by disagreements. Meanwhile, the Beijing government denied the gravity of the situation; when Zhong Nanshan, a leading Guangdong physician who clearly understood the danger of the epidemic, reported the disease, his report (which summarized important findings about the pattern of the disease's spread) was not released to the public.

SARS reached Hong Kong in late February 2003 when a visiting Guangdong physician checked himself into a Hong Kong hospital (after having first checked into a hotel), warning that he suffered from the "extremely contagious disease that he and his colleagues had been treating" (Abraham 2005, 54–55). That event began the decisive Hong Kong and international response to SARS (as it was soon to be called), for infected guests in the hotel began dispersing on international flights, while the hospital became a locus of the disease. Doctors working with the WHO in Hanoi sounded an alarm, seconded from Hong Kong. Between March 12 and 15, the WHO's headquarters in Geneva issued emergency worldwide alerts, in doing so bypassing the national health administrations through which it ordinarily worked—a measure of the extreme sense of urgency the epidemic inspired. On March 12, the number of cases known in Hong Kong and Hanoi was 55; by mid-April, 3,000 cases had been reported, involving 20 countries.

While the hunt for the cause proceeded, the emergency use of an antiviral drug, Ribavirin, became widespread before trials had determined its efficacy. A more important response was the successful WHO pressure on airlines all over the world to keep the ill from boarding their planes, thus choking off the international (as well as intranational air) diffusion of SARS. The WHO also promoted a remarkably cooperative international harnessing of virology research that ultimately confirmed that the causative organism was the previously unknown coronavirus, first identified by Malik Peiris of the University of Hong Kong.

The responses of the Chinese government in Beijing evolved from denial to cooperation with the international efforts. In the early stages of the Guangdong epidemic, news of it was suppressed, or the presence of an epidemic was denied; as some news inevitably leaked out, any disease was said to be under control. And that disease was certainly not "Asian flu" (a subject of worldwide concern); rather, it was a mild chlamydia infection. The descriptive report of Zhong Nanshan was not published. WHO enquiries were discouraged. Nevertheless, information continued to circulate, perhaps through the Internet, perhaps from cell phone texts. Discrete diplomatic pressure from the WHO and from foreign governments such as the United States played an additional role, while Chinese government statistics about SARS were released that contradicted simultaneous official denials. In mid-April, for reasons still debated, the Beijing government became an active participant in the international campaign against SARS.

UNRESOLVED ISSUES

A contemporary Chinese journalist called the SARS epidemic "our country's 9/11," in the belief that it challenged the Chinese to realize "the real meaning of globalization" (Peckham 2016, 290). That implied—among other things--that changes must occur in the Chinese health system's relative isolation from international networks. To some extent, such changes ensued; for example, the Chinese quickly adopted a more open policy about HIV/AIDS in the country, publicly acknowledging its existence and danger to the country. Some foresaw that "scientists" would replace "bureaucrats" in shaping public health policy.

Did changes also occur in therapeutic responses to epidemics? During the SARS crisis, practitioners of traditional Chinese medicine continued to act in the country, together with those who followed the course of responses discussed earlier; did the success of their respective approaches differ? Not clearly. And the epidemic was halted by an application of long-established policies: quarantine, isolation, contact epidemiology, none of them dependent on twenty-first-century biomedicine. To what extent has the Chinese public health system changed in response to SARS?

The world's, and China's, response to SARS reinforced the images of a military campaign: the disease was an "insurgent" that was to be attacked. These images joined those already employed against the contemporary H5N1 influenza epidemic. In the West, both epidemics were seen as further evidence of the dangers posed to world health by the teeming working-class cities of China. Those longstanding conceptions (or prejudices) were thus confirmed by SARS. But did SARS also contribute to raising questions about wider worldwide complicity in those teeming living conditions, such as the insatiable world demand for the cheap products of cheaply paid Asian labor?

The SARS coronavirus was clearly zoonotic, but with what animal species did it originate? For a time, civet cats were the prime suspect, and a culling of the creatures was undertaken during the epidemic. But many other species were investigated as well, including the infection from multiple animal sources, without finding an answer. And the possibility that SARS has been with humans for years remains.

REFERENCES

Abraham, Thomas. *Twenty-First Century Plague: The Story of SARS*. Baltimore, MD: Johns Hopkins University Press, 2005.

Peckham, Robert. *Epidemics in Modern Asia*. Cambridge: Cambridge University Press, 2016.

SUGGESTED ADDITIONAL READING

Davis, Mike. *The Monster at Our Door: The Global Threat of Avian Flu*. New York: New Press, 2005.

Mason, Katherine A. *Change: Reinventing Chinese Public Health after an Epidemic*. Stanford, CA: Stanford University Press, 2016.

Sipress, Alan. *The Fatal Strain: On the Trail of Avian Flu and the Coming Pandemic*. New York: Viking, 2009.

46

"Asian Flu" (H1N1) Epidemic, Asia, 2009–2010

WHEN AND WHERE

On April 21, 2009, the U.S. Centers for Disease Control (CDC) announced that two children had become infected with "swine flu," or H1N1 influenza. Three days later, it emerged that similar cases had been reported in Mexico in preceding weeks. By May 6, the same flu had been identified in 21 other countries, which drove the World Health Organization (WHO) to warn of an impending pandemic involving "sustained community level outbreaks" (quoted in Dehner 2012, 16).

From those alarms in April and May 2009, the new infection spread over most of the world and only ebbed in November. For example, in the United States nearly 61 million people were sickened by it, 275,000 hospitalized, and over 12,000 died ("CDC Estimates of 2009 H1N2 Influenza Cases, Hospitalizations and Deaths in the United States" n.d.). That number, while it represented individual tragedies, also represented about 3% of the total deaths in the country, and influenza was not numbered among the leading national causes of death. Nor did 2009's influenza toll differ significantly from its annual exactions in the United States.

The worldwide effects were similar. Across the globe estimates of the total mortality ranged between 152,000 and 575,000, again representing between 1% and 7% of the world's total deaths.

SIGNIFICANCE

This epidemic was a major cause of worldwide concern in 2009 and 2010. It has since acquired retrospective significance as an example of a dog that did not bark in the nighttime, as the feared major pandemic that did not occur and in which the death toll was typical of general flu expectations. But its relative severity for the young also refocused attention on a different demographic (see below). The epidemic also illustrated the possibilities of popular—and even technical—misunderstandings of words.

BACKGROUND

This epidemic occurred at a time when the world's public health authorities were focused on the dangers threatened by an avian "bird flu" (H5N1). Widespread concerns about such a flu had been stoked by the renewed interest in the 1918–1919 "Spanish Flu" pandemic. In 1997, the genetic code of the cause of that pandemic had been discovered, while (coincidentally) alarming cases of the new H5N1 "bird flu" appeared in China. The enormous—and domesticated—poultry population of China seemed to pose a threat to the world, further conditioned to assume that diseases of all sorts (from nineteenth-century cholera to 2002 SARS) had their origins in Asia.

Such worries led to vaccines being mobilized to confront the expected H5N1 bird flu, so when that pathogen did not in fact appear, little time remained to restock the relevant vaccine supply. The belated diagnosis of an H1N1 strain in turn called forth fears of a reappearance of the "Spanish flu" pandemic of 1918–1919.

This epidemic also coincided with a serious recession in American and many other Western economies that weakened government (and private) financing of public health institutions and reduced personnel levels.

HOW IT IS UNDERSTOOD AT PRESENT

General agreement had long been reached about many of the features of influenza: as a virus, it was very contagious, moving easily through the air from person to person; it ultimately was contracted from some other host species such as birds or mammals; it was very widespread, usually mild, but occasionally lethal. More recently, the constant mutations of the virus had been realized, and differing classes of subtypes had been recognized. In 2009 differences of opinion about the relevant subtypes, and about their animal hosts, existed. Influenza sometimes interacted with pneumonia, and in doing so posed an increased danger to the elderly; but on at least one notable occasion—1918–1919—it disproportionally affected young adults.

RESPONSES

In the early stages of the epidemic, before attention shifted to the H1N1 virus, responses characteristically followed some established routines: isolation of the sick, rigorous sanitation, face masks to contain the epidemic, together with nursing care to relieve symptoms. The possibility of closing schools (especially) or other public facilities roiled many communities. Prevention waited on the development of vaccines that would counter the unexpected H1N1 virus. Those vaccines only became available in quantity in November 2009. The vulnerability of young adults was only recognized empirically, as the epidemic unfolded.

Overlying both American and world responses to the epidemic were uncertainties about its severity, illustrated (and perhaps driven) by the WHO's labeling the epidemic as a "phase 6 pandemic." As a trio of contemporary critics argued, "Did the designation 'pandemic' refer to the pathogen's novelty, rapid transmission, geographical distribution, or to severity? Historically, the terms "epidemic" and "pandemic" have been employed interchangeably and in popular usage have come to refer to 'large-scale occurrences of infectious and chronic diseases'" (quoted in Peckham 2016, 18). How urgent should be official and popular responses? Should officials be trusted?

UNRESOLVED ISSUES

The rapid evolution of "influenza" viruses, together with the apparently increasing variety of them, remains a challenge for world public health. Can vaccines and appropriate responses keep pace? And, as Dehner says, when the warning responses of public health agencies—concerned with preventing the worst case—prove unnecessary, public opinion may turn against them, with accusations of their complicity with pharmaceutical manufacturers (Dehner 2012, 197–198).

REFERENCES AND SUGGESTED ADDITIONAL READING

"CDC Estimates of 2009 H1N1 Influenza Cases, Hospitalization and Deaths in the United States." n.d. https://www.cdc.gov/h1n1flu/estimates_2009_h1n1.htm..

The following readings supply some background:

Davis, Mike. *The Monster at Our Door: The Global Threat of Avian Flu.* New York: New Press, 2005.

Dehner, George. *Influenza: A Century of Science and Public Health Response.* Pittsburgh, PA: University of Pittsburgh Press, 2012.

Peckham, Robert. *Epidemics in Modern Asia.* Cambridge: Cambridge University Press, 2016.

Quammen, David. *Spillover: Animal Infections and the Next Human Pandemic.* New York: W. W. Norton, 2012.

Sipress, Alan. *The Fatal Strain: On the Trail of Avian Flu and the Coming Pandemic.* New York: Viking, 2009.

47

MERS Epidemic, Middle East, 2012–?

WHEN AND WHERE

In March 2012, a student in Jordan fell ill with coughing, shortness of breath, and fever; despite being in a hospital's intensive care unit, he died on April 25. Members of the hospital staff developed similar symptoms. Thus, the world met what subsequently was called Middle East Respiratory Syndrome, or MERS. Scattered cases persisted in the region throughout 2012, and then reached epidemic proportions between April and December 2013, especially in August; by year's end MERS had accounted for 84 deaths and over 200 cases. The great majority of the cases had been in Saudi Arabia, with others in Jordan, Kuwait, Qatar, United Arab Emirates, and Oman.

A new surge in MERS cases occurred in April 2014, chiefly in Saudi Arabia and the United Arab Emirates, where over 200 new cases were reported. By this time, a link between camels and the disease was being realized (see the "How It Is Understood at Present" section), and that connection was illustrated by such statistics (as of early June) as the presence in Saudi Arabia of 265,000 camels and 689 human cases of MERS.

Still another surge occurred—in the spring of 2015—not in western Asia, but in South Korea. A South Korean returned home from western Asia in May and was diagnosed with MERS shortly thereafter. By mid-June, the disease had infected 95 Koreans and 7 had died; another traveler conveyed the ailment to the Guangdong province of China, after breaking his quarantine in Korea.

SIGNIFICANCE

The outbreak of MERS in 2014 occurred in the context of the contemporary Ebola virus epidemic in west Africa. Fears generated by that joined the already-present worries following two other ominous viral infections: SARS in 2002 and "Asian flu" in 2009—especially when MERS jumped to east Asia in 2015.

BACKGROUND

The MERS epidemic illustrated the importance of international population movements of both people and animals, both enmeshed in regional interdependence. Infected people moved rapidly from west Asia to Korea; camels (see the next section) were imported from Ethiopia and Sudan to Egypt and then to Saudi Arabia. The camel population of Saudi Arabia is actually far smaller than that of many African states, which suggests the possible future magnitude of the epidemic.

HOW IT IS UNDERSTOOD AT PRESENT

From its first appearance, thinking about MERS focused on the probability that it was a viral disease found in an animal (that is, a zoonosis). But which animal? Its concentration in the Middle East brought camels to mind, since they were in frequent contact with people; among others, bats were also considered. How did the unknown pathogen jump from its animal host to its new human home? The close contacts between camels and humans suggested many possibilities: people drank camel's milk, ate camel meat, came in contact with camel urine and feces,

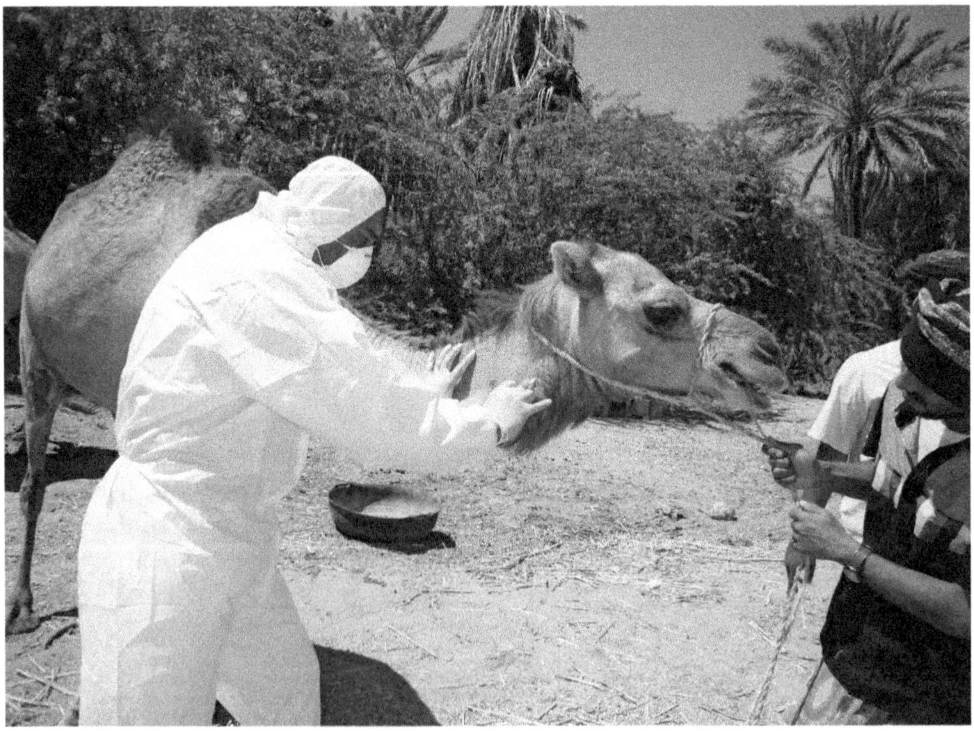

A veterinarian collects a blood sample from a camel during an investigation into the first reported MERS case in Haramout, Yemen. Scientists suspect that camels are infected with MERS by bats and then pass the virus to humans. (Centers for Disease Control and Prevention)

inhaled dust stirred up by camels, and rode on the backs of camels. But camels harboring the pathogen were apparently asymptomatic, which posed problems for any production of a vaccine. The World Health Organization (WHO) soon decided on the term "MERS-CoV," thus identifying it as a coronavirus.

In June 2014 attention shifted to Qatar, where the study of its international camel market resulted in the amassing of statistics that revealed the extent of the disease. The accompanying closer study of human–camel interactions came to focus on camel's milk as a likely infective link to people. The same studies also concluded that the number of people infected by MERS was far higher than previously realized, that many of those had had no direct contact with camels, and therefore mild versions of the disease were being passed from human to human. Such studies led to the conclusion that MERS had existed in the population long before 2012, in mild or latent forms.

RESPONSES

Responses evolved in tandem with understandings, in pursuit of cures, preventives, and environmental controls. The association with camels fed hopes that vaccines could be found for either camels themselves or at-risk human populations (Kupferschmidt December 18, 2015, 1453). The sudden appearance of MERS in Korea in 2015 vividly illustrated that human-to-human transmission was important, which demanded quarantines and isolation for those infected. Airports imposed travel restrictions. Hygiene measures were adopted around camels; camels' milk was pasteurized.

Did human responses to a disease linked to deeply loved domesticated animals in some way mirror the nineteenth-century ambivalence that complicated attitudes about rabies (to be sure a far different disease) and its association with dogs?

UNRESOLVED ISSUES

As of July 2019, the WHO reported that no successful vaccines had yet been developed. To prevent MERS from its transmission to humans, the WHO recommended hygienic practices around camels and the pasteurization of camels' milk; to prevent human-to-human transmission, isolation, quarantine, and sanitation. The obstacles to the success of those measures remained as they have been—social and/or economic resistance to their implementation. Will camel owners respect the recommended (or mandated) hygienic practices? The Saudi government has only slowly and reluctantly cooperated with international efforts. Individuals infected by the virus may remain asymptomatic (and thus unknown) or may refuse to cooperate with isolation measures. The sheer numbers and extent of the infection, among animals and people, remains unknown.

The same July 2019 report enumerated 2,461 world cases of MERS since 2012, and 851 deaths. The incidence of the disease remains at a very low level.

REFERENCES AND SUGGESTED ADDITIONAL READING

The above information has been compiled from press reports, especially those in Science *magazine, and from the reports of the WHO. The following articles in* Science *may be helpful:*

Enserink, Martin. "Mission to MERS." *Science* 344 (June 13, 2014): 1218–1220.

Kupferschmidt, Kai. "Amid Panic, a Chance to Learn about MERS." *Science* 348 (June 12, 2015): 1183–1184.

Kupferschmidt, Kai. "The Camel Connection." *Science* 343 (March 28, 2014): 1422–1425.

Kupferschmidt, Kai. "Camel Vaccine Offers Hope to Stop MERS." *Science* 350 no. 6267 (December 18, 2015): 1453.

Kupferschmidt, Kai. "MERS Surges again, but Pandemic Jitters Ease." *Science* 347 (March 20, 2015): 1296–1297.

48

Ebola Virus Epidemic, West Africa, 2013–2016

WHEN AND WHERE

The deadly Ebola virus first attracted attention in central Africa in 1976 and continued to recur there (with varying severity) in subsequent years. It then violently erupted in December 2013 in the West African state of Guinea and was confirmed in Liberia in March 2014 and Sierra Leone in May. By August 14, Ebola had resulted in 1,227 West African deaths among 2,240 reported cases. Those numbers rapidly changed; on October 3, the World Health Organization (WHO) estimated total infections as 7,470 and the dead at 3,431. In Liberia, the most severe week had been that beginning on September 21; by November 28, the number of new cases there had begun to decline.

The last known case in Liberia was recorded in mid-February 2015, but Ebola persisted in Sierra Leone and Guinea. In the former, the number of known infected had fallen to 12 by the end of April, and in the capital of Guinea (Conakry, a city of two million people) only one known Ebola patient remained. Despite that, Guinea was believed to be Ebola's last West African stronghold. On August 14, the number of Ebola cases in West Africa stood at 27,000, of whom about 11,000 had died.

The WHO suggested on October 9 that its member states could safely lift the bans that had been imposed on travel from the afflicted West African countries, a mark of the declining threat of Ebola. Liberia's last apparent case was on September 3; Sierra Leone was declared free of Ebola on November 7. The last known Ebola case in Guinea was released on November 20, 2015.

An authoritative summary of the 2013–2015 West African Ebola epidemic counted 28,644 cases, and 11,458 deaths (Oldstone and Oldstone 2017, 8–9).

SIGNIFICANCE

This Ebola epidemic was the most lethal (in terms of total mortality and morbidity) visitation of the disease in recorded history. Ebola had inspired particular

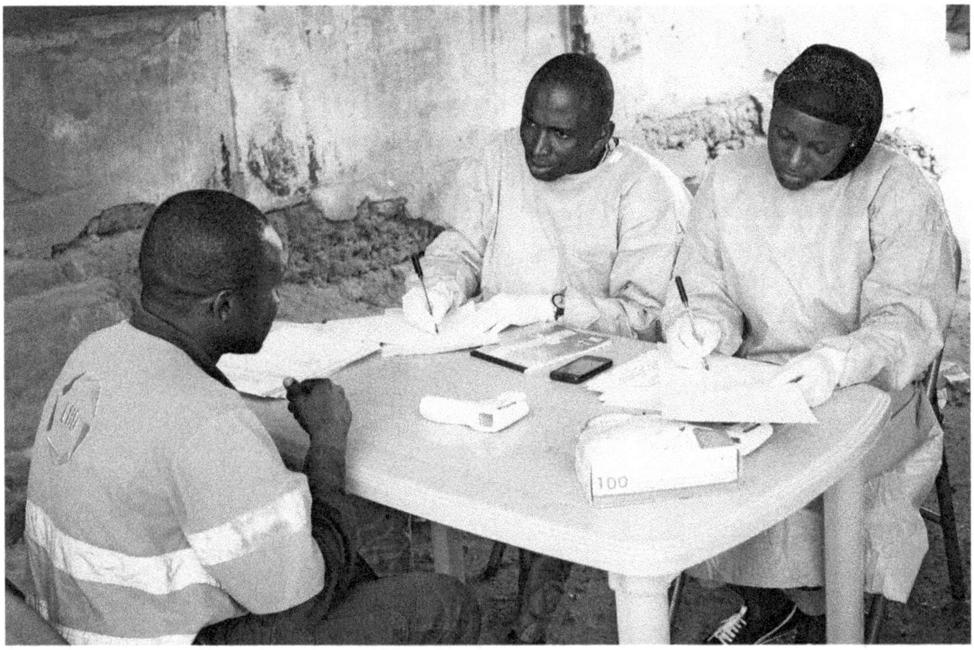

World Health Organization (WHO) Ebola vaccine trial in Guinea, July 2015. WHO vaccine trial team members follow up with a trial participant, monitoring his health after administration of the vaccine. These follow-up sessions take place 3, 9, 21, 42, 63, and 84 days after the vaccination. (WHO/S. Hawkey)

horror since it first appeared in Zaire (now the Democratic Republic of Congo, DRC) in 1976, owing both to the virus's extreme rate of contagion and its rapid and deadly onset. It was also an important example of the category of diseases known as zoonoses.

BACKGROUND

In the years before the Ebola virus appeared, a number of other "new" zoonotic viral infections had preceded it in equatorial Africa. Their emergence had followed the economic penetration of the region that brought African (and European) laborers into closer contact with wildlife, especially primates, that harbored the viruses. In addition to HIV, Marburg virus (1967) and Lassa fever (1969) had appeared, frightening populations, while HIV proceeded undetected.

The scale of the first Ebola epidemic in 1976 was far greater, and hence more frightening. In Zaire and Sudan, 602 had been infected and 431 had died. The reemergence of Ebola in Gabon and the DRC in the mid-1990s, joined by Uganda in the early 2000s, also occurred when "terrorism" began adding further international fears.

HOW IT IS UNDERSTOOD AT PRESENT

Those infected quickly showed symptoms that were common to many viral infections—diarrhea, fever, and weakness—but their distress was more extreme and their death more likely. The earlier experiences with Ebola had established the cause as a "filovirus" (so-called from its shape) that had two variants, named Ebola-Zaire and Ebola-Sudan. The Zaire variant resulted in marginally higher mortality rates. Person-to-person transmission rates were very high, both through the air and through touch. It was early understood that contagion was very likely. The known ability of the virus to remain hidden in human semen for months suggested a further possible path for contagion.

In early 2014 attention focused on fruit bats as the likely intermediate animal host, but the "natural reservoir of infection for Ebola virus is unclear"; monkeys were also likely. The route from animal to person was understood to be indirect, perhaps through eating the butchered animal (Oldstone and Oldstone 2017, 11).

RESPONSES

Responses to the epidemic focused on discovery, prevention, and cure. On one level, discovery was simple—when those affected began suffering dramatic hemorrhagic symptoms. Tracing paths of infection was complicated both by the earlier symptoms (fever, pain, vomiting) shared with other ailments, and by the rural isolation of victims. In 2014 a race began to develop reliable diagnostic tests that were inexpensive and easily applicable in remote locations, while also close enough to a laboratory sophisticated enough to analyze the findings. Several such tests were quickly developed by German and American companies, to be gradually deployed in West Africa.

Prevention relied first on successful discovery and isolation of the infected, and many obstacles existed that made that often difficult. A journalist for *Science* magazine illustrated some of them: patients who came to a hospital for an ailment who then fled into the rural vastness to avoid the fear of testing; locations reachable only by foot; when learning even the name of a possible contact is difficult; the sheer numbers of the possible contacts in cities of over one million inhabitants (Kupferschmidt 2015, 120–121).

From the beginning of the epidemic, prevention concentrated on the development of a vaccine. Development and employment of successful vaccines faced a number of obstacles. Should vaccines not yet completely tested be employed in the belief that something was better than nothing? Or would such actions endanger patients? The relative rarity of Ebola, magnified by the virus's differing subtypes, complicated the development of an effective vaccine. Would the demand for such a vaccine justify the expenses of its commercial production? In January 2015, vaccine trials were underway in Liberia, Guinea, and Sierra Leone. And by the time when "individually randomized controlled trials" (IRCT) had been perfected, the waning of the epidemic in the spring of 2015 had reduced the number of subjects for them. But the vaccines certainly contributed to the end of the West African epidemic. In December 2015, a vaccine marketed by the pharmaceutical company Merck seemed to hold promise for the future.

International responses—from both nation-states and nongovernmental agencies—played a role. The WHO took the lead, pleading for intervention; there were a variety of international responses from China, Cuba, the United States, and western Europe, involving governments, universities, and corporations. In November 2014, in response to the difficulties of treating patients in West Africa, 18 patients were airlifted to Europe or the United States. The WHO suggested that states impose travel bans from West Africa, which were widely enacted; they were lifted in October 2015.

UNRESOLVED ISSUES

As the Ebola epidemic eased in the summer of 2015, other worries arose. Would it be succeeded by (for instance) measles? Attention to Ebola had postponed plans to improve the administration of measles vaccination in the three countries, where the percentage of children vaccinated was dangerously low.

The fate of those who survived Ebola was not clear. A variety of symptoms persisted: blurred vision, hearing loss, headaches. And since (in June 2015) the WHO estimated that at least 16,000 West Africans had survived the epidemic, a sizable public health problem was ensured. The recovering sufferers also faced social isolation and stigmatization, while the discovery that the virus could linger in human semen made many fear sexual contact.

On January 14, 2016, a new Ebola case appeared in Sierra Leone, shortly after the declaration that the epidemic was over. Had the disease been eradicated? Clearly not. In May 2017, Ebola resurfaced in the DRC, and in the next year, while bats and pigs were focused on as likely reservoirs and vaccine trials proceeded, Ebola lingered on. The WHO proclaimed that Ebola was "largely contained" on July 3, 2018 (McNeil July 3, 2018, D3), only to be confronted with yet another DRC outbreak that led to a further WHO declaration of an epidemic on August 1.

As of March 4, 2020, the WHO estimated that in the DRC there had occurred 3,444 cases of Ebola, causing 2,264 deaths. This Ebola epidemic had therefore become the second most serious in the disease's history, only overshadowed by the West African events of 2013–2015.

REFERENCES AND SUGGESTED ADDITIONAL READING

An important online source for this subject: www.who.int/ebola.

Cohen, Jon, and Kai Kupferschmidt. "A Dose of Reality." *Science* 346, no. 6212 (November 21, 2014): 908–911.

Hofman, Michiel, and Sokhieng Au, eds. *The Politics of Fear: Medicins san Frontiers and the West African Ebola Epidemic.* Oxford: Oxford University Press, 2017.

Kupferschmidt, Kai. "Estimating the Ebola Epidemic." *Science* 345, no. 6201 (September 5, 2014): 1108.

Kupferschmidt, Kai. "On the Trail of Contagion." *Science* 347, no. 6218 (January 2, 2015): 120–121.

Kupferschmidt, Kai. "Surviving Ebola Survival." *Science* 348, no. 6242 (June 26. 2015): 1406–1407.

McNeil, Donald G., Jr., "Ebola Outbreak in Central Africa Is in Decline." *New York Times*, July 3, 2018, D3.

McNeil, Donald G., Jr. "New Hope for an End to Ebola's Reign of Terror." *New York Times*, August 13, 2019, A1 and A7.

Oldstone, Michael B. A., and Madeleine Rose Oldstone. *Ebola's Curse: 2013–2016 Outbreak in West Africa.* London: Academic Press, 2017.

Packard, Randall M. *A History of Global Health: Interventions into the Lives of Other Peoples.* Baltimore, MD: Johns Hopkins University Press, 2016.

Quammen, David. *Spillover: Animal Infections and the Next Human Pandemic.* New York: W. W. Norton, 2012.

49

Pneumonic Plague Epidemic, Madagascar, 2014–2017

WHEN AND WHERE

After a long period when plague had been endemic in Madagascar, an abrupt outbreak of the disease that soon became an epidemic began on August 27, 2017. What became the "index case" involved a man—apparently suffering from malaria—traveling in a "bush taxi" from the countryside into Antananarivo, the capital. During the journey, the man died, and soon 31 others who had been in contact with him fell ill, four fatally.

Between that time and mid-September, plague began a rapid spread in and around Antananarivo, but it was only identified as pneumonic plague on September 13. By October 7, the disease had infected 343 people and caused 42 deaths. The epidemic evidently peaked in the next several weeks, when the number of cases nearly doubled weekly; by October 20, the World Health Organization (WHO) put the number of cases at 1,297, with 102 deaths. Plague had also been carried to Seychelles, when an infected traveler returned there from Madagascar by air and was promptly isolated.

By early November, the WHO found that both deaths and new cases were declining, and that the epidemic might be brought under control. At that time, the estimated death toll stood at 127, from about 1,800 cases. On November 22, the Madagascar Ministry of Public Health reported that 2,348 cases had been diagnosed since August 1, and that 202 deaths had occurred. At that point, the pneumonic plague epidemic was apparently under control, but endemic levels of bubonic plague could be expected to continue until the end of the summer season in April 2018.

SIGNIFICANCE

This epidemic illustrates the persistent presence of *Yersinia pestis* in its endemic enzootic state, flourishing in rodent communities in isolated communities; in such communities, occasional endemic plague cases may erupt into epidemics when social, economic, or political conditions make proper biomedical response difficult. "Plague" still has an almost-unique power to frighten popular opinion and stimulate an international response.

BACKGROUND

The causative organism of plague, *Yersinia pestis*, reached the island of Madagascar in 1898, during the diffusion of the Third Plague Pandemic (see volume 2, chapter 31). As happened in a number of places across the globe—for example, in the western United States—a "maintenance phase" of plague infection was established in populations of burrowing rodents in Madagascar that persisted throughout the twentieth century. By 1997 (if not earlier), researchers had discovered that *Y. pestis* in Madagascar had become resistant to antibiotics, an alarming prospect for human populations.

HOW IT IS UNDERSTOOD AT PRESENT

Before this epidemic, the causes of plague had already been well understood, and convincing arguments for its phases and ecology had been advanced and applied.

RESPONSES

Initially, the health care workers on the scene in Madagascar (especially in some areas) had little or no experience with plague and so regarded it as influenza. Thirty-nine of them were quickly infected by plague. However, the Pasteur Institute in Antananarivo, the capital, began quickly ordering diagnostic tests that confirmed plague's presence, while international agencies such as the World Health Organization, the U.S. Centers for Disease Control, and UNICEF dispatched workers, who staffed regional plague centers where symptomatic people could be isolated and treated with antibiotics. Meanwhile the control—and eradication—of rats and fleas was pursued.

That the disease spread directly from person to person through the air added complications to responses. The very rapid mortality of pneumonic plague—almost certain death within two days—posed problems for the necessary isolation of those infected, isolation that would prevent further person-to-person contagion. Those difficulties were multiplied by the rural isolation of the potentially endangered population. In the capital city, schools were closed and public gatherings forbidden.

Hoping to halt the spread of plague, the WHO proclaimed a state of "very high risk" for wide swaths of East Africa and the Indian Ocean, from South Africa to Ethiopia, Comoros, Reunion, Mauritius, as well as Seychelles (where a case of plague had already occurred).

UNRESOLVED ISSUES

Both social and ecological factors that affect plague epidemics remain unresolved, and no clear end to them is likely. *Yersinia pestis* and antibiotics engage in an evolutionary struggle, as over-prescription of a drug feeds the germ's resistant response, which in turn is countered by a new antibiotic. The costs of developing those drugs may multiply, another danger to poor societies.

The difficulties of discovering cases of pneumonic plague in remote areas, where those infected may die before they are even discovered and isolated and may have (by sharing the air with neighbors) further spread the disease. The rapid burial of victims has offended some local customs of reverence for the dead and so has led to resistance to treatment, as often occurred in other societies and times.

REFERENCES AND SUGGESTED ADDITIONAL READING

As with other contemporary epidemics, this entry depends on journalistic accounts and official reports from (especially) the WHO.

McNeil, Donald G., Jr. "Deadly Plague Outbreak Appears to Wane." *New York Times*, November 7, 2017, D3.

McNeil, Donald G., Jr. "Plague Outbreak in Madagascar Spreads." *New York Times*, October 12, 2017, A9.

"Plague Rages in Madagascar." *Science* 358, no. 6360 (October 13, 2017): 152–153.

Roberts, Leslie. "Echoes of Ebola as Plague Hits Madagascar." *Science* 358, no. 6362 (October 27, 2017): 430–431.

50

Zika Virus Epidemic, Latin America and the Caribbean, 2015–2017

WHEN AND WHERE

The virus called Zika, previously occasionally found in Africa and Southeast Asia, gained widespread interest in 2007 when it suddenly infected an estimated 73% of the population of Yap, an island group in the southwest Pacific; no deaths or even serious illness resulted. In subsequent years, other Pacific Island territories experienced similar outbreaks; for example, the French Polynesian islands dominated by Tahiti suffered 30,000 Zika infections in 2013, roughly 10% of their population. In that case, some hospitalizations occurred.

In May 2015 Zika infections appeared in Brazil, and Colombia followed in October. By the end of 2015, their number began multiplying rapidly, a surge that peaked in January and February 2016, when the new infections numbered as many as 30,000 per week, chiefly but not exclusively in Brazil. On February 1, the World Health Organization (WHO) decreed a "public health emergency of international concern" in response to the alarming frequency of microcephalic brain damage found in newborn babies whose mothers had contracted Zika virus during pregnancy.

While the number of Zika cases declined steadily (or swiftly) in South America after February 2016, a corresponding increase took place in the islands of the Caribbean through the summer of that year. The decline continued across the Americas in 2017, and by the end of that year, it seemed to have ended. Statistics illustrate the trend: 205,578 cases in Brazil in 2016, only 13,253 in 2017, and all of those in the early months of the year (as of July 26).

As of August 23, 2019, the Zika infections between 2015 and 2017 numbered about 800,000; about 4,000 infants suffered brain damage ("Cuba Harbored 'hidden' Zika Outbreak" 2019).

SIGNIFICANCE

As was true of the MERS epidemic that began in 2012, Zika swept into world attention while Ebola had generated worldwide fears. Advisories warned international travelers about the dangers of West Africa (on account of Ebola) and then about the dangers of the Caribbean (on account of Zika). The very existence of inexpensive international travel made such warnings "necessary," itself a significant feature of the twenty-first century—especially for the prosperous people of Europe and North America, but also for massive populations driven in motion by economic necessities or fears of communal violence. Zika also illustrated the continuing difficulties posed by elusive viruses that hid in populations and could move rapidly, and to those variables were added the effects of climate change.

BACKGROUND

A number of viruses conveyed by *Aedes aegypti* mosquitos reached the Americas in the seventeenth century, most notably yellow fever. Zika was a member of this class of flaviviruses; its apparent clinical effects, unlike those of yellow fever, were usually so mild that it might have long remained unrecognized so that its earlier history in the Americas can only be conjectured. But its rapid movement across oceans and continents in the twenty-first century has been made possible by air travel.

HOW IT IS UNDERSTOOD AT PRESENT

Understanding of Zika followed from the long-established beliefs about other mosquito-borne flaviviruses that varied in their severity; it was thought simply to be generally milder than others. But the cases of infant microcephaly that occurred in 2015 and 2016 spurred vigorous responses.

RESPONSES

Stimulated by the World Health Organization's February 1 declaration, vaccine manufacturers responded on several fronts. The fact that vaccines existed for similar viruses, such as yellow fever and dengue, led to some belief that the development path would be an easy one. Could a vaccine for yellow fever even offer protection against Zika? Others noticed that not enough was yet known about Zika; would a single infection lead to lifelong immunity (as with yellow fever), for example? Within a few months, researchers had confronted a number of difficulties posed by Zika that complicated a vaccine's application. The scarcity of serious cases on which to test vaccines posed difficulties for any quantitative assessment of success that required placebos, and the apparent rapid waning of the epidemic further depleted the number of possible subjects for testing of vaccines.

Faced with those vaccine uncertainties, responses turned to vector control and the limitation of access to dangerous places. Pregnant women were urged to defer travel from their homes in the temperate latitudes to the Caribbean and Latin America; those already in the tropics were asked to delay pregnancies. And while eradication of *Aedes aegypti* mosquitos was possible, its spreading territorial reach, afforded by climate change, complicated the risks. Between the years 2011 and 2014, a population of such mosquitos had taken up yearlong residence in Washington, DC—deep in the temperate zone of the United States.

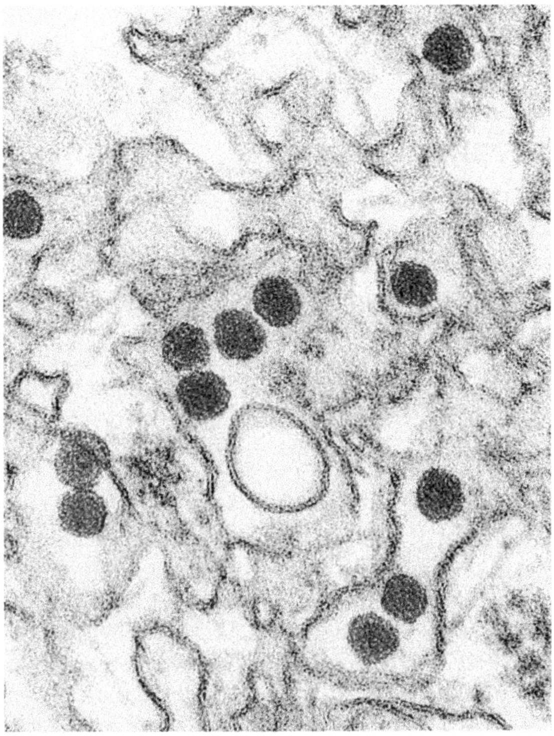

Colorized transmission electron micrograph of the Zika virus. (Centers for Disease Control and Prevention)

UNRESOLVED ISSUES

A virus that infects *people* who subsequently remain asymptomatic may conceivably remain hidden from public view, especially in populations that are for a variety of reasons—economic, social, geographical—out of the reach of analytic medical systems. Zika certainly illustrated that problem. For example, its spread to Asia and Africa (from whence it earlier came) remains likely, if not yet certain. Some evidence exists that it has established a presence in Thailand, for example (Peckham 2016, 314).

This "hidden" character of Zika also complicates understanding of its duration in a population. How do we account for its sudden disappearance from Brazil in 2016 and 2017? Had it become "endemic"? Had "herd immunity" taken hold? (That is, a certain percentage of the population gained immunity from a prior infection.)

The path of Zika infections of the body remains under study, especially explaining the complications of birth defects. Is the virus able to cross the placenta to reach the fetus? May it infect the testes, suggesting that it might be transmitted through sexual contact?

The small size of the potentially infected pregnant population has made it difficult to answer questions about the safety of vaccines. Would a Zika vaccine actually lead to an unexpected and tragic result? The 1961 thalidomide disaster still looms in vaccinators' minds (Cohen July 21, 2017).

Modern technology has also disturbed popular perceptions of the disease, complicating responses to it. For example, social media has included false information about Zika, convincing some that the disease is the product of a government conspiracy, echoing both contemporary beliefs about vaccines, older fears that arose about HIV-AIDS, and still older ones that surrounded cholera.

REFERENCES AND SUGGESTED ADDITIONAL READING

Peckham, Robert. *Epidemics in Modern Asia.* Cambridge: Cambridge University Press, 2016.

Information has been drawn from periodicals, especially Science, *and from WHO reports. These* Science *articles may be helpful:*

Cohen, Jon. "The Race for a Zika Vaccine Is On." *Science* 351, no. 6273 (February 5, 2016): 543–544.

Cohen, Jon. "Steep Drop in Zika Cases Undermines Vaccine Trial." *Science* 361, no. 6407 (September 14, 2018): 1055–1056.

Cohen, Jon. "Where Has All the Zika Gone?" *Science* 357, no. 6352 (August 18, 2017): 631–632.

Cohen, Jon. "Zika Rewrites Maternal Immunization Ethics." *Science* 357, no. 6348 (July 21, 2017): 241.

"Cuba Harbored 'Hidden' Zika Outbreak." *Science* 365, no. 6455 (August 23, 2019): 726.

Enserink, Martin. "An Obscure Mosquito-borne Disease Goes Global." *Science* 350, no. 6264 (November 27, 2015): 1012–1013.

Ferguson, Neil M., Zulma M. Cucunubá, Ilaria Dorigatti, Gemma L. Nedjati-Gilani, Christl A. Donnelly, Maria-Gloria Basáñez, Pierre Nouvellet, Justin Lessler. "Countering the Zika Epidemic in Latin America." *Science* 353, no. 6297 (July 22, 2016): 353–354.

Lessler, Justin, Lelia H. Chaisson, Lauren M. Kucirka, Qifang Bi, Kyra Grantz, Henrik Salje, Andrea C. Carcelen, et al. "Assessing the Global Threat from Zika Virus." *Science* 353, no. 6300 (August 12, 2016): 663.

Lipsitch, Marc, and Benjamin J. Cowling. "Zika Vaccine Trials." *Science* 353, no. 6304 (September 9, 2016): 1094–1095.

Vogel, Gretchen. "Evidence Grows for Zika Virus as Pregnancy Danger." *Science* 351, no. 6278 (March 11, 2016): 1123–1124.

Vogel, Gretchen. "Experts Fear Zika's Effects May Be Even Worse than Thought." *Science* 352, no. 6292 (June 17, 2016): 1375–1376.

Vogel, Gretchen. "One Year Later, Zika Scientists Prepare for a Long War." *Science* 354, no. 6316 (December 2, 2016): 1088–1089.

51

Cholera Epidemic, Yemen, 2017–?

WHEN AND WHERE

In 2017 the "worst outbreak of cholera ever documented in any country" ("Cholera Cases in Yemen Spike Again" 2019, 8) occurred in Yemen. In that year, a country with a population of 28 million experienced over one million cholera cases resulting in 2,500 deaths. The epidemic had become alarming in April 2017; by July 21, 320,000 Yemenis had been infected and 1,742 deaths had resulted, and the toll continued to soar. On October 10, the toll of infected reached about 815,000.

By the appalling standards of 2017, in 2018 cholera receded to a still-frightening total of 300,000 cases. But in 2019 cholera took an ominous turn; by April 5, 109,000 cases of a suspicious "watery diarrhea" had been recorded and 109 deaths.

SIGNIFICANCE

This epidemic is a vivid illustration of the linkages between physical infrastructures, alert public health systems, and possible epidemic outbreaks. It illustrated that the control of epidemics depends as much (or more) on social, economic, and political factors as on informed biomedical practice. Epidemics may flourish in times of war.

BACKGROUND

Yemen's recent history had been dominated by great internal tensions based on both religious and international political differences. One element of its population adhered to Shiite Islam, the other followed the Sunni interpretation. By the 1990s, the Sunni state was internationally recognized as the government, with the city of Sanaa as its capital and the support of Saudi Arabia and the United States. But the Shiite faction, the Houthis, controlled the northern sections of the country, and Sanaa itself in a rebellious region enjoyed the support of the Shiite nation of

Iran. In 2015 these two regions were engaged in a full-scale civil war, in part as proxies for a larger international struggle between (Sunni) Saudi Arabia and its ally the United States, on the one side, and (Shia) Iran, on the other. Saudi Arabia (and the United States) conducted a relentless air bombardment of Houthi territories, including Sanaa.

HOW IT IS UNDERSTOOD AT PRESENT

In the course of the twentieth century, the cause of cholera had come to be understood as the bacterium *Vibrio cholerae*, which reached the body through ingested food or water. People thus infected then became transmitters themselves when their excretions infected food and water supplies. The prevention of cholera thus depended on the continuous and reliable supply of clean water. While several different approaches to its cure had historically been pursued (including antibiotics and preventive vaccines), fluid replacement therapy to counter cholera's drastic dehydration had become surest. That technique involved an intravenous infusion.

RESPONSES

Established responses to cholera epidemics were well known, but the brutal wartime conditions hampered their effectiveness. Aerial bombing devastated infrastructures: buildings themselves collapsed; water and sewer systems broke apart, which alone made control of cholera very difficult if not impossible. When the cures of those afflicted hinged on the rehydration of body fluids administered by trained personnel, the violent conditions of war took their toll. The availability of intravenous apparatus was reduced. Death, fear, and injury affected the administering personnel and not simply by bombings, for the civil war divided local populations, and local opponents could drive caregivers away or kill them.

In this desperate situation, more hopes centered on preventive vaccines, but their administration faced multiple difficulties. The large number of Yemenis believed at risk strained the available world supply; at one point an international group mandated the delivery of one million doses to Yemen (Kupferschmidt 2017, 1316–1317), only to have Yemen's government suspend the request. The vaccines were diverted to places less beset by chaos than Yemen. It was further argued that the vaccine's presence might distract caregivers from treating those already ill ("Cholera Vaccine Plans Reversed" July 21, 2017, 232). The limited supply of vaccines led to other questions. Was it more effective to limit the doses for individuals to one, affording some protection to more people, or to give the recommended two doses, thus assuring some people of more certain immunity?

Expanding world supplies of cholera vaccines began to have an effect in 2018, and by April 2019, over 700,000 Yemenis had been vaccinated against cholera.

UNRESOLVED ISSUES

As long as civil discord persists, disrupting safe water supplies and crippling public health infrastructure, cholera will be hard to control. Among the countries that have continued to suffer seriously have been Zimbabwe (Moyo and Perez-Pena 2018, A4) and the Democratic Republic of Congo.

Vaccines continue to improve, as does their availability. They also have made single-dose application more effective. Such improvements may lead to successful preventive, as opposed to reactive, vaccines in countries such as Bangladesh where cholera has been endemic.

But countering those improvements may be the continuing evolutionary struggle between vaccine development and pathogen adaptive variation. The El Tor variant of *Vibrio cholerae* has already shown its capacity to mutate, and the development of strains that resist vaccines remains likely.

REFERENCES AND SUGGESTED ADDITIONAL READING

These articles in Science *may be helpful:*

"Cholera Cases in Yemen Spike Again." *Science* 364, no. 6435 (April 5, 2019): 8.

"Cholera Vaccine Faces Major Test in Yemen." *Science* (June 30, 2017): 1316–1317.

"Cholera Vaccine Plans Reversed." *Science* 357, no. 6348 (July 21, 2017): 232.

"How Today's Cholera Pandemic Was Born." *Science* 354, no. 6314 (November 18, 2016): 810.

Kupferschmidt, Kai. "Cholera Vaccine Faces Major Test in Yemen." *Science* 356, no. 6345 (June 30, 2017): 1316–1317.

Kupferschmidt, Kai. "Use of Cholera Vaccines Expands, Raising Hopes." *Science* (February 9, 2018): 620–621.

Moyo, Jeffrey, and Richard Perez-Pena. "Zimbabwe Tries to Stem an Outbreak of Cholera." *New York Times*, September 12, 2018, A4.

See also the sources listed in volume 2, chapter 40.

52

Contemporary Measles Outbreaks, United States

WHEN AND WHERE

In 2013 the incidence of measles in the United States—where it had been declared eradicated in 2000—had reached a total of 187 cases, and it had remained over 100 in most subsequent years. Then in October 2018 an alarming surge began in one state, New York, and soon became an epidemic. Its center was in Rockland County, an outer suburban area for New York City, and particularly in the community called "New Square," an ethnic enclave settled by Hasidic Orthodox Jews whose community had close ties with both Israel and Ukraine. The initial case involved an Israeli teenager who had traveled to Israel and there met another person who had just returned from Ukraine conveying the infection. The circumstances of the worship center in New Square—a large enclosed hall—made diffusion of the airborne virus very likely. Driven by those Rockland County events, the national measles cases rose to 375 by the end of 2018.

In 2019 the epidemic continued and spread, still focused on New York. By the end of that year, the national total had reached 1,282, New York state numbering 1,046, with 296 of those in Rockland County and a further 358 elsewhere in the immediate New York City area. California was another state with significant measles activity in 2019. In that year, there were 73 confirmed measles cases in that state, including 41 cases associated with six outbreaks (defined as three or more cases). As of May 7, 2020, there have been only 12 additional cases.

SIGNIFICANCE

The escalation of measles in the United States since 2000 and especially since 2013 had been shocking to a nation that had become accustomed to regarding measles as a forgotten and common childhood ailment. The epidemic illustrated how frail some public health systems were; if the United States could endure such blow, was nowhere safe? World attention could realize afresh that, in fact, measles was still a worldwide scourge.

BACKGROUND

Measles had long been an almost universal childhood disease in the United States, rarely fatal. Vaccines had developed between 1949 and 1963 to prevent it; in the latter year, the number of annual cases there had fallen to between three and four million (still a large number), but then vaccinations had taken hold and in 2000 measles was declared eradicated.

Vaccinations, however, were never universal. Vaccines had been resisted since the early nineteenth century when smallpox vaccines first appeared. Some people objected to the power of state mandatory vaccination being imposed on parents of children; others feared vaccines were not safe or had unwanted effects; still others called on religious beliefs that seemed to be violated by the manner or substance being used. To mollify some such objections nations and states (at different times and in different places) allowed religious or moral exemptions from mandatory vaccinations. It was only in 1902 that France even attempted to compel smallpox vaccination; by the 1930s four American states went so far as to forbid local authorities from requiring the vaccinations of schoolchildren. By the beginning of 2019, 47 U.S. states had laws on the books allowing such exemptions.

A variety of American communities had taken advantage of these exemptions from vaccination: Amish farmers in Ohio, Indiana, Pennsylvania; Somali immigrants in Minnesota; and free spirits in California private schools proclaimed freedom from restraint. A number of media celebrities had become outspoken "anti-vaxxers." In 1998 their cause was given—briefly—authoritative scientific support in an article in the prestigious British medical journal *The Lancet* by the physician Andrew Wheeler, in which he claimed a connection between the measles vaccine and autism. The article's flaws were quickly exposed, its publication was revoked, and Wheeler was stripped of his medical privileges, but the damage persisted as anti-vaxxers seized on the thoroughly debunked idea.

The Hasidic communities in New York were vulnerable targets for the anti-vaxx movement. Some rabbis (not all) looked on vaccines as violations of purity. The isolation (and resulting ignorance) imposed on Hasidic women made them more likely to react to rumors and false ideas found on social media. In addition, international links of communities such as that in New Square (which had 15 "sister cities") regularly drew visitors from Ukraine and elsewhere.

The reemergence of American measles occurred in the larger context of world disease and health. While advanced and prosperous states had greatly reduced or eradicated measles, it remained very widespread elsewhere. In 1985 the world still recorded over one million cases of measles. Ten years later, the gradual progress of vaccination reduced that to about 400,000; in 2015 the number had reached 145,000. By 2018 measles cases in Europe more than tripled since the previous year, rising from 25,500 to 83,000. Ukraine (significantly for Rockland County) accounted for 54,000 cases, 16 of whom died (Wadman February 2019, 677–678).

Some world religious practitioners continued to resist measles vaccination. In Indonesia in 2018, Islamic clerics pronounced a *fatwa* on a combined measles/rubella vaccine, arguing that it contained pork products.

HOW IT IS UNDERSTOOD AT PRESENT

In the course of the twentieth century, the epidemiological path of the measles virus had come to be clearly understood. It was a highly contagious infection that passed through the air; the droplets that carry it may reach a whole room and the virus may linger for hours, so that one already infected may be a danger to many. Such transmissions may begin up to eight days during which the carrier has remained asymptomatic, without the characteristic rash. Victims may remain contagious for nine days after symptoms appear. Therefore, the chain of infections—between the infection of the first case and the onset of the second—may vary from 8 days to 21.

The disease may result in very high morbidity rate, but a very low mortality rate; that is perhaps a week of discomfort, but only rare hospitalizations and very rare deaths. The low death rates have characterized modern measles epidemics in part because one case of the disease almost always confers subsequent immunity, and the incidence has been nearly universal. But measles has been deadly in virgin soil epidemics (see, e.g., volume 2, chapter 27), and the point of vaccines is to ensure immunity. When a society or nation achieves the benchmark of 95% of the population immunized, it is said to have "herd immunity," meaning that any stray case of measles most likely will be contained without meeting another susceptible victim.

RESPONSES

Responses in the United States and elsewhere largely centered on the promotion of vaccines and accompanying fervid opposition to anti-vaccination beliefs. In New York, the city's health commissioner mandated vaccinations in some sections of Brooklyn, to be met with legal challenges based on the religious exemption statutes. Of those infected, a minority (128) were hospitalized, which involved for them well-established medical curative responses.

UNRESOLVED ISSUES

While measles and its epidemiology have been long-studied and widely understood, new research continues and may add to that knowledge. A recent example of that: such infections in unvaccinated children may compromise the immune system for a length of time, weakening the different immunities to other past pathogens (Frederick 2019, 560–561).

The extremely contagious nature of the measles virus makes its total eradication very difficult. Some of the difficulties are rooted in the vaccination procedure itself; for greatest effectiveness two doses, in separate injections, are needed. Thus, the likelihood of error is increased, especially in poorer societies, which may lack trained vaccinators. A recent case in Samoa illustrates the problem; in July 2018 a contaminated measles vaccine injection led to the deaths of two infants, in turn sparking off resistance to vaccination. By December 2019, there had occurred 4,819 measles cases in a population of about 200,000, and 70 deaths. The World Health Organization estimated that the percentage of vaccinated Samoan children had fallen from 90% to 31%.

World social, economic, and political factors remain uncertain. The gulf between rich and poor nations persists. Poverty limits training; the persistence and depth of religious beliefs, perhaps overlain by superstitions and ignorance, lead to distrust of medical authority. Madagascar had more than 126,000 cases of measles between January and April 2019; the Democratic Republic of Congo, about 269,000 by December. Shrinking the gulf between rich and poor nations will be crucial.

In the United States and elsewhere in the rich world, perceptions and beliefs may still regard measles frivolously, as either a disease of the past and/or a trivial matter. The apparent omnipresence of social media may subvert medical and other forms of authority.

REFERENCES AND SUGGESTED READINGS

Crucial for this subject are these websites: www.cdc.gov *and* www.who.int.

Cliff, Andrew, Peter Haggett, and Matthew Smallman-Raynor. *Deciphering Global Epidemics: Analytical Approaches to the Disease Records of World Cities, 1888–1912.* Cambridge: Cambridge University Press, 1998.

McNeil, Donald G., Jr. "Once Tamed, Measles Rears Its Ugly Head." *New York Times*, April 4, 2019, A1 and A8.

Offit, Paul. *Deadly Choices: How the Anti-Vaccine Movement Threatens Us All.* New York: Basic Books, 2011.

Paumgarten, Nick. "The Message of Measles." *The New Yorker*, September 2, 2019, 38–47.

The following articles in Science *magazine may be of particular interest:*

Frederick, Eva. "How Measles Causes the Body to 'Forget' Past Infections." *Science* 366, no. 6465 (November 1, 2019): 560.

Graham, Matthew, et al. "Measles and the Canonical Path to Elimination." *Science* 364, no. 6440 (May 10, 2019): 584–587.

Roberts, Leslie. "Is Measles Next?" *Science* 348, no. 6238 (May 29, 2015): 959–961.

Rochmyaningsih, Dyna. "Indonesian Fatwa Causes Immunization Rates to Drop." *Science* 362, no. 6415 (November 9, 2018): 628–629.

"Samoa Battles Measles, Vaccine Fears." *Science* 366, no. 6471 (December 13, 2019): 1292.

"Suit Challenges Measles Order." *Science* 364, no. 6437 (April 19, 2019): 216.

Wadman, Meredith. "Measles Epidemic in Ukraine Drove Troubling European Year." *Science* 363, no. 6428 (February 15, 2019): 677–678.

Wadman, Meredith. "Measles Resurgent." *Science* 366, no. 6472 (December 20, 2019): 1442–1443.

Glossary

Antibiotic
A substance that destroys (or inhibits) bacteria. Most often, an antibiotic is derived from other organic substances, such as molds and fungi. The first antibiotic, penicillin, was extracted by Alexander Fleming in 1928, produced in testable quantities in 1940, and introduced in use against bacterial diseases during World War II. Other antibiotics followed shortly thereafter and revolutionized human ability to cure many diseases.

Asymptomatic
Showing no symptoms. A person who is infected by a disease microorganism but who shows no symptoms is asymptomatic; the word is used to describe healthy carriers, among others.

Bacteria
Microorganisms, usually one-celled, many of them found in animals (including humans) and plants. Some bacteria are responsible for diseases. *Bacteria* is a plural word; a single such microorganism is a *bacterium.*

Construction of a disease
The way a particular society or individual interprets a disease. Claiming that moral failure is responsible for AIDS is, for example, one construct of it; another would be attributing the disease to a retrovirus.

Contagion
Disease passing from one person to another by direct contact.

Diagnosis
The process of identifying a disease in a particular case. In the past, different pieces of evidence have been used to diagnose diseases: examining external symptoms, consulting omens, blood tests for microorganisms are examples.

Divination
Consultation of signs from the supernatural, for example, to forecast the outcome of a disease.

Early modern period
In Western history, that period between about 1500 and about 1800.

Endemic
Of a disease, found usually or habitually in an area or among a population. The common cold, for example, is endemic.

Enzootic
An endemic disease in an animal population.

Epidemic
Of a disease, resulting in levels of sickness and/or death above those ordinarily expected, an excessively prevalent disease.

Epidemiology
The study of epidemics, which measures their incidence and distribution and tries to understand why they spread where and when they do.

Epizootic
An epidemic disease in an animal population.

Etiology
The study of the causes of a disease or a statement of the causes of it.

Galen
A Greco-Roman physician (c. 130–c. 210) whose ideas about human anatomy and physiology and about the causes of disease influenced the medieval Christian and Muslim worlds for many centuries.

Germ theory
The belief that disease is produced by the actions of microorganisms ("germs"). The theory, while in some respects centuries old, was given its modern shape in the 1870s by the work of Louis **Pasteur** and Robert **Koch**.

Hippocrates
An ancient Greek physician, of the fifth century BCE. His writings (and likely those of others), collected in the "Hippocratic Corpus," had great later influence. They lay behind Galen and the humoral theory.

Host
An organism (a plant or animal) in which a pathogen lives. For example, plague bacteria may live in burrowing rodents; the Ebola virus may live in monkeys.

Humoral theory
The belief that disease resulted from an imbalance of the essential humours of the body. The *humours* were most often associated with specific fluids: blood, phlegm, yellow bile, and black bile. Disease was treated by restoring those humours to proper balance, often by removing excess blood and/or bile, through bleeding and purging the bowels. The theory continued to influence Western and Muslim approaches to disease through the medieval and early modern periods.

Immunity
Ability to resist a specific disease. In some cases, immunity may be inherited, acquired by a previous exposure to the disease, or gained by the administration of inoculation or vaccination.

Inoculation
The deliberate introduction of a disease into a body with the goal of conferring later immunity to it.

Jenner
Edward Jenner (1749–1832), an English surgeon who developed a vaccination for smallpox in 1798. Although what exactly he did remains controversial, his smallpox vaccine became the first deliberately prepared preventive measure that did not involve an inoculation of the disease itself, and it became the model for other vaccines.

Koch
Robert Koch (1843–1910), a German physician and one of the pioneers of modern germ theory. His experiments (in the 1870s) first demonstrated the role of germs in the animal disease anthrax, and he later isolated the germs responsible for cholera and tuberculosis.

Medicalization
The acceptance by a population or an individual of the authority of medical explanations and experts. A medicalized view of a problem refers the solution of the problem to physicians. A medicalized view of crime, for example, would urge that criminals needed hospital treatment, not incarceration.

Medieval period
In history, the period between about 500 and about 1500. Primarily refers to Western history but is usually applied to the Muslim world and sometimes to other civilizations in the same years.

Miasma
A pollution of the atmosphere held responsible for diseases. Thus, miasmatic theory would argue that bubonic plague, for example, resulted from a miasma, perhaps generated from volcanoes and caves in the earth or perhaps a product of celestial influences on the atmosphere.

Modern period
In history, the period since about 1800. The most recent decades are sometimes called contemporary history.

Morbidity
The incidence of a disease in a particular time and place. A morbidity rate is the rate of incidence of a disease; the level of sickness in a population. Morbidity rate is often expressed as a ratio, for example, 500 per 100,000 population means that in a population of one million, 5,000 people are sick. Some epidemics (most influenzas) have very high morbidity rates and low mortality rates; that is, many are sick, but relatively few die.

Mortality
The incidence of death in a particular time and place. A mortality rate is the death rate in a disease. Mortality rate is also often expressed as a ratio; a disease with a mortality rate of 100 per 100,000 per year is one in which in a population of one

million, 1,000 deaths will occur in a year from the disease. Some epidemics, notably those of plague and cholera, have mortality rates that approach their morbidity rates, meaning that a majority of the sick die of the disease.

Omens
Supernatural signs taken as evidence of a disease's future course.

Outbreak
A significant rise in the number of cases of a specific disease in a specific location.

Paleomicrobiology
Methods that use molecular diagnoses of surviving tissues of past disease victims to identify the responsible pathogen. For example, the presence of plague bacteria in the dental pulp of fourteenth-century Italian skeletons.

Pandemic
An epidemic on a very large geographical scale, involving several regions, continents, or the whole world.

Pasteur
Louis Pasteur (1822–1895), French chemist and pioneer of germ theory. His experiments traced germs through a number of animal diseases and led him to prepare a successful vaccination against rabies in 1885.

Prognosis
The forecast or prediction of a disease's likely outcome.

Prophylaxis, or Prophylactic
A measure used by a person to avoid contracting a specific disease.

Quarantine
Isolation of a person (or persons, on a ship, for example) to prevent the spread of disease (real or suspected) to others; can also mean isolating products and goods from a place where disease is suspected by forbidding their trade with others. Originally the word literally meant a forty-day period of isolation (as in Italian, *quaranta*, forty).

Rickettsial diseases
Diseases caused by organisms that are smaller and less complex than bacteria but unlike viruses are visible in microscopes. Typhus is perhaps the most prominent such disease.

Sacrifices
Offerings to the gods, perhaps the killing of an animal victim, in the hope of pleasing the gods and thus (in the case of an epidemic) diverting their anger.

Signs
The outward manifestations of a disease apparent to another person, such as a doctor.

Spells
Words spoken to invoke magic or supernatural powers, for example, in response to disease.

Sulfa drugs
Drugs introduced in the 1930s that had a *bacteriostatic* effect on bacteria; that is, they inhibited bacteria from multiplying in the body. Generally supplanted by antibiotics, which usually killed the bacteria outright.

Symptoms
Manifestations of a disease felt or perceived by the patient, which may or may not be perceptible to an outside person, such as a doctor.

Therapy
Measures taken to alleviate or cure a disease.

Vaccination
Administration of an agent of a disease or of a synthetically prepared substitute for it to promote a body's immunity to the disease. Originally used specifically for the process developed in 1798 by Jenner to prevent smallpox. Because Jenner used material from the animal disease cowpox, he named the process from the Latin word *vacca*, cow. The word has subsequently been extended to preventive treatments for any disease. Vaccine is the material used.

Vector
An organism that conveys a pathogen from one host to another. For example, fleas may convey plague bacteria from a rodent to a person.

Virgin soil epidemic
An epidemic of a disease in a population that has not experienced the disease before and so has no inherited or acquired immunity to it. Such epidemics can be very severe.

Virus
An extremely simple, submicroscopic organism. Some viruses are responsible for important diseases, including smallpox, poliomyelitis, influenzas, AIDS, and the common cold. Such ailments are therefore called viral diseases. Antibiotics have no effect on viruses.

Bibliography

Aberth, John. *Plagues in World History.* Lanham, MD: Rowman & Littlefield, 2011.

Ackerknecht, Erwin H. *A Short History of Medicine.* Rev. ed. Baltimore, MD: Johns Hopkins University Press, 1982.

Adams, Lisa V., and John R. Butterly. *Diseases of Poverty: Epidemiology, Infectious Diseases, and Modern Plagues.* Hanover, NH: Dartmouth College Press, 2015.

Alchon, Suzanne Austin. *A Pest in the Land: New World Epidemics in a Global Perspective.* Albuquerque: University of New Mexico Press, 2003.

Amundsen, Darrel. *Medicine, Society and Faith in the Ancient and Medieval Worlds.* Baltimore, MD: Johns Hopkins University Press, 1996.

Apple, Rima D., ed. *Women, Health, and Medicine in America: A Historical Handbook.* New Brunswick, NJ: Rutgers University Press, 1992.

Arnold, David. *Colonizing the Body: State Medicine and Epidemic Disease in Nineteenth-century India.* Berkeley: University of California Press, 1993.

Ayalon, Yaron. *Natural Disasters in the Ottoman Empire: Plague, Famine, and Other Misfortunes.* New York: Cambridge University Press, 2015.

Barrett, Ron, and George J. Armelagos. *An Unnatural History of Emerging Infections.* New York: Oxford University Press, 2013.

Bollet, Alfred Jay. *Plagues and Poxes: The Impact of Human History on Disease.* New York: Demos, 2004.

Bray, R. S. *Armies of Pestilence: The Impact of Disease on History.* New York: Barnes and Noble, 2000.

Brunton, Deborah. *Health and Wellness in the 19th Century.* Santa Barbara, CA: Greenwood Press, 2014.

Burnham, John C. *Health Care in America: A History.* Baltimore, MD: Johns Hopkins University Press, 2015.

Byrne, Joseph P., ed. *Encyclopedia of Pestilence, Pandemics, and Plague.* Westport, CT: Greenwood Press, 2008.

Byrne, Joseph P. *Health and Wellness in the Renaissance and Enlightenment.* Santa Barbara, CA: Greenwood Press, 2013.

Cliff, Andrew D., and Peter Haggett. *Atlas of Disease Distribution: Analytic Approaches to Epidemiological Date.* Oxford: Basil Blackwell, 1988.

Cliff, Andrew D., Peter Haggett, and Matthew Smallman-Raynor. *Deciphering Global Epidemics: Analytical Approaches to the Disease Records of World Cities, 1888–1912.* New York: Cambridge University Press, 1998.

Cohn, Samuel K. *Epidemics: Hate and Compassion from the Plague of Athens to AIDS.* New York: Oxford University Press, 2018.

Conrad, Lawrence I., Michael Neve, Roy Porter, Vivian Nutton, and Andrew Wear. *The Western Medical Tradition, 800 B.C.–A.D. 1800.* New York: Cambridge University Press, 1995.

Curtin, Philip D. *Disease and Empire: The Health of European Troops in the Conquest of Africa.* New York: Cambridge University Press, 1998.

Diamond, Jared. *Guns, Germs, and Steel: The Fates of Human Societies.* New York: W. W. Norton, 1997.

Esch, Gerald W. *Parasites and Infectious Disease: Discovery by Serendipity, and Otherwise.* New York: Cambridge University Press, 2007.

Farmer, Paul. *Infections and Inequalities: The Modern Plagues Updated.* Berkeley: University of California Press, 2001.

Fields, Sherry. *Pestilence and Headcolds: Encountering Illness in Colonial Mexico.* New York: Columbia University Press, 2008.

Gilman, Sander L. *Picturing Health and Illness: Images of Identity and Difference.* Baltimore, MD: Johns Hopkins University Press, 1995.

Gordis, Leon. *Epidemiology.* 5th ed. New York: W. B. Saunders, 2013.

Green, Monica. "The Globalization of Disease." In *Human Dispersal and Species Movement: From Prehistory to the Present*, edited by Nicole Boivin, Rémy Crassard, and Michael Petraglia, 494–520. New York: Cambridge University Press, 2017.

Grob, Gerald N. *The Deadly Truth: A History of Disease in America.* Cambridge, MA: Harvard University Press, 2002.

Hahn, Robert A. *Sickness and Healing: An Anthropological Perspective.* New Haven, CT: Yale University Press, 2002.

Hall, William, Anthony McDonnell, and Jim O'Neill. *Superbugs: An Arms Race against Bacteria.* Cambridge, MA: Harvard University Press, 2018.

Harper, Kyle. *The Fate of Rome: Climate, Disease, and the End of an Empire.* Princeton, NJ: Princeton University Press, 2017.

Harrison, Mark. *Contagion: How Commerce Has Spread Disease.* New Haven, CT: Yale University Press, 2013.

Harrison, Mark. *Disease and the Modern World: 1500 to the Present Day.* Malden, MA: Polity, 2004.

Harrison, Mark. *Medicine in an Age of Commerce and Empire: Britain and Its Tropical Colonies, 1660–1830.* New York: Oxford University Press, 2010.

Hays, J. N. *The Burdens of Disease: Epidemics and Human Response in Western History.* Rev. ed. New Brunswick, NJ: Rutgers University Press, 2009.

Israelowich, Ido. *Patients and Healers in the High Roman Empire.* Baltimore, MD: Johns Hopkins University Press, 2015.

Karlin, Arno. *Man and Microbes: Disease and Plagues in History and Modern Times.* New York: Simon & Schuster, 1995.

Kasper, Dennis L., and Anthony S. Fauci, eds. *Harrison's Infectious Diseases*. 3rd ed. New York: McGraw Hill, 2016.

Khan, Ali S. *The Next Pandemic: On the Front Lines against Humankind's Gravest Dangers*. New York: Public Affairs, 2016.

Kiple, Kenneth F., ed. *The Cambridge World History of Human Disease*. New York: Cambridge University Press, 1993.

Kleinman, Arthur. *The Illness Narrative: Suffering, Healing, and the Human Condition*. New York: Basic Books, 1988.

Koch, Tom. *Cartographies of Disease: Maps, Mapping, and Medicine*. Redlands, CA: ESRI Press, 2005.

Kunitz, Stephen J. *Disease and Social Diversity: The European Impact on the Health of Non-Europeans*. New York: Oxford University Press, 1994.

Matossian, Mary Kilbourne. *Poisons of the Past: Molds, Epidemics, and History*. New Haven, CT: Yale University Press, 1989.

McKeown, Thomas. *The Origins of Human Disease*. New York: Basil Blackwell, 1988.

McNeill, John Robert. *Mosquito Empires: Ecology and War in the Greater Caribbean, 1620–1914*. New York: Cambridge University Press, 2010.

McNeill, William H. *Plagues and Peoples*. Garden City, NY: Anchor/Doubleday, 1976.

Newson, Linda A. *Conquest and Pestilence in the Early Spanish Philippines*. Honolulu: University of Hawai'i Press, 2009.

Numbers, Ronald L., and Judith Walzer Leavitt, eds. *Sickness and Health in America: Readings in the History of Medicine and Public Health*. 2nd ed. Madison: University of Wisconsin Press, 1985.

Osterfeld, Richard S., Felicia Keeting, and Valerie T. Eviner, eds. *Infectious Disease Ecology: Effects of Ecosystems on Disease and of Disease on Ecosystems*. Princeton, NJ: Princeton University Press, 2008.

Packard, Randall M. *A History of Global Health: Interventions into the Lives of Other Peoples*. Baltimore, MD: Johns Hopkins University Press, 2016.

Pearson, Jessica Lynne. *The Colonial Politics of Global Health: France and the United Nations in Postwar Africa*. Cambridge, MA: Harvard University Press, 2018.

Porter, Dorothy. *Health, Civilization and the State: A History of Public Health from Ancient to Modern Times*. New York: Routledge, 1999.

Porter, Roy, ed. *The Cambridge Illustrated History of Medicine*. New York: Cambridge University Press, 1996.

Porter, Roy. *The Greatest Benefit to Mankind: A Medical History of Humanity*. New York: W. W. Norton, 1998.

Porter, Roy. *Madness: A Brief History*. New York: Oxford University Press, 2002.

Ranger, Terence, and Paul Slack, eds. *Epidemics and Ideas: Essays on the Historical Perception of Pestilence*. New York: Cambridge University Press, 1992.

Rhodes, John. *The End of Plague: The Global Battle against Infectious Disease*. New York: Macmillan, 2013.

Riley, James C. *The Eighteenth-Century Campaign to Avoid Disease*. New York: St. Martin's Press, 1987.

Riley, James C. *Low Income, Social Growth, and Good Health: A History of Twelve Countries*. Berkeley: University of California Press, 2008.

Risse, Guenter B. *Mending Bodies, Saving Souls: A History of Hospitals*. New York: Oxford University Press, 1999.

Rosenberg, Charles E. *Explaining Epidemics and Other Studies in the History of Medicine*. New York: Cambridge University Press, 1992.

Rosenberg, Charles E., and Janet Golden, eds. *Framing Disease: Studies in Cultural History*. New Brunswick, NJ: Rutgers University Press, 1992.

Rothman, David J., Steven Marcus, and Stephanie A. Kiceluk, eds. *Medicine and Western Civilization*. New Brunswick, NJ: Rutgers University Press, 1995.

Santer, Melvin. *Confronting Contagion: Our Evolving Understanding of Disease*. New York: Oxford University Press, 2015.

Selin, Helaine, and Hugh Shapiro, eds. *Medicine across Cultures: History and Practice of Medicine in Non-Western Cultures*. Dordrecht: Kluwer, 2003.

Shah, Sonia. *Pandemic: Tracking Contagion from Cholera to Ebola and Beyond*. New York: Picador, 2016.

Sherman, Irwin W. *The Power of Plagues*. 2nd ed. Washington, DC: ASM Press, 2017.

Shryock, Richard Harrison. *The Development of Modern Medicine: An Interpretation of the Social and Scientific Factors Involved*. Madison: University of Wisconsin Press, 1979. (Reissue of a 1936 edition by Alfred A Knopf.)

Stearns, Justin. *Infectious Ideas: Contagion in Premodern Islamic and Christian Thought in the Western Mediterranean*. Baltimore, MD: Johns Hopkins University Press, 2011.

Tomes, Nancy. *The Gospel of Germs: Men, Women, and the Microbe in American Life*. Cambridge, MA: Harvard University Press, 1995.

Wald, Priscilla. *Contagious: Cultures, Carriers, and the Outbreak Narrative*. Durham, NC: Duke University Press, 2008.

Watts, Sheldon. *Disease and Medicine in World History*. New York: Routledge, 2003.

Wear, Andrew, ed. *Medicine in Society: Historical Essays*. New York: Cambridge University Press, 1992.

York, William H. *Health and Wellness in Antiquity through the Middle Ages*. Westport, CT: Greenwood Press, 2012.

Index

Note: Numbers in **bold** indicate volume numbers. Page numbers in *italics* indicate photos and illustrations. Page numbers followed by *t* indicate tables.

About the Authors

Joseph P. Byrne holds a doctorate in medieval and early modern European history from Indiana University and taught in the honors program and history department at Belmont University from 1998 to 2020. He has published five books and numerous articles on the Black Death and early medical history, including the *Encyclopedia of the Black Death* (ABC-CLIO, 2012) and *Health and Wellness in the Renaissance and Enlightenment* (Greenwood, 2013). Most recently, his *The World of Renaissance Italy: A Daily Life Encyclopedia* was published by Greenwood in 2017.

Jo N. Hays received his PhD in history and the history of science from the University of Chicago in 1970. He is now professor emeritus of history at Loyola University Chicago. His fields of teaching at Loyola included the histories of science, medicine, and disease; medical humanities, in the university's medical school; the histories of modern Britain and the British Empire; and environmental history. He earlier published articles and book chapters on popular science in nineteenth-century Britain. His recent publications include the second edition of his *The Burdens of Disease* (2009); *Epidemics and Pandemics* (ABC-CLIO, 2005); and "Historians and Epidemics: Simple Questions, Complex Answers" in L. K. Little, ed., *Plague and the End of Antiquity: The Pandemic of 541–750* (2007).